THE WASHINGTON MANUAL®

Allergy, Asthma, and Immunology

THIRD EDITION

Editors

Andrew L. Kau, MD, PhD

Assistant Professor
Division of Allergy and Immunology
Department of Medicine
Washington University School of
   Medicine
St. Louis, Missouri

Jennifer Marie Monroy, MD

Assistant Professor
Division of Allergy and Immunology
Department of Medicine
Washington University School of
   Medicine
St. Louis, Missouri

Brooke Ivan Polk, MD, FACAAI

Assistant Professor
Division of Allergy and Pulmonary
   Medicine
Department of Pediatrics
Washington University School of
   Medicine
St. Louis, Missouri

Christopher J. Rigell, MD

Assistant Professor
Division of Allergy and Immunology
Department of Medicine
Washington University School of Medicine
St. Louis, Missouri

Executive Editor

Thomas M. Ciesielski, MD

Associate Professor of Medicine
Division of General Medicine
Department of Internal Medicine
Washington University School of Medicine
St. Louis, Missouri

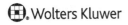 **Wolters Kluwer**

Philadelphia · Baltimore · New York · London
Buenos Aires · Hong Kong · Sydney · Tokyo

Executive Editor: Sharon Zinner
Development Editor: Thomas Celona
Editorial Coordinators: Katie Sharp, Tim Rinehart
Marketing Manager: Kirsten Watrud
Production Project Manager: Catherine Ott
Design Coordinator: Stephen Druding
Manufacturing Coordinator: Beth Welsh
Prepress Vendor: S4Carlisle Publishing Services

Third Edition

Library of Congress Cataloging-in-Publication Data

Names: Kau, Andrew L., editor. | Monroy, Jennifer M., editor. | Polk,
   Brooke I., editor. | Rigell, Christopher J., editor. | Ciesielski,
   Thomas, other. | Washington University (Saint Louis, Mo.). Department of
   Medicine.
Title: The Washington manual allergy, asthma, and immunology subspecialty
   consult / editors, Andrew L. Kau, Jennifer M. Monroy, Brooke I. Polk,
   Christopher J. Rigell; executive editor, Thomas Ciesielski.
Other titles: Washington manual subspecialty consult series.
Description: Third edition. | Philadelphia: Wolters Kluwer Health, [2022]
   | Series: Washington manual subspecialty consult series | Includes
   bibliographical references and index.
Identifiers: LCCN 2020055484 | ISBN 9781975113261 (paperback)
Subjects: MESH: Hypersensitivity—diagnosis | Hypersensitivity—therapy |
   Handbook
Classification: LCC RC584 | NLM QW 539 | DDC 616.97—dc23
LC record available at https://lccn.loc.gov/2020055484

Contents

Contributors

Abeer S. Algrafi, MBBS
Fellow
Division of Allergy and Immunology
Department of Medicine
Washington University School of Medicine
St. Louis, Missouri

Danielle F. Atibalentja, MD, PhD
Fellow
Division of Allergy and Immunology
Department of Medicine
Washington University School of Medicine
St. Louis, Missouri

Leonard B. Bacharier, MD
*Robert C. Strunk Endowed Chair for Lung
and Respiratory Research*
Professor of Pediatrics and Medicine
Department of Pediatrics
Washington University School of Medicine
St. Louis, Missouri

Tiffany Dy, MD
Assistant Professor of Medicine
Division of Allergy and Immunology
Department of Medicine
Washington University School of Medicine
St. Louis, Missouri

Stacy Ejem, MD
Fellow
Division of Allergy and Immunology
Department of Medicine
Washington University School of Medicine
St. Louis, Missouri

Alysa G. Ellis, MD
Associate Professor of Pediatrics
Division of Allergy and Pulmonary Medicine
Department of Pediatrics
Washington University School of Medicine
St. Louis, Missouri

Caroline Horner, MD
Associate Professor of Pediatrics
Division of Allergy and Pulmonary Medicine
Department of Pediatrics
Washington University School of Medicine
St. Louis, Missouri

Maya Jerath, MD, PhD
Professor and Clinical Director
Division of Allergy and Immunology
Department of Medicine
Washington University School of Medicine
St. Louis, Missouri

Nora Kabil, MD
Assistant Professor
Division of Allergy and Pulmonary Medicine
Department of Pediatrics
Washington University School of Medicine
St. Louis, Missouri

**Watcharoot Kanchongkittiphon,
MD, PhD**
Fellow
Division of Allergy and Immunology
Department of Medicine
Washington University School of Medicine
St. Louis, Missouri

Andrew L. Kau, MD, PhD
Assistant Professor
Division of Allergy and Immunology
Department of Medicine
Washington University School of Medicine
St. Louis, Missouri

Jeffrey A. Kepes, MD
Fellow
Division of Allergy and Immunology
Department of Medicine
Washington University School of Medicine
St. Louis, Missouri

Maleewan Kitcharoensakkul, MD, MSCI
Assistant Professor
Divisions of Allergy and Pulmonary Medicine
and Rheumatology
Department of Pediatrics
Washington University School of Medicine
St. Louis, Missouri

Anthony Kulczycki, Jr., MD
Associate Professor
Division of Allergy and Immunology
Department of Medicine
Washington University School of Medicine
St. Louis, Missouri

Christina G. Kwong, MD
Assistant Professor
Division of Allergy and Pulmonary Medicine
Department of Pediatrics
Washington University School of Medicine
St. Louis, Missouri

Hung Le, MD
Resident Physician
Division of Allergy and Immunology
Department of Medicine
Washington University School of Medicine
St. Louis, Missouri

Jennifer Marie Monroy, MD
Assistant Professor
Division of Allergy and Immunology
Department of Medicine
Washington University School of Medicine
St. Louis, Missouri

Kelsey Ann Childs Moon, MD
Physician
Division of Allergy and Immunology
Department of Medicine
Washington University School of Medicine
St. Louis, Missouri

Mark Alan Pinkerton, II, MD
Instructor
Division of Hospital Medicine
Department of Medicine
Washington University School of Medicine
St. Louis, Missouri

Brooke Ivan Polk, MD, FACAAI
Assistant Professor
Division of Allergy and
Pulmonary Medicine
Department of Pediatrics
Washington University School of Medicine
St. Louis, Missouri

Zhen Ren, MD, PhD
Instructor
Division of Allergy and Immunology
Department of Medicine
Washington University School of Medicine
St. Louis, Missouri

Christopher J. Rigell, MD
Assistant Professor
Division of Allergy and Immunology
Department of Medicine
Washington University School of Medicine
St. Louis, Missouri

Benjamin D. Solomon, MD, PhD
Fellow
Division of Allergy and Immunology
Department of Medicine
Washington University School of Medicine
St. Louis, Missouri

Jeffrey R. Stokes, MD
Professor
Division of Allergy and
Pulmonary Medicine
Department of Pediatrics
Washington University School of Medicine
St. Louis, Missouri

Niharika Thota, MD
Fellow
Division of Allergy and Immunology
Department of Medicine
Washington University School of Medicine
St. Louis, Missouri

Aaron M. Ver Heul, MD, PhD
Instructor of Medicine
Division of Allergy and Immunology
Department of Medicine
Washington University School of Medicine
St. Louis, Missouri

Xiaowen Wang, MD
Instructor
Department of Medicine
Washington University School of
  Medicine
St. Louis, Missouri

H. James Wedner, MD, FACP, FAAAI
Dr. Phillip and Arleen Korenblat Professor
Division of Allergy and Immunology
Department of Medicine
Washington University School of Medicine
St. Louis, Missouri

Roseanna F. Zhao, MD
Fellow
Division of Rheumatology
Department of Medicine
Washington University School of Medicine
St. Louis, Missouri

Ofer Zimmerman, MD
Instructor in Medicine
Division of Allergy and Immunology
Department of Medicine
Washington University School of Medicine
St. Louis, Missouri

Chairman's Note

It is a pleasure to present the new edition of *The Washington Manual*® Subspecialty Consult Series: *Allergy, Asthma, and Immunology Subspecialty Consult*. This pocket-size book continues to be a primary reference for medical students, interns, residents, and other practitioners who need ready access to practical clinical information to diagnose and treat patients with a wide variety of allergy, asthma, and immunologic disorders. Medical knowledge continues to increase at an astounding rate, which creates a challenge for physicians to keep up with the biomedical discoveries and novel therapeutics that can positively impact patient outcomes. This *Washington Manual*® Subspecialty Consult Series edition addresses this challenge by concisely and practically providing current scientific information for clinicians to aid them in the diagnosis, investigation, and treatment of allergy, asthma, and immunologic conditions.

I want to personally thank the authors, who include fellows, residents, and faculty from the Washington University School of Medicine and Barnes-Jewish Hospital. Their commitment to patient care and education is unsurpassed, and their efforts and skill in compiling this manual are evident in the quality of the final product. In particular, I would like to acknowledge our editors, Drs. Andrew L. Kau, Jennifer Marie Monroy, Brooke Ivan Polk, and Christopher J. Rigell, and Executive Editor Thomas M. Ciesielski, MD, who have worked tirelessly to produce another outstanding edition of this manual. I would also like to thank Dr. Tom De Fer, interim chief of the Division of General Medicine in the Department of Medicine at Washington University School of Medicine, for his advice and guidance. I believe this edition of the *Allergy, Asthma, and Immunology Subspecialty Consult* will meet its desired goal of providing practical knowledge that can be directly applied at the bedside and in outpatient settings to improve patient care.

Victoria J. Fraser, MD
Adolphus Busch Professor of Medicine
Chair, Department of Medicine
Washington University School of Medicine

Preface

This is the third edition of the *Allergy, Asthma, and Immunology Subspecialty Consult*, which incorporates many significant updates to the prior edition, reflecting current clinical practices and understanding of allergic and immunologic diseases. Since its inception nearly 80 years ago, *The Washington Manual*® has been written with the goal of conveying relevant and up-to-date medical information in a clear and concise manner. Like the preceding edition, this edition of the *Allergy, Asthma, and Immunology Subspecialty Consult* was written in the tradition of *The Washington Manual*®, with the intent of informing the reader about current practice in allergy and immunology.

The content of this third edition was written by fellows and faculty of the Washington University Departments of Medicine and Pediatrics. We have written this manual as a reference tool for interested students, residents, and primary care physicians. Fellows-in-training and other health care professionals will also find it to be a succinct but thorough reference tool.

We would like to acknowledge our appreciation for the excellent work of the authors and editors of the preceding edition of the *Allergy, Asthma, and Immunology Subspecialty Consult*. We would also like to thank the administrators, especially Katie Sharp, and past and present executive editors, Drs. Tom De Fer and Thomas M. Ciesielski, for their patience and input throughout this project. Finally, we would like to thank our excellent mentors, including Drs. H. James Wedner, Anthony Kulczycki, Jr., Philip E. Korenblat, Leonard B. Bacharier, and Caroline Horner, for their advice and assistance that made this work possible.

—Andrew L. Kau,
Jennifer Marie Monroy,
Brooke Ivan Polk, and Christopher J. Rigell

Approach to the Allergic Patient

Hung Le and H. James Wedner

GENERAL PRINCIPLES

Definition

- The term **allergy** is credited to the pediatrician Clemens von Pirquet, who in 1906 used it to describe an "altered biologic reactivity." This was in reference not only to immunity against disease but also to hypersensitivity leading to tissue damage.[1]
- The modern definition of *allergy* is an overreaction or abnormal response of the immune system to innocuous substances.[1]

DIAGNOSIS

Clinical Presentation

History

- As with most disorders in medicine, the most important component in diagnosing allergic disorders is taking a thorough history.
- Identify the symptom location, character, and frequency, as well as the alleviating and exacerbating factors.
- Exacerbating or alleviating factors
  - Seasonal variation of symptoms
  - Prior response to medications
  - Reactions to specific and nonspecific exposures
    - Pets
    - Smoke, perfume, irritant fumes
    - Change in temperature
    - Foods, medications, etc.
- Environmental history
  - Common relevant environmental exposures may not be obvious to the patient.
  - Typical questions that may help to identify relevant exposures include
    - Location of home: rural, urban, suburban
    - Work exposures
    - Hobbies, sports, etc.
    - Presence of water damage or visible mold at home or workplace
    - Presence of pets
    - Age of mattress/bedding
    - Age of carpeting at home
- Family history
  - Allergic diseases have a strong hereditary link.
  - A parental history of allergic rhinitis increases a 6-year-old's odds of allergic rhinitis by 1.84 (1.16–2.94).[2]
  - A parental history of asthma increases a 6-year-old's odds of asthma by 2.72 (1.19–6.18).[2]

- A maternal history of eczema or atopy increases a 6-month-old's risk of eczema by 1.58 (1.01–2.47) and 1.99 (1.43–2.78), respectively.[3]
- The Asthma Predictive Index (API), a validated clinical model for childhood asthma, includes parental asthma as a major clinical criteria to predict asthma later in childhood. A positive API at age 3 had a sensitivity (SN) of 15–28%, specificity (SP) of 96–97%, positive predictive value (PPV) of 48–52%, and negative predictive value (NPV) of 84–92%.[4]

- Food allergy history
  - Although allergies to food are thought to be much more common in children, they are also seen in adults in comparable numbers.[5]
  - Food allergies are often self-reported (prevalence of 3–35%),[5] more often than they are proven to be true (actual prevalence rate of 1–10.8% after oral food challenge).[5,6] A thorough history can lead to appropriate testing, which may further help to confirm or exclude suspected foods.
  - Food diaries are written records of everything that is ingested by a patient, including all foodstuffs, beverages, condiments, and candies. Although rarely diagnostic on their own, food diaries occasionally may be helpful in identifying a food that was overlooked by the patient, a food containing hidden ingredients, or patterns of reactions (e.g., in association with exercise, alcohol, or anti-inflammatory medications).

Physical Examination

- **General appearance**
  - Nasal congestion can lead to a "nasal" or "adenoidal" sounding voice as well as mouth breathing.
  - Nasal tissue edema may lead to compression of the draining veins under the eyes. This can manifest as dark regions under the eyes often called **allergic shiners**.
  - Infraorbital folds or **Dennie–Morgan lines** may be present.
  - Patients may be observed to rub upward across their nose with the palm of the hand. This is known as the **allergic salute** and may cause a transverse line across the lower portion of the nose or nasal crease.
- **Head and neck**
  - Eyes are commonly noted to have conjunctival injection and watering because of allergic disease.
  - Common allergic features of the nose include swollen, edematous turbinates that are pale blue in color.
  - Nasal polyps, which often appear like clear whitish sacs hanging from the underside of a turbinate, may be present.
  - Close examination of nasal septum to assess the presence of perforations or deviations
  - Tympanic membranes may be dull with the presence of effusion behind them.
  - **Flexible rhinoscopy** is helpful in looking closer at the turbinate anatomy and vocal cords to assess for the presence of nasal polyps, sinusitis, or vocal cord dysfunction.
- **Pulmonary**
  - A thorough lung examination is required, including auscultation of all lung fields, to listen for any evidence of wheezing or an increased expiratory phase.
  - If wheezing cannot be heard during a standard examination, a forced expiratory maneuver may be helpful.
- **Skin**
  - **Urticaria**, or hives, is a circumscribed, raised erythematous eruption in the cutaneous tissue. These can range from pinpoint size to multiple inches in diameter and are typically pruritic and blanch with pressure.
  - **Angioedema** is edema of the subcutaneous tissue; it is nonpruritic and often painful.
  - **Dermatographism** is the tendency to form a wheal-and-flare response when firm pressure is applied to the skin.

- **Atopic dermatitis** is associated with allergic disease. This presents as dry, scaly, pruritic papules and plaques occurring at typical locations depending on the age of the patient.
- **Darier sign** is defined as the development of localized urticaria and erythema following rubbing, scratching, or stroking skin or skin lesions that are heavily infiltrated by mast cells. This is present in various forms of cutaneous mastocytosis.

Diagnostic Testing

- As with all testing, the results must be interpreted with appropriate clinical context as to distinguish between sensitization and symptomatic allergy.
- **Skin testing**
  - This is the most rapid and sensitive method to test for allergic sensitization.
  - Two methods are commonly used, and both are discussed in Chapter 3:
    - Epicutaneous testing
    - Intradermal testing
- **In vitro testing**
  - In vitro testing (radioallergosorbent test [RAST] and ImmunoCAP) is designed to screen for the presence of allergen-specific IgE in the patient's serum.
  - These methods have lower SN and SP compared to epicutaneous skin testing but are helpful in instances where skin testing cannot be performed.
- **Pulmonary testing**
  - When a history of breathing difficulties, wheezing, or coughing is reported, pulmonary function tests are often needed to evaluate for asthma.
  - Occasionally, a plain CXR is helpful.
  - When standard pulmonary function tests are normal, but there is still a high suspicion for asthma, modifications may be needed.
    - Exercise spirometry
    - Bronchoprovocation challenge (i.e., methacholine or mannitol)
  - The peak expiratory flow rate (PEFR) correlates reasonably well with FEV_1. Documentation of PEFR variability may be used to support the diagnosis of asthma. Within-day or between-day variability in PEFR of >20% is characteristic of asthma. Monitoring the PEFR is also useful for detecting changes or trends in a patient's asthma control.

REFERENCES

1. Jamieson M. Imagining "reactivity": allergy within the history of immunology. *Stud Hist Philos Biol Biomed Sci.* 2010;41:356–66.
2. Alford SH, Zoratti E, Peterson E, et al. Parental history of atopic disease: disease pattern and risk of pediatric atopy in offspring. *J Allergy Clin Immunol.* 2004;114:1046–50.
3. Moore MM, Rifas-Shiman SL, Rich-Edwards JW, et al. Perinatal predictors of atopic dermatitis occurring in the first six months of life. *Pediatrics.* 2004;113:468–74.
4. Castro-Rodriguez JA. The Asthma Predictive Index: a very useful tool for predicting asthma in young children. *J Allergy Clin Immunol.* 2010;126:212–6.
5. Rona RR, Keil T, Summers C, et al. The prevalence of food allergy: a meta-analysis. *J Allergy Clin Immunol.* 2007;120:638–46.
6. Lieberman JA, Sicherer SH. Diagnosis of food allergy: epicutaneous skin tests, in vitro tests, and oral food challenge. *Curr Allergy Asthma Rep.* 2011;11:58–64.

Basic Immunology Underlying Hypersensitivity, Allergy, and Inflammation

2

Roseanna F. Zhao and Andrew L. Kau

GENERAL PRINCIPLES

Definitions

- The immune system helps us navigate among the billions of microbes that we interact with daily through contact, inhalation, and ingestion. On the one hand, it is responsible for protecting us from bacterial, viral, fungal, and helminthic pathogens. However, it must also learn to tolerate self-derived antigens as well as potential antigens present on commensal organisms, in food, and in the environment.
  - **Immunodeficiency** refers to the inability of the immune system to adequately respond to pathogens, resulting in a predisposition to infection and cancer (see Chapter 21).
  - **Autoimmunity** results when there is loss of immunologic tolerance to self-antigens.
  - **Allergy** stems from loss of tolerance to environmental or food antigens.
- Components of the immune system include a physical barrier, the innate immune response, and the adaptive immune response.[1] These systems work together to maintain homeostasis.

Physical Barriers

- Skin and mucosal surfaces are the initial sites of interaction with potential pathogens and the first line of defense against infection.
- Fatty acids and lactic acid in sebaceous secretions, as well as low pH on skin, in the stomach, and in the urogenital tract inhibit bacterial growth.
- Tears, saliva, and other secreted body fluids contain bactericidal components such as lysozyme.
- Mucus blocks direct adhesion of microbes to epithelial cells and helps eliminate them by ciliary action, coughing, or sneezing.
- Colonization by commensal flora, also known as the **human microbiota or microbiome**, suppresses overgrowth of potentially pathogenic microbes. Disruption of the normal protective flora can lead to opportunistic infections by organisms such as *Clostridium difficile* and *Candida*.

Immune Cells

Immune cells derive from a common CD34+ hematopoietic stem cell progenitor in the bone marrow, which gives rise to myeloid and lymphoid progenitors; these stem cells further differentiate into different cell types based on the activation of different transcriptional programs.

Innate Immune System

- The innate immune system is comprised primarily of myeloid-derived cells, including neutrophils, monocytes, macrophages, dendritic cells, eosinophils, mast cells, and basophils.
- These cells are able to identify pathogens through **pattern recognition receptors (PRRs)**, such as **toll-like receptors (TLRs)**, that recognize conserved features of pathogens, termed **pathogen-associated molecular patterns (PAMPs)**. They have poor specificity but can mount a rapid response to a wide range of foreign molecules.

- **Macrophages** are specialized tissue-resident cells, differentiated from monocyte precursors circulating in the blood, that phagocytose and kill microbes upon recognition of PAMPs. They also generate cytokines, chemokines, and other soluble mediators to recruit other immune cells and help amplify the immune response. They are known by different names based on their associated tissue (e.g., alveolar cells in lung, microglia in brain, Kupffer cells in liver).
- **Mast cells** migrate to peripheral tissue where they mature near blood vessels and nerves, and beneath epithelia. They have round nuclei with cytoplasmic granules containing acidic proteoglycans that bind to basic dyes and vary in shape. Along with macrophages, they are often the first to detect pathogens and help recruit other immune cells through secretion of cytokines, chemokines, and vasoactive amines. They play a key role in protecting against infection by parasites and are involved in allergic diseases.
- **Granulocytes** circulate in the bloodstream and are recruited to sites of inflammation under the direction of cytokines and chemokines.
  - **Basophils** make up <1% of blood leukocytes. They have a similar function as mast cells, can synthesize many of the same mediators, and are important in defense against parasites. Their name is derived from the ability of their granules to bind to basic dye.
  - **Eosinophils** protect against intracellular parasites and are commonly involved in allergic diseases. They are normally seen in peripheral tissue and are recruited to sites of inflammation, mainly in the late-phase reaction. Eosinophil maturation is promoted by granulocyte macrophage colony-stimulating factor (GM-CSF), interleukin (IL)-3, and IL-5. Eosinophils have receptors for IgG, IgA, and IgE. Once activated, eosinophils can release major basic protein, eosinophil cationic protein, and eosinophil peroxidase, which are toxic to bacteria, helminths, and normal tissue. They can also release lipid mediators that aid in the allergic response.
  - **Neutrophils** (also known as **polymorphonuclear [PMN] cells**) account for about 97% of the granulocyte population. They have high phagocytic activity against bacteria and yeast.
- **Dendritic cells** are antigen-presenting cells that bridge the innate and adaptive immune systems. They continuously sample the environment through micropinocytosis and phagocytosis of extracellular material. On detection and processing of a PAMP, they undergo maturation and migrate to lymph nodes where they present antigen to T cells.
- **Natural killer (NK) cells** are lymphoid-derived cells, in contrast to most other innate immune cells, and provide a rapid response to virally infected or tumor cells. They recognize and kill cells that have downregulated major histocompatibility complex class I (MHC-I) (major HLA-A, HLA-B, HLA-C or minor HLA-D, HLA-E, HLA-F) via the release of cytolytic granules containing perforin and granzymes. They can also regulate the adaptive immune response by affecting T cells.

Adaptive Immune System

The adaptive immune response is delayed but highly specific and results in immunologic memory. It is mediated by lymphoid-derived cells, including T and B cells.

Cell-Mediated Immunity

- Involves antigen-specific T cells
- **CD4+ helper T cells** recognize antigen presented in the context of MHC-II receptors (major HLA-DP, HLA-DQ, HLA-DR or minor HLA-DM, HLA-DO) on the surface of antigen-presenting cells, such as dendritic cells, macrophages, and B cells. Naïve CD4+ T cells differentiate into helper cells, which are classified by the subset of cytokines that they secrete.
  - T_H1 cells produce cytokines such as interferon-γ (IFN-γ) to activate macrophages in response to intracellular pathogens, such as bacteria, viruses, mycobacteria, and some parasites.

- ○ **T$_H$2 cells** produce cytokines like IL-4, IL-5, and IL-13 and protect from parasitic infections. They also help promote IgE class switching.
- ○ **T$_H$17 cells** produce IL-17 to promote neutrophil recruitment in response to extracellular pathogens.
- ○ Follicular helper T cells (**Tfh cells**) can produce IFN-γ or IL-4 and stimulate immunoglobulin class switching.
- ○ Regulatory T cells (**Tregs**) mediate immune tolerance through expression of immunoregulatory cytokines such as IL-10 and transforming growth factor (TGF)-β. Their differentiation is dependent on the FOXP3 transcription factor. Absent or impaired Treg function leads to hypersensitivity and autoimmunity.
  - ▪ Natural Tregs (nTregs) arise in the thymus and primarily mediate tolerance to self-antigens, like insulin.
  - ▪ Inducible Tregs (iTregs) arise in peripheral lymphoid tissues from naïve conventional CD4+ T cells exposed to antigen in the presence of TGF-β. They primarily mediate tolerance to peripheral or exogenous antigens at environmental interfaces and are found in abundance in the lungs, gastrointestinal tract, and skin. They also promote healing of tissues injured by inflammation.
- • **CD8+ cytotoxic T cells** recognize antigen presented in the context of MHC-I. Activated effector CD8+ T cells kill virally infected or tumor cells through the release of cytolytic granules.

Humoral Immunity
- • Mediated by immunoglobulins (antibodies) produced by plasma cells. Upon recognition of the specific antigen by surface immunoglobulin (also known as **B-cell receptor [BCR]**), naïve B cells internalize and process antigen before returning it to the cell surface as peptides presented by MHC-II. Antigen-specific CD4+ helper T cells recognize these complexes and interact with B cells to stimulate B-cell proliferation, differentiation into plasma cells, and direct immunoglobulin class switching from IgM.
  - ○ IgM is the first immunoglobulin expressed on the surface of B cells, where it functions as the BCR. The secreted form helps to neutralize a variety of viral and bacterial pathogens.
  - ○ IgD is present on the surface of mature naïve B cells and often coexpressed with IgM. The function of the secreted form remains elusive but is thought to augment immunity in plasma and at mucosal surfaces.
  - ○ IgG is present primarily in plasma and helps protect from viral and bacterial pathogens.
  - ○ IgA is found primarily at mucosal surfaces, protects against pathogens, and helps maintain homeostasis with colonizing microbes.
  - ○ IgE is thought to protect from parasitic infections and is responsible for most allergic reactions.

Classification of Hypersensitivity Reactions

Gell–Coombs provides a classification for immune-mediated hypersensitivity reactions that is divided into four main types, as presented in Table 2-1.

Etiology of Allergy

- • Allergic diseases likely develop from a combination of environmental factors acting on genetically susceptible individuals.
- • The exact reasons for breakdown of immune tolerance are unknown.
- • The **hygiene hypothesis** was formulated to explain the rising incidence of allergic and autoimmune disease in developed countries. It postulates that reduced exposure to pathogenic infections in early childhood resulting from improved living standards, hygiene, and smaller family size results in less T$_H$1 stimulation and an increase in T$_H$2-mediated

TABLE 2-1	HYPERSENSITIVITY REACTIONS	
Type	**Mechanism**	**Examples**
I (Immediate)	IgE-mediated mast cell degranulation and activation	Allergic rhinitis, anaphylaxis, acute urticaria, atopic dermatitis, food allergy, insect sting allergy, allergic asthma
II (Cytotoxic)	IgG or IgM binds antigen on cell surface, causing phagocytosis or complement-mediated cellular destruction	Autoimmune or drug-induced hemolytic anemia or thrombocytopenia
III (Immune complex)	IgG or IgM binds to antigen to cause immune complex–mediated disease	Serum sickness, hypersensitivity pneumonitis
IV (Delayed)	T cell mediated	
IVa	T_H1 cells activate macrophages (IFN-γ, IL-1, IL-2)	Tuberculin reaction
IVb	T_H2 cells activate eosinophils (IL-4, IL-5, IL-13)	Allergic asthma
IVc	CD8+ cytotoxic T cells (perforin, granzyme B, Fas ligand)	Contact dermatitis, Stevens–Johnson syndrome, toxic epidermal necrolysis
IVd	CD4+ and CD8+ T cells activate neutrophils (IL-8, GM-CSF)	Acute generalized exanthematous pustulosis (AGEP)

GM-CSF, granulocyte macrophage colony-stimulating factor; IFN-γ, interferon-γ; IL, interleukin.

diseases (associated with skewing toward IgE responses). Since its original development, this idea has undergone modifications to reflect nuances afforded by more recent epidemiologic data.

- For example, the **"biodiversity" hypothesis** states that early exposure to a diverse range of common microbes (not necessarily pathogenic) is important to educate the immune system to tolerate self, environment, and food exposures.[2] This is mediated through a combination of both innate and adaptive immune modulation.
- The **microbiome** is shaped by prenatal factors (maternal microbiota, mode of delivery) and postnatal factors (diet, environmental exposure, antibiotic use, genetics). Imbalance in early-life microbiome composition is associated with the development of food intolerance, asthma, allergy, and autoimmunity.
- Prenatal exposure to a microbe-rich environment, such as farming, leads to upregulation of receptors of innate immunity and protects against atopic sensitization.[3] This may be mediated through epigenetic changes.
- Children living in rural areas with heavy exposure to animals have a lower prevalence of allergy and asthma compared to children living in the same area without exposure to animals.[4,5]
- Among Amish and Hutterite farm children with similar genetic ancestries and lifestyles, exposure to a microbe-rich environment was associated with distinct immune profiles (with profound effects on innate immunity) and protection against asthma.[6]

- Environmental pollutants may contribute to asthma and allergic reactions. Some may disrupt the physical barrier, allowing easier access of allergens to body surfaces and increasing inflammation, whereas others can elicit epigenetic changes or act as adjuvants that alter the immune response.[7,8]

Mechanisms of Allergy

- Allergy results from specific immune-mediated hypersensitivity reactions. They can be IgE mediated (type I) or cell mediated (type IV) or have features of both.[9] **Atopy** is the genetic predisposition to become sensitized and produce IgE in response to common antigens in the environment.
- Antigens that mediate allergic reactions (also called **allergens**) comprise a wide variety of molecules, including chemicals and proteins commonly encountered in the environment. Examples include dust mite, pollen, and animal dander. Allergens have diverse molecular features, such as specific oligosaccharide moieties, protease activity, and lipid-binding properties, which can facilitate their recognition by immune and nonimmune cells; these features contribute to their "allergenicity."
- Haptens are small molecules that are not capable of eliciting an immune response alone but can do so by binding to self-proteins to create a hapten–carrier conjugate. This is seen in penicillin allergy (may cause type I, II, or III hypersensitivity).
- In IgE-mediated allergic reactions, initial allergen exposure induces **sensitization** and **memory** through a process that includes differentiation of naïve CD4 T cells to T_H2 cells, secretion of IL-4 and IL-13, and stimulation of B cells to differentiate into IgE-producing plasma cells.
- Reexposure to the allergen triggers an allergic response that is composed of two phases: immediate and late.
  ○ The **immediate-phase** response is a type I reaction that occurs when antigen binds to mast cell–associated IgE and stimulates mast cells to release preformed granules. Local histamine and prostaglandin increase vascular permeability and smooth muscle contraction. This reaction can appear within 5–10 minutes after the administration of antigen and usually subsides in an hour. The wheal-and-flare response seen during allergy skin testing (see Chapter 3) is an example of an immediate allergic response.
  ○ The **late-phase** reaction of allergic inflammation occurs in about 50% of cases and is mediated by cytokines and lipid mediators produced by mast cells along with neutrophils, eosinophils, basophils, and T_H2 cells that are recruited to the site. The late-phase reaction occurs 2–4 hours after the immediate response, and the inflammation is maximal by 24 hours before it subsides. Late-phase allergic inflammation can be reduced with corticosteroids but not antihistamines. Long-term sequelae of chronic inflammation include development of asthma.
- Clinical symptoms depend on the route of allergen entry, dose of allergen, and amount of allergen-specific IgE present.

IgE Sensitizes Cells to Allergens

- In contrast to the other immunoglobulin isotypes, IgE is primarily produced at the site of antigen stimulation and passively diffuses through tissues until it is bound by a receptor, where it has a long half-life of weeks to months. Only small amounts of IgE are found in systemic circulation.
- There are two main types of IgE receptors: the high-affinity FcɛRI receptor and the low-affinity FcɛRII receptor. The high-affinity receptor is expressed abundantly on mast cells and basophils, as well as in lower concentrations on dendritic cells, Langerhans cells, eosinophils, macrophages, neutrophils, platelets, and intestinal epithelium.
  ○ On mast cells and basophils, the high-affinity FcɛRI receptor is a tetramer composed of an α-chain that binds to the Fc portion of IgE, two γ-chains, and a β-chain that is involved with intracellular signaling and degranulation.

- Other cell types, where the receptor is involved in antigen presentation rather than degranulation, do not contain the β-chain.
- IgE upregulates FcεRI expression.
- Once bound to a cell surface Fc receptor, IgE sensitizes the cell to allergen. Presence and binding of allergen to surface IgE cause aggregation and cross-linking of the high-affinity FcεRI, which activates protein tyrosine kinases associated with the β-chains and downstream signaling, leading to degranulation in mast cells and basophils.
- Atopic individuals with higher IgE levels need a smaller trigger to induce mast cell activation.

Mast Cells Orchestrate IgE-Mediated Allergic Reactions
- Activated mast cells are a key component to allergic reactions. They secrete various mediators that are either stored preformed in granules or synthesized upon activation. This helps to promote recruitment of other immune cells to the site of inflammation and regulate adaptive immunity. Mast cells can be stimulated to release their mediators by:
  - Allergens binding to surface IgE on mast cells causing cross-linking
  - Antibody binding to IgE or FcεR1 receptor causing cross-linking
  - Histamine-releasing factors that include chemokines such as macrophage inflammatory protein (MIP)-1, complement factors C3a and C5a, and neuropeptides such as substance P
  - Drugs (morphine, codeine) and IV contrast dye
  - Physical stimuli such as pressure, heat, cold, and sunlight
- Preformed granules consist of biogenic amines (histamine), neutral proteases (tryptase, chymase, carboxypeptidase), acid hydrolases, proteoglycans (heparin, chondroitin sulfate), and tumor necrosis factor (TNF)-α. These are released within minutes of cross-linking of surface-bound IgE.
- Histamine acts upon release on the four different histamine receptors. Its actions are short-lived, because it is rapidly removed from the extracellular space.
  - Through the H_1 receptor, histamine causes smooth muscle contraction (bronchospasm), pruritus, vasodilation, and vasopermeability. This creates the wheal-and-flare response on the skin.
  - The H_2 receptor is responsible for gastric acid secretion and increased mucus production in the airways.
  - The H_3 receptor is found in the nervous system and controls the release of histamine and other neurotransmitters.
  - The H_4 receptor aids in chemotaxis of mast cells.
- Tryptase is found only in mast cells and is a marker of mast cell activation. Tryptase cleaves fibrinogen and activates collagenase, causing tissue damage. Tryptase is found in two forms, α-tryptase and β-tryptase.
  - α-Tryptase is constitutively secreted. Levels are elevated in mastocytosis.
  - β-Tryptase is released upon mast cell degranulation. It is stabilized by heparin. Blood levels peak 30 minutes after anaphylactic reaction but may remain above baseline level for 6–12 hours after inciting event.
- Synthesized mediators are made by mast cells minutes to hours after activation and include arachidonic acid metabolites and cytokines.
- Lipid metabolites are created from arachidonic acid via the cyclooxygenase or lipoxygenase pathways and are mediators in allergic reactions.
  - Prostaglandin D_2 (PGD_2) is synthesized through the cyclooxygenase pathway. PGD_2 acts on smooth muscle cells to mediate vasodilation and bronchoconstriction. It also promotes neutrophil chemotaxis.
  - Leukotrienes are created via the lipoxygenase pathways. Leukotriene C_4 (LTC_4) is made by mucosal mast cells and is degraded to LTD_4 and LTE_4. These are important mediators of asthmatic bronchoconstriction. In addition, they also increase vascular permeability and mucus secretion.

○ Platelet-activating factor (PAF) causes bronchoconstriction and vascular permeability, relaxes vascular smooth muscle, and can activate leukocytes. PAF has a short half-life as it is rapidly destroyed. It received its name as it causes rabbit platelet aggregation.
- Mast cell–synthesized cytokines that contribute to allergic inflammation include the following:
  ○ IL-3 induces mast cell proliferation and stimulates basophil development/activation.
  ○ IL-4 and IL-13 promote IgE isotype switching and mucus secretion.
  ○ IL-5 activates and induces eosinophil proliferation.
  ○ IL-6 promotes B-cell differentiation.
  ○ TNF-α activates endothelial expression of adhesion molecules that aid in leukocyte recruitment.

Eosinophils, Basophils, and Neutrophils Amplify Inflammation and Tissue Damage in Allergic Reaction
- **Eosinophils** produce and release many of the same mediators as mast cells and are able to modulate both innate and adaptive immunity. Their accumulation in the blood and recruitment to tissues are associated with disease severity in many inflammatory and allergic conditions,[10] including atopic dermatitis, allergy, asthma, eosinophilic pneumonia, eosinophilic esophagitis, and hypereosinophilic syndrome. Therapies targeting eosinophils are effective in many allergic diseases.
- **Basophils** migrate to tissues and have a nonredundant role in the development of T_H2-mediated inflammation via release of histamines, leukotrienes, and T_H2 cytokines, as well as modulation of adaptive immunity.[11] They are involved in immediate hypersensitivity reactions, asthma, atopic and contact dermatitis, and drug reactions. They also produce PAF and are critical for IgG- (but not IgE-)mediated anaphylaxis such as that induced by penicillin–antibody complexes.[12] The basophil activation test (BAT) has shown high accuracy in detecting allergy to foods, drugs, and pollens.
- **Neutrophils** are recruited to sites of inflammation, such as airways, where they contribute to allergic inflammation. They release chemokines and inflammatory cytokines such as IL-8. They are the most abundant cell type in the airway of noneosinophilic asthma and are associated with severity of disease and steroid resistance.

Tregs Modulate Allergic Responses
- Absence of Tregs because of FOXP3 deficiency causes immune dysregulation, polyendocrinopathy, enteropathy, X-linked (IPEX) syndrome, which is characterized by autoimmunity and severe allergic inflammation with increased IgE, peripheral eosinophilia, atopic dermatitis, food allergy, and asthma.[13,14]
- Tregs mediate tolerance through multiple mechanisms[15]
  ○ Blocking of mast cell degranulation via direct cellular interaction
  ○ IL-2 depletion
  ○ Downmodulation of antigen-presenting cells
  ○ Granzyme-mediated cytolysis
  ○ Production of inhibitory cytokines such as IL-10, which inhibits mast cells, T_H2 cells, eosinophils, and dendritic cells
- Tregs play an important role in controlling allergic inflammation by suppressing T_H2 responses.

REFERENCES

1. Murphy K, Weaver C. *Janeway's Immunobiology.* 9th ed. New York, NY and London: Garland Science, Taylor & Francis Group, LLC, 2017.
2. Tamburini S, Shen N, Wu HC, et al. The microbiome in early life: implications for health outcomes. *Nat Med.* 2016;22:713–22.
3. Ege MJ, Bieli C, Frei R, et al. Prenatal farm exposure is related to the expression of receptors of the innate immunity and to atopic sensitization in school-age children. *J Allergy Clin Immunol.* 2006;117(4):817–23.
4. Von Ehrenstein OS, Mutius EV, Illi S, et al. Reduced risk of hay fever and asthma among children of farmers. *Clin Exp Allergy.* 2000;30(2):187–93.
5. Ege MJ, Mayer M, Normand A-C, et al. Exposure to environmental microorganisms and childhood asthma. *N Engl J Med.* 2011;364(8):701–9.
6. Stein MM, Hrusch CL, Gozdz J, et al. Innate immunity and asthma risk in Amish and Hutterite farm children. *N Engl J Med.* 2016;375:411–21.
7. Bégin P, Nadeau KC. Epigenetic regulation of asthma and allergic disease. *Allergy Asthma Clin Immunol.* 2014;10:27.
8. Ji H, Biagini Myers JM, Brandt EB, et al. Air pollution, epigenetics, and asthma. *Allergy Asthma Clin Immunol.* 2016;12:51.
9. Johansson SG, Bieber T, Dahl R, et al. Revised nomenclature for allergy for global use: report of the Nomenclature Review Committee of the World Allergy Organization, 2003. *J Allergy Clin Immunol.* 2004;113(5):832–6.
10. Fulkerson PC, Rothenberg ME. Targeting eosinophils in allergy, inflammation and beyond. *Nat Rev Drug Discov.* 2013;12(2):117–29.
11. Siracusa MC, Kim BS, Spergel JM, et al. Basophils and allergic inflammation. *J Allergy Clin Immunol.* 2013;132(4):789–801.
12. Tsujimura U, Obata K, Mukai K, et al. Basophils play a pivotal role in immunoglobulin-G-mediated but not immunoglobulin-E-mediated systemic anaphylaxis. *Immunity.* 2008;28(4):581–9.
13. Chatila TA, Blaeser F, Ho N, et al. JM2, encoding a fork head-related protein, is mutated in X-linked autoimmunity-allergic dysregulation syndrome. *J Clin Invest.* 2000;106:R75–81.
14. Torgerson TR, Linane A, Moes N, et al. Severe food allergy as a variant of IPEX syndrome caused by a deletion in a noncoding region of the FOXP3 gene. *Gastroenterology.* 2007;132:1705–17.
15. Rivas MN, Chatila TA. Regulatory T cells in allergic diseases. *J Allergy Clin Immunol.* 2016;138:639–52.

Diagnostics in Allergy and Immunology

Ofer Zimmerman and Aaron M. Ver Heul

3

GENERAL PRINCIPLES

- **Allergy** is defined as immune sensitization leading to clinically observed symptoms, whereas **tolerance** is a lack of response upon exposure to an antigen. Allergic sensitization (i.e., the presence of antigen-specific IgE) can occur without associated clinical symptoms.
- Diagnostics in allergy focus on elucidation of antigen-specific sensitizations that correlate with symptoms. Testing can only identify sensitization, whereas clinical judgment is required to diagnose allergy vs. sensitization without clinical symptoms.
  - Testing for antigen-specific IgE helps determine culprit allergens responsible for immediate hypersensitivity, including drug allergies and atopic diseases such as allergic rhinitis, asthma, and food allergies.
  - Testing for antigen-specific delayed hypersensitivity helps determine agents responsible for conditions such as contact dermatitis or delayed drug reactions.

DIAGNOSIS

Immediate Hypersensitivity Skin Testing

- Measures the presence of **antigen-specific IgE** in vivo
- The most sensitive and cost-effective method to determine existing IgE sensitivities that may be responsible for clinical symptoms

Indications

Documentation of allergic sensitivity to specific allergens in patients with the following conditions:

- Asthma (aeroallergens and/or occupational allergens) (see also Chapters 5 and 6)
- Rhinitis (see also Chapter 9)
- Conjunctivitis (see also Chapter 10)
- Food allergy (see also Chapter 15)
- Certain drug allergies (see also Chapter 17)
- Insect hypersensitivity (see also Chapter 18)
- Allergic bronchopulmonary aspergillosis (see also Chapter 5)

Contraindications

- Results are unreliable in patients with a history of **recent severe allergic reaction** (i.e., anaphylaxis). Testing is usually deferred until 4–6 weeks after the event.[1]
- Tests are difficult to interpret in patients who have **severe eczema or dermatographism**.
- **Intradermal testing is never performed for food allergy**.
- Patients with a history of severe hypersensitivity reactions (i.e., to venom, foods, or drugs) are at higher risk for adverse reactions to testing.
- Patients taking β-adrenergic blocking agents or angiotensin-converting enzyme inhibitors are at higher risk for serious reactions to food and environmental aeroallergens or venom testing, respectively.

- Many medications can interfere with skin testing, **usually because of antihistaminic effects** (Table 3-1). Although most of these medications can be safely held prior to testing, others, such as atypical antipsychotics or tricyclic antidepressants, can precipitate serious events when discontinued without alternate therapy.

TABLE 3-1 DRUGS THAT INTERFERE WITH ALLERGY SKIN TESTING	
Medication generic name	Mean days suppressed
First-generation antihistamines	
Chlorpheniramine	2–6
Clemastine	5–10
Cyproheptadine	9–11
Dexchlorpheniramine	4
Diphenhydramine	2–5
Hydroxyzine	5–8
Promethazine	3–5
Tripelennamine	3–7
Second-generation antihistamines	
Azelastine nasal	2
Cetirizine	3
Fexofenadine	2
Loratadine	7
Levocabastine nasal	0
Levocabastine opth	0
Tricyclic antidepressants	
Desipramine	2
Imipramine	>10
Doxepin	6
Doxepin topical	11
Histamine2 antihistamines	
Ranitidine	<1
Cysteinyl leukotriene antagonists	
Montelukast	0
Zafirlukast	0
Oral corticosteroids	
≤30 mg prednisone <1 week	No suppression
>20 mg prednisone >1 week	Possible suppression
Topical corticosteroids (high potency)	3 weeks to area of application

Adapted from Bernstein IL, Li JT, Bernstein DI, et al. Allergy diagnostic testing: an updated practice parameter. *Ann Allergy Asthma Immunol.* 2008;100(3 suppl 3):S1–148.

Methods

- Antigens are applied to the skin surface by epicutaneous or intradermal methods.[1]
- If present, antigen-specific IgE bound to resident mast cells recognizes cognate antigen, leading to cross-linking and activation of the cells, which, in turn, release mediators such as histamine or tryptase.
- Skin mast cell activation manifests as a **"wheal-and-flare" reaction**.
  - The wheal is the area of swelling and **edema** surrounding the site of allergen exposure.
  - The **flare** refers to the **erythema** around a site of allergen exposure resulting from vasodilation.
  - Wheal size is more specific than flare size and correlates better with clinical symptoms.
  - The maximal diameter of both the wheal and the flare is recorded in millimeters for interpretation. Grading systems (e.g., 1+, 2+, ...) are not recommended owing to high variability between practitioners.
  - Results should be measured at the peak of the reaction.
    - The peak time for histamine reaction is 8–10 minutes.
    - The peak time for mast cell activators such as opiates is 10–15 minutes.
  - The peak time for most allergens is 15–20 minutes.
- Skin testing is not valid without proper controls.[1]
  - A common positive control is **histamine** (1 mg/mL for epicutaneous and 0.1 mg/mL for intradermal skin testing). Other compounds leading to mast cell degranulation, such as codeine or morphine sulfate, may also be used.
  - Possible causes of a negative response to a histamine control include medications (see later) and certain skin conditions. Diluents used to preserve the allergen extracts are used as negative controls. Possible causes of a positive response to diluents include problems with technique, possible skin irritation reaction, or dermatographism.
- **Positive reactions are any wheals that measure >3 mm in diameter more than the negative control.**
- Skin testing **should be performed by a trained professional who is familiar with possible adverse reactions** and the implications of a positive or a negative test result as it relates to the patient's clinical presentation.
- **Epicutaneous skin tests**
  - Performed by introducing antigen into the epidermis through various techniques, including prick, puncture, or scratch[1]
    - **Prick skin testing**
      - Performed by placing a small drop of antigen on the cleansed skin surface and passing a 25- or 26-gauge needle through the antigen at a 45-degree angle
      - The needle should be lightly pressed into the epidermis and then lifted, creating a break in the epidermis without causing bleeding.
      - Test antigens should be placed >2 cm from one another.
      - Various hollow and solid bore needles and blood lancets are available under different trade names.
    - **Puncture skin testing**
      - Performed by placing a small drop of the allergen extract on the cleansed skin surface and puncturing the skin with a device at a perpendicular angle, penetrating 1–1.5 mm into the skin
      - Each test antigen site should be placed >2 cm apart.
      - Disposable, commercially available devices made of plastic allow for placement of multiple antigen test sites at one time. Results may not be comparable between different device manufacturers.
    - **Scratch skin test**
      - Performed by making abrasions on the skin and then applying the allergen extract to the site, allowing it to diffuse through the skin
      - Because of its **poor standardization and reproducibility**, this method has fallen out of favor and is rarely used.

- Preferred areas for testing are the upper back and/or volar aspect of the arm.
- Some sensitizations are not detectable by this method, and intradermal testing may be necessary.
- **Intradermal skin tests**
  - Performed using 25- to 27-gauge needles to inject a small amount of allergen extract into the dermis, creating a small bleb 2–3 mm in diameter
  - **More sensitive,** but **less specific,** than the epicutaneous skin tests[1]
  - **Generally, only performed if the epicutaneous test is negative because of the risk of severe reaction**
  - Spaces between each injection site should be >2 cm.
  - The concentration of extract for intradermal testing should be between 100- and 1,000-fold more dilute than the concentration used for epicutaneous testing.
  - **Variability in test results** is often due to common errors, including injecting too deeply, using too much extract, or causing bleeding. Injecting the extract too deeply may hide the response, thereby giving a false-negative result. On the other hand, use of too much extract or bleeding from the prick or puncture may give false-positive results.
  - Set point titration (Rinkel method)
    - Involves placement of serial dilutions of allergenic extract, increasing in fivefold concentrations, using the intradermal method
    - A **set point** is defined as the dose that initiates an incremental 2 mm increase in the wheal with the fivefold increase in concentration.
    - Although this method is still in use today, its **scientific validity is controversial**, and there is evidence that its use in determining subsequent immunotherapy doses leads to underdosing and **inferior efficacy.**[2]

Clinical Use of Skin Tests
- **Aeroallergen testing**
  - Antigens typically come in the form of extracts derived from the allergen source (e.g., pollens, fungal spores, animal hair or epithelium, or arthropods).[3]
  - Crude aqueous extracts are the most commonly used. They are complex mixtures of allergenic and nonallergenic compounds, including proteins, glycoproteins, polysaccharides, lipids, nucleic acids, low-molecular-weight metabolites, salts, and pigments.[3,4]
  - Commercial allergen extracts can vary significantly in the types, quantities, and potencies of antigens both between manufacturers and even batch to batch from the same manufacturer.[3,4]
  - Glycerin and human serum albumin are often added to stabilize the extracts and increase shelf life.[3,4]
  - **Several aeroallergen extracts are standardized** (Table 3-2).
  - Using Food and Drug Administration (FDA) guidelines,[5] allergen extracts are standardized by the intradermal dilution for 50 mm sum of erythema (ID50EAL) method. This uses a series of threefold dilutions of a candidate reference extract, injected in 0.05 mL intradermal volumes to "highly sensitive" allergic subjects. The dilution that results in an erythema with the sum of the longest diameter and midpoint (orthogonal) diameter equaling 50 mm is considered the end point (D50). The mean D50 is calculated, and the potency of the extract is assigned.
  - Concentrations are reported in allergen units (AU) or bioequivalent allergen units (BAU).[3,4]
  - Nonstandardized extracts are reported as weight/volume of starting crude allergen to final extracted volume, or in protein nitrogen units (PNU).[3,4]
  - Epicutaneous tests are typically done with undiluted extracts, whereas intradermal tests use extracts diluted between 1:100 and 1:1,000. Aeroallergen intradermal tests have lower specificity but higher sensitivity and are warranted in situations where clinical suspicion is high but relevant epicutaneous testing is negative.[1]

TABLE 3-2	STANDARDIZED ALLERGEN EXTRACTS
Allergen	**Stock concentrations**
Cat hair	5,000 and 10,000 BAU/mL
Cat pelt	
Mite *D.f.*	3,000, 5,000, 10,000, and
Mite *D.p.*	30,000 AU/mL
Bermuda grass	100,000 BAU/mL
Kentucky bluegrass	
Meadow fescue grass	
Orchard grass	
Redtop grass	
Perennial rye grass	
Sweet vernal grass	
Timothy grass	
Short ragweed	100,000 AU/mL
Honey bee venom	100 µg/mL
Wasp venom protein	
White-faced hornet venom protein	
Yellow hornet venom protein	
Yellow jacket venom protein	
Mixed vespid venom protein (yellow jacket, yellow hornet, and white-faced hornet)	300 µg/mL

Adapted from Nelson MR, Cox L. Allergen immunotherapy extract preparation manual. In: *AAAAI Practice Management Resource Guide.* 2012 ed. Milwaukee, WI: American Academy of Allergy, Asthma, and Immunology, 2012:1–39.

- ○ Skin testing is the preferred method of determining sensitivities for prescribing immunotherapy because most immunotherapy is formulated with the same extracts used for testing (see Chapter 11).
- **Stinging insect testing**
  - ○ All **Hymenoptera extracts are standardized** to the protein content of the relevant allergen (phospholipase A or hyaluronidase). These are derived directly from venom, either through stimulated stinging or through removal of venom sacs.[3,4]
  - ○ Imported fire ant extract is derived from the crushed whole insects and contains relevant venom proteins. Despite not being standardized, fire ant extract has shown efficacy in both diagnosis and treatment.[6]
  - ○ **If venom epicutaneous testing is negative, subsequent intradermal testing is necessary** to attain maximal negative predictive value. It should typically start with a 1:1,000 dilution of that used for epicutaneous testing.
  - ○ In vitro testing will demonstrate venom-specific IgE for up to 15% of patients with negative skin tests.[1,6]
- **Food testing**
  - ○ There are no standardized food extracts.
  - ○ **Commercially available extracts rapidly lose potency**, so many clinicians prepare fresh abstracts or test using the prick–prick method.[1,7] The prick–prick method

involves first pricking the food to be tested to inoculate the device with allergen, then proceeding with the prick test as usual on the patient's skin.

- **Intradermal testing should never be performed with food allergen extracts** owing to high risk of systemic reactions and high false-positive rates.[1,7]
- **Drug testing**
  - The only standardized drug testing components are for the penicillin.[1]
  - As with venoms, **intradermal testing is necessary for complete evaluation if epicutaneous tests are negative**. It should typically start with a 1:1,000 dilution of that used for epicutaneous testing.
  - It is important to be aware of the maximal **nonirritating concentrations for drugs** being tested to avoid false positives. The European Network and European Academy of Allergy and Clinical Immunology (EAACI) Interest Group on Drug Allergy has compiled a large list of nonirritating concentrations for drug testing.[8]
  - Some drugs (e.g., ciprofloxacin) can directly activate mast cells through the MRGPRX2 receptor and thus cannot be reliably skin tested. Activation of this receptor may be involved in non–IgE-mediated anaphylaxis ("anaphylactoid" reactions), making it difficult to properly rule out antigen-specific IgE because of false positives in skin testing.[9]
- **Other testing**

Autologous serum skin tests are used to detect autoantibodies in chronic autoimmune urticaria. A patient's blood is drawn and centrifuged to separate out the serum. The serum is then tested similarly to any other allergen extract, first with epicutaneous prick tests and then with a series of intradermal dilutions. There is no evidence that this testing identifies any particular subset of chronic urticaria patients, and this test is not recommended for routine use.[10]

Delayed Hypersensitivity Skin Testing

Delayed hypersensitivity skin testing measures the presence of **antigen-specific T cells** in vivo.

Indications
- Commonly used to diagnose allergic contact dermatitis (patch testing)
- Also used to screen for latent TB (tuberculin skin test or purified protein derivative [PPD])

Contraindications
- The presence of active lesions where skin testing is performed can interfere with testing.
- Pregnancy is a relative contraindication because of associated immunologic changes that can interfere with testing.[11]
- Concurrent immunosuppressive therapy can affect testing, but does not absolutely preclude diagnostic utility of results.[1]

Patch Testing
- Small amounts of diluted testing materials are loaded onto small aluminum discs (Finn chambers) and then placed on the patient's back under nonocclusive dressing with hypoallergenic tape. The concentration of each test material should be sufficiently dilute to minimize the chance of an irritant reaction.[12] Standard testing kits are also available commercially.
- The patient should not bathe, shower, or participate in strenuous activities until the test site is graded.
- **Two days after placing patch tests, the patient should return for removal of the discs and grading of the test areas.**

- **The patient should return for a late reading 4–5 days after original application.** This second reading increases the sensitivity of testing because some reactions are not evident at the first reading.[12]
- **Precautions**
  - The application of the patch test may itself sensitize the patient or cause a flare-up in an already sensitized patient.
  - Patients should be instructed to remove any patch that causes severe irritation. Repeated patch testing should be avoided. For drugs, the patch should be assessed 20 minutes after application before the patient leaves to rule out immediate hypersensitivity.
  - Standardized concentrations of test material should be used to avoid an inflammatory reaction, which can lead to a false-positive result.[12]
- **Allergen panels**
  - Only 35 commercially prepared allergens are FDA approved in the United States.
  - There are several patch test kits containing these allergens; one is described in Table 3-3.[13] Note that one of the components is a negative control.
  - Although these commercially prepared allergens are convenient to use, they only detect 25–30% of all cases of allergic contact dermatitis. As a result, the North American Contact Dermatitis Group commonly tests for 65 allergens, but most of these are not FDA approved and, therefore, cannot be commercially purchased.
- **Grading**
  - Each reagent is graded on a scale of 0–3 (Table 3-4). Grades 1+ and above are considered positive.
  - False-positive test results may be due to the following:
    - Skin may be hypersensitive to one of the antigens, and, therefore, the entire back can become inflamed.
    - Irritation due to factors other than antigen (i.e., the tape used)
  - False-negative test results may be due to the following:
    - Low antigen concentration
    - Technical errors in applying the antigen patches
    - Failure to acquire a late reading at 3–7 days
- **Clinical application of test results**
  - It is important to remember that a positive patch skin test result does not mean diagnosis of causative agent for contact dermatitis.
  - The antigen could be a secondary aggravating factor.
  - Positive test results should be correlated with clinical history, and, when possible, the patient should avoid the antigens that caused a positive reaction.

TABLE 3-3	THIN-LAYERED RAPID USE EPICUTANEOUS TEST PANEL OF ALLERGENS
Allergen	**Environmental occurrences**
Nickel sulfate	Jewelry, metal
Wool alcohols (lanolin)	Cosmetics, soaps, topical medications
Neomycin sulfate	Topical antibiotics
Potassium dichromate	Cement, cutting oils
Caine mix	Topical anesthetics
Fragrance mix	Toiletries, scented household products
Colophony	Cosmetics, adhesives

TABLE 3-3	THIN-LAYERED RAPID USE EPICUTANEOUS TEST PANEL OF ALLERGENS (continued)

Allergen	Environmental occurrences
Paraben mix	Preservative in topical formulations and foods
Negative control	—
Balsam of Peru	Foods, cosmetics
Ethylenediamine dihydrochloride	Topical medicines, industrial solvents
Cobalt dichloride	Metal-plated objects, paints
p-tert-Butylphenol formaldehyde resin	Waterproof glues, bonded leather
Epoxy resin	Two-part adhesives, paints
Carba mix	Rubber products, glues for leather, vinyl
Black rubber mix	All black rubber products, some hair dyes
Cl+ Me− isothiazolinone	Cosmetics, topical medicines
Quaternium-15	Preservative in cosmetics, household cleaners
Methyldibromo glutaronitrile	Coolants, glues, and adhesives
p-Phenylenediamine	Hair dyes, dyed textiles
Formaldehyde	Fabric finishes, plastics, synthetic resins
Mercapto mix	Rubber products, glues for leather/plastics
Thimerosal	Preservative in contact lens solutions and injectable drugs
Thiuram mix	Rubber products, adhesives
Diazolidinyl urea	Cosmetics, cleaning agents, liquid soaps, pet shampoos
Quinoline mix	Topical antibiotic and antifungal preparations; animal food
Tixocortol-21-pivalate	Anti-inflammatory agents such as nasal spray, lozenges, and rectal suspensions
Gold sodium thiosulfate	Gold or gold-plated jewelry, dental restorations, electronics
Imidazolidinyl urea	Cosmetics, cleaning agents, liquid soaps, moisturizers
Budesonide	Topical, inhaled, and rectal anti-inflammatory agent
Hydrocortisone-17-butyrate	Topical and rectal anti-inflammatory agent
Mercaptobenzothiazole	Rubber products, adhesives
Bacitracin	Topical antibiotics
Parthenolide	Found in certain plants, as well as supplements, tinctures, or teas derived thereof
Disperse Blue 106	Textiles, fabrics, and clothing
Bronopol	Antimicrobial found in many common products, such as cosmetics, cleaning agents, water-based paints, topical medications

Adapted from Smart Practice. T.R.U.E. TEST® Ready-to-Use Patch Test Panels. Last Accessed 10/23/20. https://www.smartpractice.com/shop/category?cn=Products-T.R.U.E.-TEST&id=50 8222&m=SPA

TABLE 3-4	GRADING OF PATCH TEST READINGS
Grade	**Findings**
0	Negative reaction
1+	Weak positive reaction with nonvesicular erythema, infiltration, possible papules
2+	Strong positive reaction with vesicular erythema, infiltration, papules
3+	Extreme positive reaction with intense erythema and infiltration, coalescing vesicles, bullous reaction
Irritant	Possible pustular, mild erythema, minimal-to-no pruritus

Adapted from Fonacier L, Bernstein DI, Pacheco K, et al. Contact dermatitis: a practice parameter-update 2015. *J Allergy Clin Immunol Pract.* 2015;3:S1–39.

In Vitro Testing

Assays for Immediate-Type Hypersensitivity

- These test for *sensitization*, which is the presence of IgE to specific antigens.
  - **The confirmation or exclusion of an allergy to a specific allergen cannot be based solely on a laboratory result and should rely on relevant history and sometimes on the combination of both in vivo and in vitro tests.**[14]
  - A positive test can usually be used for the confirmation of allergy in patients with a clear history of allergic reaction to the same specific allergen.
  - A negative test result in the setting of a strongly suggestive history **does not** exclude allergy.
- **The advantages of skin testing over in vitro tests are lower cost, rapid results, and higher sensitivity.**[1]
- The advantages of in vitro testing
  - **No patient risk** (e.g., anaphylaxis in patients with latex allergy or patients with severe reactions to small amount of allergen)
  - **Not affected by medications** and does not require discontinuation of medications prior to the test (e.g., antihistamine or antidepressant)
  - Can be performed immediately after anaphylaxis
  - Not influenced by skin integrity or skin diseases. Can be performed in patients with severe and disseminated **eczema or patients with dermatographism**
  - Reliable in infants starting at the age of 6 weeks, compared with skin testing that is reliable only from the age of 12 months
  - Does not require prolonged testing time and clinic visits
  - Better positive predictive value for some type of testing (i.e., food allergy)
- **Types of in vitro immediate hypersensitivity tests**
  - **Immunoassays**
    - Are qualitative and quantitative tests that are based on interaction of a patient's serum antibodies with specific antigens[14]
    - Available for: insect venoms, foods, aeroallergens such as pollens (trees, grasses, and weeds), molds, animal dander and dust mite, latex (natural rubber), β-lactam antibiotics, and occupational allergens[1,14]
    - Are often incorrectly referred to collectively as **radioallergosorbent test (RAST),** which involves anti-IgE antibodies that are coupled to radioactive tags and seldom used today[1]

- Enzyme-linked immunosorbent assay (ELISA) makes use of anti-IgE antibodies linked to enzymes. When the substrate of the enzyme is added, the reaction generates a colored product. Fluorescent enzyme immunoassays (FEIAs) and chemiluminescent immunoassays are additional assays that are similar to the basic ELISA and are based on reactions that generate a fluorescent or chemiluminescent product.[14]
  - Solid-phase method is the most used method. In this method, allergens are bound to an "immunosorbent" or "allergosorbent"—a specific matrix, such as a plastic plate, cellulose, disc, bead, or other substrate. Patient serum is incubated with the immunosorbent, and if specific IgE to the antigen is present in the serum, it will attach to the allergen–immunosorbent complex. Any unbound components of the serum are washed away. Then anti-human IgE secondary antibodies are added and create a complex of allergen patient-specific IgE–anti-human IgE antibodies. This complex is detected and measured by ELISA or RAST as described earlier.
  - **Liquid-phase immunoassays** are performed with solutions of allergens and antibodies. **Competitive binding technique** can be used with both liquid and solid assays. It measures specific IgE level, by quantifying the inhibitory effect of the measured patient-specific IgE antibody on the attachment of a control antibody with a known concentration.
- **Component-resolved diagnostics (CRDs)** are relatively new testing methods that allow for more specific identification of the precise antigenic epitopes of an allergen that a given patient is allergic to. It helps in identifying patients with allergy to component of different allergens that cross-react and share structural similarity with each other, such as PR10 family of allergens (e.g., **Bet v 1—birch, Mal d 1—apple, Pru p 1—peach, Gly m 4—soybean, Ara h 8—peanut, Api g 1—celery, Dau c 1—carrot**).[14]
  - CRDs are in clinical use mainly for the diagnosis of food allergy, especially peanut allergy. In peanut allergy, patients sensitized to pollen-related components, such as the peanut allergen Ara h 8 (which is related to some birch pollen allergens), usually experience no or very mild oral symptoms, whereas those who are sensitized to more stable components, such as seed storage proteins (e.g., Ara h 2), are more likely to experience systemic reactions to peanut. CRD assays for foods in addition to peanut include tree nuts, wheat, vegetables, fruits, milk, and hen's egg.[7,15]
  - They can help to predict cross-reactivity between food and pollen allergens and the type of reaction that a patient will have. This is an important advance because standard IgE immunoassays may detect IgE against clinically irrelevant epitopes that are not associated with any symptoms, causing false-positive results in patients who are not clinically reactive to the allergen in question.
  - A commercially available example of CRD is the ImmunoCAP, which allows detection of IgE against >100 individual components of allergens, derived from >50 allergen sources.
- Different immunoassay technique and tests for specific allergens have **a wide range of sensitivity (60–95%) and specificity (30–95%)**, a range that is wider than the expected in skin allergy testing.[1,16]
- Concordance among different immunoassay systems is reported to be approximately 75–90% for well-characterized allergens.[1,16,17]
- The best available tests are for pollens of common grasses and trees, dust mites, and cat allergens, with sensitivity, specificity, and predictive values of >90%. In children, some of the major food allergen tests have very high positive predictive value (ImmunoCAP assay).[1,18] In general, less accurate assays include those from venoms, foods, weed pollens, latex, drugs, dogs, and molds.[1]
- **Results are usually reported in kUA/L for allergen-specific IgE (or kIU/L for total IgE measurements),**[14] whereas other immunoassays are reported in nanograms of IgE/mL. **The conversion is 1 kIU/L = 2.4 ng IgE/mL.**

- ○ **Newer tests can analytically detect IgE antibody levels as low as 0.1 kUa/L (0.244 ng/mL)**, which is lower compared to the past lower threshold of detection, that is, 0.35 kUa/L. **The clinical significance of antigen-specific IgE levels between 0.1 and 0.35 kUa/L is unknown**, because most clinical data and research work are based on the previous 0.35 kUa/L threshold. **A level of ≥0.35 kUa/L has been shown to be more consistently related to symptoms upon exposure, whereas asymptomatic sensitization may occur in some individuals having <0.35 kUa/L level of allergen-specific IgE.**[1]
- ○ Positive specific IgE level <0.35 kUa/L has little utility in the diagnosis and management of allergies because they require skin testing or a challenge for the specific antigen and cannot help in ruling out or verifying allergy to a specific allergen.
- ○ Predicting whether a patient will react after an exposure to the allergen is influenced by the degree of positivity, the allergen in question, and the patient's clinical history, as mentioned earlier.
  - ▪ **The level of the antibody is the most reliable predictor for allergic reaction. The higher the level, the higher the likelihood for reaction.** High specific IgE level does not predict severe reaction or the type of reaction. **Anaphylaxis is not more likely than any other type of IgE-mediated reaction, such as urticaria in patients with high specific IgE level.**[19]
  - ▪ With the exception of some foods (see Chapter 15), threshold levels above which most patients will react clinically have not been determined.
- ○ **False-positive** results of allergen-specific IgE can occur in patients with extremely elevated total IgE levels. As an example, patients with eczema can have a markedly elevated total IgE level and test positive for IgE to food allergens to which there is no history of clinical reactivity.[20]
- ○ Another important cause of false-positive allergy testing is **cross-reactive carbohydrate determinants (CCDs)**. Allergen extract used in allergy in vitro testing, such as latex, some foods, venom, and pollen allergens, and the cellulose sponges used in some of the assays (ImmunoCAP) contain glycoprotein-carrying CCD epitopes that react with human IgE.[21] Anti-CCD IgE does not cause noticeable clinical symptoms, but can lead to false-positive results in up to 30% of tested patients. Use of in vivo testing such as skin-prick test or placebo-controlled food challenges or using *refined in vitro* testing methods can overcome this problem.[21]
- • Total IgE levels
  - ○ IgE is one of the five isotypes of human immunoglobulins.[22]
  - ○ IgE is a monomer and consists of four constant regions in contrast to other immunoglobulins that contain only three constant regions. Owing to this extra region, the weight of IgE is 190 kDa compared with 150 kDa for IgG. The variable regions of IgE possess an estimated 10^6–10^8 allergen-binding specificities. Its Fc binds to mast cell and basophil Fcε receptor. IgE has the lowest serum concentration of all of the immunoglobulins, approximately 150 ng/mL (about 62 IU/mL), which is approximately 66,000-fold less abundant in serum compared to IgG (typically 10 mg/mL).[23,24]
  - ○ Total IgE levels are frequently measured by a sandwich-type assay as described earlier and are reported as IU or ng/mL (1 IU/mL = 2.44 ng/mL).[25] Laboratory techniques used for the assessment of immunoglobulin concentration for other classes of immunoglobulin (i.e., IgG, IgA, IgM), such as radial immunodiffusion, cannot be used to measure IgE concentrations because serum IgE levels are normally too low.
  - ○ Normal serum levels range from approximately 0 to 100 IU/mL (sometimes expressed in kU/L, depending upon the laboratory).
  - ○ IgE does not cross the placenta. Allergens can be passed transplacentally, and the fetus can produce allergen-specific IgE. Total IgE levels increase from birth and peak during adolescence.[26] Preschool levels do not correlate well with those at older ages.

- Factors associated with increased levels of total IgE include male gender, African American race, poverty, increased serum cotinine (reflecting tobacco smoke exposure), <12th-grade education, and obesity.[26]
- In atopic individuals, total serum IgE levels may fluctuate. For example, in pollen-sensitized individuals, serum IgE levels peak 4–6 weeks after the height of pollen season and subsequently decline until the next pollen season.[23]
- The half-life of free IgE in the serum is about 2 days, although once IgE has bound to mast cells, the half-life is extended to about 2 weeks because of the high affinity of this interaction.[23]
- Although IgE deficiency (defined as levels <2.5 IU/mL) has been associated with low levels of other immunoglobulins, recurrent infection, and inflammatory diseases, it is unclear if isolated IgE deficiency in humans is a clinically relevant immunodeficiency or a marker of more general immune dysregulation.
- Increased total serum IgE is seen in a variety of pathologic states
  - Allergic diseases: atopic dermatitis, allergic bronchopulmonary aspergillosis, and asthma.[23,26] Total IgE has clinical implication in determining the eligibility of patients with moderate-to-severe asthma for treatment with omalizumab (Xolair, see Chapter 5).
  - Immunodeficiencies including hyper-IgE syndromes; immune dysregulation, polyendocrinopathy, enteropathy, X-linked (IPEX); Wiskott–Aldrich syndrome; Omenn syndrome; and a rare phenotype of DiGeorge syndrome[14,23,26] (see Chapter 21)
  - Infections
    - In the developing world, parasitic infection is the most common cause of elevations in IgE.[23,26] Peripheral blood eosinophilia is usually also present. Parasites known to increase serum IgE include *Strongyloides*, *Toxocara*, *Trichuris*, *Ascaris*, *Echinococcus*, hookworms, filaria, and *Schistosoma*. Increased IgE levels reflect both parasite-specific IgE and total IgE.[26]
    - Viral infections associated with elevated IgE levels include HIV, Epstein–Barr virus (EBV), and cytomegalovirus.[26]
    - Elevated IgE levels may be seen in infections with *Mycobacterium tuberculosis* and leprosy.[26]
  - Inflammatory diseases: eosinophilic granulomatosis with polyangiitis (EGPA) and Kimura disease[26]
  - Malignancies: Hodgkin and non-Hodgkin lymphoma, especially nodular sclerotic histology, cutaneous T-cell lymphoma/Sézary syndrome, and, very rarely, IgE myeloma[26,27]
  - Other disorders: bone marrow transplantation, glomerulonephritis with nephrotic range proteinuria, cigarette smoking, and alcohol abuse[26]
- Evaluation of anaphylaxis
  - Anaphylaxis results from massive activation of mast cells and basophils.[28]
  - Serum tryptase and plasma histamine released from basophil and mast cells may be detectable for minutes to hours after episodes of anaphylaxis and can be used to support the diagnosis of anaphylaxis. Elevations in these mediators are short-lived, and blood or other fluids must be collected as soon as possible after the event.
  - Metabolites of mast cell mediators, such as *N*-methyl histamine and prostaglandin compounds, can be assayed in 24-hour urine samples collected shortly after a clinical event or in patients with suspected mast cell disorders. The use of laboratory tests to support the diagnosis of anaphylaxis and mast cell disorders is reviewed in detail separately.

Assays for Delayed-Type Hypersensitivity
- Most lab tests for delayed-type allergic reactions to medication are available only in research settings.

- ○ Lymphocyte transformation testing (LTT), enzyme-linked immunospot (ELISpot), and intracellular cytokine staining (ICS) are in vitro tests that are used to assess for drug delayed-type hypersensitivity in patients with suspected drug allergy following ex vivo exposure to a specific drug.[29]
- ○ LLT measures cell proliferation reflected by H-thymidine level. Interferon (IFN)-γ is usually the marker used for measuring activation of CD8-positive cell by ELISpot assay.
- ○ Flow cytometry can be used to measure various intracellular cytokines in different types of immune cells, by combining intracellular staining for cytokines with surface staining for immune cell markers.
- ○ These ex vivo tests can be helpful in identifying the causing agent of different disorders such as maculopapular drug eruptions, drug reaction with eosinophilia and systemic symptoms (DRESS), Stevens–Johnson syndrome (SJS), and toxic epidermal necrolysis (TEN).
- There is some evidence that combining in vivo skin testing with the ex vivo ELISpot might have a better yield in recognizing the causative agent in antibiotic-associated severe cutaneous adverse reactions.[30]
- The only commercially available in vitro assays in clinical use are the various **HLA typing tests**.
  - ○ These assays are used both for identifying the culprit drug in patients with delayed hypersensitivity drug reaction and for screening patients prior to the initiation of medications with a known strong association between HLA type and specific reaction.
  - ○ **HLA-B*5701** is associated with abacavir hypersensitivity with severe drug eruption in patients with HIV. The inexpensive polymerase chain reaction (PCR)-based screening assay is used widely and has a 100% negative predictive value. **Abacavir treatment is safe for patients who are HLA-B*5701 negative.**
  - ○ Multiple HLA types were associated with various types of delayed drug reaction, such as **B*5801 and allopurinol** (commercially available), **B*1502 and carbamazepine** (commercially available), or **B*38 sulfamethoxazole-induced SJS or TEN**.

Other Unproven Allergy Tests

- There are many other forms of testing available for diagnosing allergic conditions that provide no clear clinical benefit.
- Specific allergen IgG and IgG4 tests
  - ○ These tests are often performed for the evaluation of food allergy and typically yield positive results. **However, IgG antibodies against specific foods represent normal immune response and are not pathologic.** They do not predict true food hypersensitivity.
  - ○ The formation of allergen-specific IgG4 and IgG "blocking antibodies" is one of several immunologic changes that are **associated with effective immunotherapy**, and their measurement is performed in research studies of immunotherapy.[31] Venom-specific IgG correlates with the efficacy of immunotherapy in patients with venom allergy and can be measured to evaluate if a patient treatment was adequate.
- There are several other tests for allergy that have been shown in blinded studies to perform no better than placebo, including provocation/neutralization tests, kinesiology, and cytotoxic.

REFERENCES

1. Bernstein IL, Li JT, Bernstein DI, et al. Allergy diagnostic testing: an updated practice parameter. *Ann Allergy Asthma Immunol.* 2008;100(3 suppl 3):S1–148.
2. Van Metre TE, Adkinson NF, Lichtenstein LM, et al. A controlled study of the effectiveness of the Rinkel method of immunotherapy for ragweed pollen hay fever. *J Allergy Clin Immunol.* 1980;65:288–97.

3. Hauck PR, Williamson S. The manufacture of allergenic extracts in North America. *Clin Rev Allergy Immunol.* 2001;21:93–110.
4. Nelson MR, Cox L. Allergen immunotherapy extract preparation manual. In: *AAAAI Practice Management Resource Guide.* 2012 ed. Milwaukee, WI: American Academy of Allergy, Asthma, and Immunology, 2012:1–39.
5. U.S. Food and Drug Administration. Allergenics. 2020. Last Accessed 7/31/20. https://www.fda.gov/vaccines-blood-biologics/allergenics
6. Golden DBK, Demain J, Freeman T, et al. Stinging insect hypersensitivity: a practice parameter update 2016. *Ann Allergy Asthma Immunol.* 2017;118:28–54.
7. Sampson HA, Aceves S, Bock SA, et al. Food allergy: a practice parameter update-2014. *J Allergy Clin Immunol.* 2014;134(5):1016–25.e1043.
8. Brockow K, Garvey LH, Aberer W, et al. Skin test concentrations for systemically administered drugs—an ENDA/EAACI Drug Allergy Interest Group position paper. *Allergy.* 2013;68:702–12.
9. McNeil BD, Pundir P, Meeker S, et al. Identification of a mast-cell-specific receptor crucial for pseudo-allergic drug reactions. *Nature.* 2015;519:237–41.
10. Bernstein JA, Lang DM, Khan DA, et al. The diagnosis and management of acute and chronic urticaria: 2014 update. *J Allergy Clin Immunol.* 2013;133:1270–77.e1266.
11. Lazzarini R, Duarte I, Ferreira AL. Patch tests. *An Bras Dermatol.* 2013;88:879–88.
12. Fonacier L, Bernstein DI, Pacheco K, et al. Contact dermatitis: a practice parameter-update 2015. *J Allergy Clin Immunol Pract.* 2015;3:S1–39.
13. Smart Practice. T.R.U.E Test® Ready-to-use Patch Test Panels. 2020. Last Accessed 7/31/20. www.truetest.com/panelallergens.aspx
14. Hamilton RG. Laboratory tests for allergic and immunodeficiency diseases. In: Adkinson NF, Bochner BS, Burks WA, et al., eds. *Middleton's Allergy: Principles and Practice.* 8th ed. Philadelphia, PA: Elsevier/Saunders, 2014:1187–204.
15. Sicherer SH, Wood RA. Advances in diagnosing peanut allergy. *J Allergy Clin Immunol Pract.* 2013;1(1):1–13; quiz 14.
16. Nolte H, DuBuske LM. Performance characteristics of a new automated enzyme immunoassay for the measurement of allergen-specific IgE. Summary of the probability outcomes comparing results of allergen skin testing to results obtained with the HYTEC system and CAP system. *Ann Allergy Asthma Immunol.* 1997;79(1):27–34.
17. Wood RA, Segall N, Ahlstedt S, et al. Accuracy of IgE antibody laboratory results. *Ann Allergy Asthma Immunol.* 2007;99(1):34–41.
18. Sampson HA. Update on food allergy. *J Allergy Clin Immunol.* 2004;113(5):805–19; quiz 820.
19. Simons FE, Frew AJ, Ansotegui IJ, et al. Risk assessment in anaphylaxis: current and future approaches. *J Allergy Clin Immunol.* 2007;120(suppl 1):S2–24.
20. Yousef E, Haque AS. A pilot study to assess relationship between total IgE and 95% predictive decision points of food specific IgE concentration. *Eur Ann Allergy Clin Immunol.* 2016;48(6):233–6.
21. Hemmer W, Altmann F, Holzweber F, et al. ImmunoCAP cellulose displays cross-reactive carbohydrate determinant (CCD) epitopes and can cause false-positive test results in patients with high anti-CCD IgE antibody levels. *J Allergy Clin Immunol.* 2018;141(1):372–81.e373.
22. Schroeder HW Jr, Cavacini L. Structure and function of immunoglobulins. *J Allergy Clin Immunol.* 2010;125(2 suppl 2):S41–52.
23. Stone KD, Prussin C, Metcalfe DD. IgE, mast cells, basophils, and eosinophils. *J Allergy Clin Immunol.* 2010;125(2 suppl 2):S73–80.
24. Dullaers M, De Bruyne R, Ramadani F, et al. The who, where, and when of IgE in allergic airway disease. *J Allergy Clin Immunol.* 2012;129(3):635–45.
25. Hamilton RG, Williams PB, Specific IgE Testing Task Force of the American Academy of Allergy, et al. Human IgE antibody serology: a primer for the practicing North American allergist/immunologist. *J Allergy Clin Immunol.* 2010;126(1):33–8.
26. Smith JK, Krishnaswamy GH, Dykes R, et al. Clinical manifestations of IgE hypogammaglobulinemia. *Ann Allergy Asthma Immunol.* 1997;78(3):313–8.
27. Scala E, Abeni D, Palazzo P, et al. Specific IgE toward allergenic molecules is a new prognostic marker in patients with Sezary syndrome. *Int Arch Allergy Immunol.* 2012;157(2):159–67.
28. Brown SGA, Kemp SF, Lieberman PL, et al. Anaphylaxis. In: Adkinson NF Jr, Bochner BS, Burks WA, et al., eds. *Middleton's Allergy: Principles and Practice.* 8th ed. Philadelphia, PA: Elsevier/Saunders, 2014:1237–59.

29. Rive CM, Bourke J, Phillips EJ. Testing for drug hypersensitivity syndromes. *Clin Biochem Rev.* 2013;34(1):15–38.

30. Trubiano JA, Strautins K, Redwood AJ, et al. The combined utility of ex vivo IFN-γ release enzyme-linked immunospot assay and in vivo skin testing in patients with antibiotic-associated severe cutaneous adverse reactions. *J Allergy Clin Immunol Pract.* 2018;6(4):1287–96.e1.

31. Nelson HS, Nolte H, Creticos P, et al. Efficacy and safety of timothy grass allergy immunotherapy tablet treatment in North American adults. *J Allergy Clin Immunol.* 2011;127(1):72–80; 80.e1–2.

Anaphylaxis

4

Danielle F. Atibalentja and Alysa G. Ellis

GENERAL PRINCIPLES

Anaphylaxis is a life-threatening disease with multisystem involvement, including airway, breathing, circulation, as well as mucosal and skin changes. **Anaphylaxis is a medical emergency.**

Definition

According to an international consensus statement of specialists, **anaphylaxis** is "a serious, generalized or systemic, allergic or hypersensitivity reaction that can be life-threatening or fatal."[1,2]

Classification

- Historically, the causes of anaphylaxis were subdivided based on the mechanism of the reaction as either IgE dependent (allergic anaphylaxis) or IgE independent (nonallergic anaphylaxis).[3]
- Attempts are underway to refine the classification of anaphylaxis in a way that combines both phenotype and endotypes (cellular and molecular mechanisms).[3–5]
- A proposed classification system stratifies anaphylactic reactions into four categories: type I reactions (IgE and non-IgE), cytokine release reactions, mixed reactions, and bradykinin or complement-mediated reactions.[3]

Epidemiology

- The true incidence of anaphylaxis has been difficult to assess owing to several factors, including underdiagnosis, underreporting, differences in coding among institutions, and lack of a consensus definition. Depending on the study, incidence rates have ranged from 50–2,000 episodes/100,000 person-years.[6,7]
- The prevalence of anaphylaxis varies among studies depending on methodology. Among adults in the United States, a recent national survey estimates the lifetime prevalence of anaphylaxis at 1.6–5.1%.[8]
- Recent epidemiologic data suggest an increase in both the incidence and prevalence of anaphylaxis over the past 10 or more years. This could be attributable to consensus definition and improved diagnosis, reporting, and awareness.[9]
- Death from anaphylaxis is rare, with incidence estimated at 0.12–1.06 deaths per million person-years.[8,9] There are an estimated 1,500 fatal anaphylactic reactions per year in the United States.[10] Food, insect bites, and drugs account for the top causes of death from anaphylaxis.[9]

Etiology

- The most common causes of anaphylaxis include the following[7,11]:
  - Ingested foods (e.g., peanuts, tree nuts, fish, shellfish, milk, eggs)
  - Medications (e.g., opiates, antibiotics, aspirin, NSAIDs)
  - Insect bites and stings
  - Other triggers include exposure to latex, allergen immunotherapy, seminal fluid, radiocontrast, blood products (e.g., in IgA-deficient patients), and mast cell disorders (e.g., mastocytosis).[4,11]
- In idiopathic anaphylaxis, a clear cause or trigger is not clearly identifiable.[4] Idiopathic causes account for 6–27% cases of anaphylaxis.[10]

Pathophysiology

- Anaphylaxis caused by an allergen is a severe, life-threatening immediate or type I hypersensitivity (IgE-mediated) reaction.
  - In the classical pathway of anaphylaxis, exposure to allergens results in the production of allergen-specific IgE antibodies by B cells, which bind to the surface of mast cells and basophils via the high-affinity FcεR1 receptor. This is the **sensitization** phase.[2,3,5]
  - In subsequent exposures, the allergen binds to the receptor–antibody complex, resulting in the **cross-linking of the FcεR1-bound allergen-specific IgE. This interaction** leads to the immediate release of preformed and synthesized vasoactive amines and lipid mediators, including histamine, tryptase, carboxypeptidase A, chymase, and proteoglycans.[3,5,12] These factors act on vascular smooth muscles, increasing vascular permeability and smooth muscle contractions leading to the symptoms seen in an anaphylactic reaction. The initial reaction is further amplified by the recruitment of more inflammatory cells, such as eosinophils, which release even more mediators, creating a positive feedback loop that worsens symptoms if left untreated.
  - In a minority of patients, a biphasic reaction is observed wherein a late-phase reaction occurs over a period of 2–6 hours. This late phase is thought to be mediated by the recruitment of T cells, eosinophils, and neutrophils with the **synthesis of** leukotrienes, sphingosine-1-phosphate, platelet-activating factor, cytokines, interleukin (IL)-6, IL-33, and tumor necrosis factor (TNF)-α, resulting in further tissue injury.[3,5,12]
- The presence of allergen-specific IgE antibodies alone does not account for all anaphylactic reactions.[2,3] **Several observations suggest the existence of IgE-independent pathways that lead to reactions that are clinically indistinguishable from anaphylaxis.**
  - Some individuals will develop severe anaphylactic reactions in the absence of detectable allergen-specific IgE antibodies.[2]
  - Tissue injury in anaphylaxis can also be mediated by activation of the complement cascade, resulting in the production of C3a, C4a, and C5a (also called **anaphylatoxins**), which causes mast cell and basophil activation.[2,5] Anaphylaxis to vancomycin and contrast media is thought to occur through complement activation.[3]
  - Other mechanisms of anaphylaxis include activation of the bradykinin pathway.[3,5] High-molecular-weight heparin anaphylactic reactions are thought to be mediated by this pathway.[5]

Risk Factors

- History of prior anaphylaxis
- Parenteral exposure to antigen is associated with higher risk of anaphylaxis compared to ingestion.
- Intermittent exposure to antigen
- Large-dose exposure
- In children aged <15 years, males are at higher risk. For adults, females are at higher risk.
- Adults are at higher risk for anaphylaxis because of penicillin and Hymenoptera, whereas children are at higher risk for food-induced anaphylaxis.
- Atopy does not appear to increase the risk of anaphylaxis, but it may place an individual at risk for more severe expressions of anaphylaxis, including death.
- β-Blocker and angiotensin-converting enzyme inhibitor (ACEi) therapy places an individual at risk for a more severe anaphylaxis reaction and may make resuscitation more difficult.[3]
- Risk factors for fatal food-induced anaphylaxis
  - Adolescents
  - Patients with a history of reaction
  - Patients allergic to peanut or tree nuts
  - Patients with a history of asthma
  - Those presenting without cutaneous symptoms[13]

- Genetic risk factors
  - Patients with mastocytosis who have a KIT mutation are at higher risk of anaphylaxis.[2,5]
  - Drug and latex anaphylaxis have been linked to polymorphisms in cytokines involved in the T_H2 signaling pathway, IL-4Rα, IL-10, and IL-13.[2]

Prevention

- Secondary prevention is predicated on **identification and avoidance of the inciting agent.**
- Accidental ingestion of allergic foods in the form of condiments and prepared foods is a well-known hazard, particularly for food-allergic children.
- **If a known trigger is identified, a comprehensive avoidance strategy and action plan should be provided to the patient.**[8]
- Medical identification (i.e., bracelet) may help health care professionals recognize a patient with a known history of anaphylaxis promptly.
- **Patients with a history of anaphylaxis because of food or Hymenoptera sting should carry self-administered epinephrine.**
- **Desensitization** in the case of certain drugs or **immunotherapy** in the case of venom should be considered if future exposure to putative agent is unavoidable.[3]

DIAGNOSIS

The diagnosis of anaphylaxis is made clinically. History should include an extensive review of exposures and activities leading up to the reaction. The clinical presentation of anaphylaxis is on a spectrum from cutaneous reaction to severe anaphylactic shock.

Clinical Presentation

- Onset of symptoms is typically within minutes of exposure to antigen. In rare circumstances, it can be delayed for hours. **A delayed reaction can occur in some individuals (biphasic reaction),** leading to recurrence of symptoms 4–8 hours after the initial event.[8] Up to 20% of people are thought to experience a biphasic reaction.[8]
- The clinical manifestations of anaphylaxis are highly variable. Signs and symptoms include any combination of the following (listed in order of frequency) ranging from a mild to life-threatening severe reaction.[14]
  - **Dermatologic** (80–90%): flushing, urticaria, angioedema, and pruritus
  - **Respiratory** (up to 70%): rhinorrhea/sneezing, cough, choking, stridor, wheeze, bronchospasm, and laryngeal edema
  - **Cardiovascular** (up to 45%): hypotension, tachycardia, arrhythmia, myocardial infarction, and syncope
  - **Gastrointestinal/genitourinary** (up to 45%): abdominal or uterine cramping, diarrhea, nausea, and vomiting
- Although cutaneous symptoms are common in anaphylaxis, they are not necessary to confirm the diagnosis.[15]
- Similarly, hypotension may not be present.[15]
- Onset of symptoms tends to be more rapid for parenterally administered agents compared to food exposures.
- **Protracted anaphylaxis** requiring many hours of active resuscitation occurs in as many as 28% of patients.[16] Risk factors for prolonged anaphylaxis are oral ingestion of the allergen, onset of symptoms >30 minutes after exposure to the stimulus, and lack of epinephrine administration.
- Anesthetic drugs during surgical procedures may blunt the signs and symptoms of anaphylactic shock requiring particular high vigilance in these settings.

Diagnostic Criteria

The 2005 Second Symposium on the definition and management of anaphylaxis by the National Institute of Allergy and Infectious Diseases (NIAID) and Food Allergy and Anaphylaxis Network (FAAN) developed a set of three criteria, which were felt to capture >95% of anaphylaxis cases, thereby improving identification and risk stratification in the acute care setting (Table 4-1).[15] These guidelines were adopted by the World Allergy Organization and the 2010 Task Force Practice Parameter for Anaphylaxis.[15] Based on these consensus criteria:

- A diagnosis of anaphylaxis should be considered when there is an acute onset of symptoms in two or more organ systems, especially in the setting of an exposure to a possible provoking antigen.
- If the patient has a known allergy to a particular allergen, hypotension after exposure to that antigen is enough to make the diagnosis of anaphylaxis.

Differential Diagnosis

- The differential diagnosis of anaphylaxis[13] is presented in Table 4-2.
- If all other diagnoses are excluded, **idiopathic anaphylaxis** should be considered.[4,8]
  - Idiopathic anaphylaxis is a **diagnosis of exclusion** with no causative factor identified and is thought to be the result of **nonimmunologic mast cell activation**.
  - Clinical presentation and treatment are the same as for anaphylaxis because of known allergens.
- **Recurrent episodes** of anaphylaxis without a known cause warrant consideration of other diagnoses.
- **Systemic mastocytosis** can present with recurrent anaphylaxis. Total tryptase will be elevated persistently even when patient is asymptomatic.

TABLE 4-1 CLINICAL DIAGNOSIS OF ANAPHYLAXIS

Anaphylaxis is likely when one of the three criteria occurs

Acute skin and/or mucosal symptoms (e.g., hives, pruritus, flushing, lip/tongue/uvula swelling) and one of the following:
- Respiratory symptoms (e.g., wheezing, stridor, shortness of breath, hypoxia)
- Hypotension or associated end-organ dysfunction (e.g., hypotonia, syncope, incontinence)

Exposure to probable allergen for the patient and ≥2 of the following:
- Skin-mucosal tissue involvement
- Respiratory symptoms
- Hypotension or end-organ dysfunction
- Persistent gastrointestinal symptoms (e.g., emesis, abdominal pain)

Decreased blood pressure after exposure to known allergen for the patient
- Adults: Systolic blood pressure <90 mm Hg or >30% decrease
- Infants and children: Hypotension for age or >30% decrease in systolic blood pressure

Adapted from Sampson HA, Muñoz-Furlong A, Campbell RL, et al. Second symposium on the definition and management of anaphylaxis: summary report—Second National Institute of Allergy and Infectious Disease/Food Allergy and Anaphylaxis Network symposium. *J Allergy Clin Immunol.* 2006;117:391–7.

TABLE 4-2	DIFFERENTIAL DIAGNOSIS OF ANAPHYLAXIS
Cardiovascular	Cardiogenic shock
	Arrhythmia
Endocrine	Hypoglycemia
	Adrenal insufficiency
Flushing syndromes	Carcinoid syndrome
	Serotonin syndrome
	Mastocytosis/mast cell–activation disorder
Other	Scombroid
	Hereditary angioedema
Nonorganic disease	Vocal cord dysfunction
	Panic attack
	Somatoform disorder

Diagnostic Testing

Diagnostic testing for anaphylaxis can be helpful to confirm the diagnosis of anaphylaxis and identify the culprit antigen. However, these tests are not helpful at predicting the severity of the anaphylactic response or the risk of recurrence.[9]

Laboratories

- Laboratory testing can aid in the diagnosis of anaphylaxis, but use may be limited by institutional availability and rapidity of symptom presentation.
- Serum β-tryptase and histamine are the most commonly tested serologic markers in anaphylaxis.[4,8]
Measurement of **serum β-tryptase** after patient stabilization can help confirm the diagnosis of anaphylaxis. Serum β-tryptase corresponds to acute mast cell–mediator release. Serum tryptase peaks at 60–90 minutes following mast cell degranulation and is present for up to 5–8 hours after a putative anaphylactic reaction.[4,17] In the case of an insect sting anaphylaxis, β-tryptase blood levels are maximal 15–120 minutes after anaphylaxis and decline with a half-life of 1.5–2.5 hours.[17] **β-Tryptase levels may not always be elevated after anaphylaxis, especially if mediated by food.**[2]
- Serum histamine is the earliest marker of mast cell degranulation but has limited usefulness owing to its short half-life, with rise within 5–10 minutes, and peaks at 15–60 minutes.[2,4] It is also produced by basophils and neutrophils and is, therefore, not specific to mast cells.[2]

Diagnostic Procedures

- Skin testing/serum IgE testing
  - Patients are often referred to an allergist after an episode of presumed anaphylaxis. If a careful history unveils the causative agent, the anaphylaxis can be confirmed with skin testing, in vitro testing for allergen-specific IgE, or challenge testing.
  - **Skin testing is the test of choice for IgE-dependent anaphylactic reactions.**
  - **Skin tests are not reliable for up to 4–6 weeks after an episode of anaphylaxis because of generalized mast cell degranulation and temporary loss of cutaneous activity.**[3]
  - A single episode of anaphylaxis with no obvious causative antigen by history does not warrant random skin testing or in vitro testing.

- In vitro antigen-specific IgE can be tested immediately after an episode of anaphylaxis but is less sensitive than skin testing.
- Basophil activation testing (BAT)
- BAT is a flow cytometry–based blood test used to identify sensitized IgE-bound basophils.[3] On reexposure to a specific allergen, basophils become activated with upregulation of surface markers, which are detected by flow cytometry.[3]
- This test is commercially available for use in diagnosing IgE-mediated reactions to food, drugs, and Hymenoptera venom.[3,5]
- However, it is not recommended in patients who have chronically elevated histamine at baseline (e.g., food allergies, recurrent reactions, or NSAID hypersensitivities).
- BAT has not yet been validated or approved by the Food and Drug Administration (FDA) for use in patients.[3]

TREATMENT

- Regardless of severity, all anaphylactic episodes deserve treatment and observation, because any mild reaction can rapidly degrade into a more serious reaction.
- Cardiac and respiratory arrest can develop in as early as 5 minutes.[8] In one report, 50% of the fatalities occurred within the first 60 minutes of symptom onset.[14] Therefore, for **acute treatment**, the initial assessment is paramount for prompt recognition of symptoms and immediate institution of treatment.
- The **first line of therapy is epinephrine**, and it should be administered immediately.[8]
- The patient may require cardiopulmonary resuscitation to support the airway and maintain adequate oxygenation and circulation.
- Treatment also includes long-term risk management. Physicians should take steps to reduce long-term risk: assess and treat comorbidities (asthma, cardiovascular disease, mastocytosis, and others); assess for comedications such as nonselective β-blockers; identify triggers; and avoid known allergens.

Medications

First Line
- **Epinephrine is the only known medication that can prevent or reverse obstruction to airflow in the upper and lower airways and prevent or reverse cardiovascular collapse.**[8] Epinephrine acts on vascular smooth muscle as a vasoconstrictor, increasing systemic blood pressures. It also acts on the mucosa to reduce edema.
- **There are no absolute contraindications to the use of epinephrine in anaphylaxis.**[18] Failure to inject epinephrine in a timely manner is reported to contribute to fatality.[8,18]
- **It should be administered immediately using a dose of 0.3–0.5 mg IM** (0.3–0.5 mL of a 1:1,000 solution) in the anterolateral thigh preferentially.
- Epinephrine dose may be repeated at 5-minute intervals PRN.
- Smaller doses may be needed in the elderly (0.2 mg).
- In children, the dose is 0.01 mg/kg (1:1,000) IM to a maximum of 0.5 mg with repeated doses every 5 minutes PRN.
- Larger doses may be needed in patients receiving β-blockers. **Glucagon** (1–2 mg IV push) may be needed in these patients.
- Administration via central line (3–5 mL of **1:10,000 solution**) or through endotracheal tube (3–5 mL of a **1:10,000 solution diluted in 10-mL normal saline**) may be necessary in cases of severe hypotension or respiratory failure.
- A continuous infusion of 1:10,000 epinephrine may be necessary in patients with protracted symptoms, a bolus of 100 μg/70 kg over a period of 5–10 minutes may be given (1:10,000 concentration). A continuous infusion of 1–5 μg/min/70 kg is usually sufficient to maintain systemic perfusion.

Second Line
- **Glucocorticosteroids**
  - **Glucocorticosteroids do not have an immediate effect, and their use is currently considered ancillary.**
  - Glucocorticosteroids have the theoretical ability to prevent a relapse of symptoms based on management of acute asthma and the abrogation of the late-phase response. However, the ability to prevent an anaphylactic biphasic reaction has not been proven in a controlled study.
  - Patients with idiopathic anaphylaxis may also require long-term glucocorticoid treatment. Patients who have more than six episodes per year may be considered for placement on maintenance prednisone therapy.
  - **Antihistamines**
  - **Antihistamines also do not have an immediate effect but may shorten the duration of symptoms.**
  - **Diphenhydramine** can be administered IV (25–100 mg over 5–10 minutes), IM, or PO. It can be given every 6 hours for 24–48 hours after the reaction.
  - **H2 antagonists** (i.e., ranitidine, cimetidine) may also be added.[14]
- **Bronchodilators**
  - **In patients with asthma who are undergoing anaphylaxis-associated wheezing, epinephrine remains the first line of therapy.**
  - However, if wheezing persists, bronchodilators such as albuterol (nebulized every 20 minutes or continuously) or theophylline may be considered.
- Omalizumab: In patients with food, venom, or idiopathic anaphylaxis, anti-IgE monoclonal antibody (omalizumab) may be an effective preventative medication. In idiopathic anaphylaxis, the use of omalizumab reduces the frequency of attacks and improves quality of life.[3,19]

Nonpharmacologic Therapies

- Airway management
  - Airway management may require endotracheal intubation if marked stridor or respiratory failure occurs.
  - **Racemic epinephrine** may be useful in treating laryngeal edema.
  - **If laryngeal edema is severe and not immediately responsive to epinephrine, consider a cricothyroidotomy or tracheotomy.**
- Volume expansion
  - Significant third spacing of fluid may occur in anaphylaxis, and the intravascular volume may decrease by up to 50%.
  - Volume expansion with IV fluids, beginning with a 500–1,000 mL bolus, should be titrated to blood pressure and urine output.
  - Colloid solutions, such as albumin, may be beneficial in cases of refractory hypotension or shock. The risk–benefit profile of each solution should be carefully weighed, as albumin may precipitate pulmonary edema and is rather costly.

COMPLICATIONS

- Complications from anaphylaxis may arise from the uncontrolled reaction or from the treatment.
- Untreated anaphylaxis can lead to circulatory and respiratory collapse, leading to anaphylactic shock, severe airway obstruction, angioedema, cardiac arrhythmias, myocardial infarction, cardiac arrest, and, in rare cases, death.[18] Patients with sustained airway obstruction may require ventilator assistance.
- The risk of mortality is higher with any delays in rapid use of epinephrine.[4,11] Improper use of auto-injectable epinephrine by patients because of lack of training, failure to carry

epinephrine, and lack of access of epinephrine in public spaces are also risk factors for higher mortality.[3,20]

- Potential risks of treatment with IV epinephrine include myocardial ischemia and infarction, arrhythmias, and hypertensive crisis.

REFERRAL

Consider referral to an allergy/immunology specialist for consideration for allergen-specific and allergen nonspecific immunomodulation. Allergen-specific therapy includes immunotherapy with insect venom and desensitization to β-lactam antibiotics, NSAIDs, and others.[3]

PATIENT EDUCATION

Prepare for emergencies with an **anaphylaxis emergency action plan** (see www.aaaai.org), **auto-injector, and medical identification.**

MONITOR/FOLLOW-UP

- Patients with mild reactions limited to flushing, urticaria, angioedema, cramping, or mild bronchospasm should be monitored in the emergency department for a minimum of 6–8 hours for possible biphasic reaction.
- All other reactions warrant admission to the hospital for 24-hour observation.

OUTCOMES/PROGNOSIS

- There are scant data regarding recurrence of anaphylaxis. It is estimated that at least 30% of patients will experience one or more recurrence after the initial episode.[11]
- Patient with a history of atopy are more likely to have recurrent episodes.
- An emphasis on prevention and avoidance strategies are key in preventing future episodes.

SPECIAL CONSIDERATIONS

- **Latex allergy (LA)** is a type of immediate hypersensitivity reaction caused by exposure to products containing natural rubber latex in persons with latex-specific IgE.
  - Clinical presentation includes **urticaria, asthma, rhinoconjunctivitis, or, at its most, severe anaphylaxis.**[21]
  - It is estimated that **LA occurs in 4–5% of the health care worker population, which is three times more prevalent in LA than in the general population.**[22]
  - Increased prevalence of LA has been reported among patients with spina bifida and those with a history of multiple surgeries early in life.[23]
  - Although there was a dramatic increase in reported LA with the institution of universal precautions in the 1980s, more recent years have seen a decrease in the incidence of LA, likely because of improvements in the manufacturing process and creation of latex-safe environments.[3]
- Latex-related anaphylaxis occurs when sensitized individuals are exposed to latex products.
  - It is a rare phenomenon, and most episodes occur during surgical procedures, childbirth, gynecologic examinations, or dental procedures.

○ In patients undergoing surgical procedures, latex was the second most common cause of anaphylaxis occurring after muscular blockade.[3,24]

○ Anaphylaxis has also been associated with inhalational exposure.

• **Diagnosis of LAs** relies on measurement of latex-specific serum IgE.[3] None of the assays can demonstrate complete diagnostic reliability, and results must be interpreted in the context of the clinical suspicion for LA.

○ Skin testing poses a high risk of anaphylactic reactions and is, therefore, not recommended in the United States.[3]

○ Provocational challenge studies have been performed on patients with negative results from serologic or skin prick testing when they have strong clinical histories that support LA.

• **Treatment and prevention**

○ **Treatment of anaphylaxis secondary to LA is similar to other types of anaphylactic reactions with epinephrine.**

○ Most IgE-mediated reactions to latex occur in health care workers or latex-sensitive individuals undergoing medical procedures. Creation of "latex-safe" clinics and hospitals has been successful in decreasing latex-induced symptoms.[25]

▪ Prior to hospital admission and surgical procedures, screening questions should be asked to identify patients with possible latex sensitization.

▪ Once LA is detected, documentation and education regarding latex avoidance are imperative.

REFERENCES

1. Simons FE, Ardusso LR, Bilo MB, et al. International consensus on (ICON) anaphylaxis. *World Allergy Organ J.* 2014;7:9.

2. Reber LL, Hernandez JD, Galli SJ. The pathophysiology of anaphylaxis. *J Allergy Clin Immunol.* 2017;140:335–48.

3. Jimenez-Rodriguez TW, Garcia-Neuer M, Alenazy LA, et al. Anaphylaxis in the 21st century: phenotypes, endotypes, and biomarkers. *J Asthma Allergy.* 2018;11:121–42.

4. Samant SA, Campbell RL, Li JT. Anaphylaxis: diagnostic criteria and epidemiology. *Allergy Asthma Proc.* 2013;34:115–19.

5. Muraro A, Lemanske RF Jr, Castells M, et al. Precision medicine in allergic disease-food allergy, drug allergy, and anaphylaxis-PRACTALL document of the European Academy of Allergy and Clinical Immunology and the American Academy of Allergy, Asthma and Immunology. *Allergy.* 2017;72:1006–21.

6. Decker WW, Campbell RL, Manivannan V, et al. The etiology and incidence of anaphylaxis in Rochester, Minnesota: a report from the Rochester Epidemiology Project. *J Allergy Clin Immunol.* 2008;122:1161–5.

7. Lieberman P, Camargo CA Jr, Bohlke K, et al. Epidemiology of anaphylaxis: findings of the American College of Allergy, Asthma and Immunology Epidemiology of Anaphylaxis Working Group. *Ann Allergy Asthma Immunol.* 2006;97:596–602.

8. Lieberman PL. Recognition and first-line treatment of anaphylaxis. *Am J Med.* 2014;127(1 suppl):S6–11.

9. Simons FE, Ebisawa M, Sanchez-Borges M, et al. 2015 update of the evidence base: World Allergy Organization anaphylaxis guidelines. *World Allergy Organ J.* 2015;8:32.

10. Wood RA, Camargo CA Jr, Lieberman P, et al. Anaphylaxis in America: the prevalence and characteristics of anaphylaxis in the United States. *J Allergy Clin Immunol.* 2014;133:461–7.

11. Tejedor Alonso MA, Moro Moro M, Mugica Garcia MV. Epidemiology of anaphylaxis. *Clin Exp Allergy.* 2015;45:1027–39.

12. Ditto AM, Harris KE, Krasnick J, et al. Idiopathic anaphylaxis: a series of 335 cases. *Ann Allergy Asthma Immunol.* 1996;77:285–91.

13. Lieberman P, Nicklas RA, Randolph C, et al. Anaphylaxis—a practice parameter update 2015. *Ann Allergy Asthma Immunol.* 2015;115:341–84.

14. Lieberman P. Anaphylaxis. In: Adkinson NF Jr, ed. *Middleton's Allergy Principles and Practice.* Vol 2. 7th ed. Philadelphia, PA: Elsevier Inc., 2009:1027–49.

15. Sampson HA, Munoz-Furlong A, Campbell RL, et al. Second symposium on the definition and management of anaphylaxis: summary report—Second National Institute of Allergy and Infectious Disease/Food Allergy and Anaphylaxis Network symposium. *J Allergy Clin Immunol.* 2006;117:391–7.

16. Stark BJ, Sullivan TJ. Biphasic and protracted anaphylaxis. *J Allergy Clin Immunol.* 1986;78:76–83.

17. Schwartz LB, Irani AM. Serum tryptase and the laboratory diagnosis of systemic mastocytosis. *Hematol Oncol Clin North Am.* 2000;14:641–57.

18. Greenberger PA. Fatal and near-fatal anaphylaxis: factors that can worsen or contribute to fatal outcomes. *Immunol Allergy Clin North Am.* 2015;35:375–86.

19. Warrier P, Casale TB. Omalizumab in idiopathic anaphylaxis. *Ann Allergy Asthma Immunol.* 2009;102:257–8.

20. Song TT, Worm M, Lieberman P. Anaphylaxis treatment: current barriers to adrenaline auto-injector use. *Allergy.* 2014;69:983–91.

21. Poley GE Jr, Slater JE. Latex allergy. *J Allergy Clin Immunol.* 2000;105:1054–62.

22. Bousquet J, Flahault A, Vandenplas O, et al. Natural rubber latex allergy among health care workers: a systematic review of the evidence. *J Allergy Clin Immunol.* 2006;118:447–54.

23. Niggemann B. IgE-mediated latex allergy—an exciting and instructive piece of allergy history. *Pediatr Allergy Immunol.* 2010;21:997–1001.

24. Yunker NS, Wagner BJ. A pharmacologic review of anaphylaxis. *Plast Surg Nurs.* 2016;36:173–9.

25. Bernstein DI, Karnani R, Biagini RE, et al. Clinical and occupational outcomes in health care workers with natural rubber latex allergy. *Ann Allergy Asthma Immunol.* 2003;90:209–13.

Asthma

5

Watcharoot Kanchongkittiphon and
Leonard B. Bacharier

GENERAL PRINCIPLES

Definition

- Asthma is a **chronic inflammatory disorder of the airways associated with airway hyperresponsiveness**, which leads to recurrent wheezing, coughing, chest tightness, and difficulty breathing.[1]
- **Variable, reversible airflow obstruction** is a hallmark of asthma.
- **Asthma exacerbations** are periods of worsening symptoms between periods of relative symptom stability.

Classification

Asthma classification is based on symptom frequency and severity at diagnosis and prior to initiation of controller therapy (Table 5-1),[2] while the level of disease control is assessed at follow-up visits and is reflected by symptom frequency and frequency of exacerbations (Table 5-2).[2]

Epidemiology

- Asthma usually begins in childhood. Adult-onset asthma occurs less often and should raise consideration for occupational asthma.[3]
- As of 2018, an estimated 8.3% of U.S. residents have asthma.[4]
- The increase in asthma prevalence has correlated with atopic sensitization, also reflected in the increase in allergic rhinitis and eczema.[5,6]
- The United States initially had an increase in asthma-specific mortality rate between 1982 and 1995. Since then, the death rate has decreased.[7] In Canada, asthma-specific mortality rates per 100,000 asthma population decreased by 54.4%, from 13.6% in 1999 to 6.2% in 2008.[8]
- **Socioeconomic considerations**
  - A higher rate of asthma prevalence has been seen in blacks and Hispanics than in whites.[7]
  - In people living in poverty and in the inner city, greater asthma mortality may be associated with the lack of adherence to asthma treatment complicated by a decreased or lack of access to medical care or insurance.[9]
  - According to the Centers for Disease Control and Prevention (CDC), asthma costs in the United States total $56 billion annually, which includes medical expenditures such as hospitalizations, emergency department (ED) visits, outpatient care, and medications.
  - Asthma is also responsible for significant work and school absenteeism and losses in productivity.

Etiology

- The pathogenesis of asthma is complex and results from a combination of factors including **genetic, environmental, immunologic, and developmental**.
- Airway narrowing causing obstruction of airflow results in a combination of bronchoconstriction **and airway inflammation,** which are the dominant physiologic factors leading to clinical symptoms.[1]

TABLE 5-1 CLASSIFICATION OF ASTHMA SEVERITY

Level of severity[a]			Persistent		
Components of severity		Intermittent	Mild	Moderate	Severe
Impairment	Symptoms	≤2 days/week	>2 days/week, but not daily	Daily	Throughout the day
	Nighttime awakenings	≤2×/month	3–4×/month	>1×/week, but not nightly	Often 7×/week
	SABA use for symptom control (not prevention of EIB)	≤2 days/week	>2 days/week, but not daily and not >1× on any day	Daily	Several times per day
	Interference with normal activity	None	Minor limitation	Some limitation	Extremely limited
	Lung function[b]	Normal FEV$_1$ between exacerbations FEV$_1$ >80% predicted FEV$_1$/FVC normal	FEV$_1$ >80% predicted FEV$_1$/FVC normal	FEV$_1$ >60% but <80% predicted FEV$_1$/FVC reduced 5%	FEV$_1$ <60% predicted FEV$_1$/FVC reduced >5%
Risk	Exacerbations requiring oral systemic corticosteroids	0–1/year	≥2/year	≥2/year	≥2/year
Recommended starting step (see Table 5-5)		Step 1	Step 2	Step 3	Step 4 or 5 Consider short course of OSC

[a]For patients ≥12 years.

[b]Normal FEV$_1$/FVC: 8–19 years, 85%; 20–39 years, 80%; 40–59 years, 75%; 60–80 years, 70.

EIB, exercise-induced bronchospasm; FEV$_1$, forced expiratory volume in 1 second; FVC, forced vital capacity; OSC, oral systemic corticosteroids; SABA, short-acting β$_2$-agonist.

Adapted from National Institutes of Health. National Heart, Lung, and Blood Institute. National Asthma Education and Prevention Program. Expert Panel Report 3 (EPR-3): Guidelines for the Diagnosis and Management of Asthma. Summary Report 2007. NIH Publication 08-5846. Bethesda, MD. August 2007.

TABLE 5-2 CLASSIFICATION OF ASTHMA CONTROL

Components of control		Well controlled	Not well controlled	Very poorly controlled
Impairment	Symptoms	≤2 days/week	>2 days/week	Throughout the day
	Nighttime awakenings	≤2×/month	1–3×/week	≥4×/week
	Interference with normal activity	None	Some limitation	Extremely limited
	SABA use for symptom control (not prevention of EIB)	≤2 days/week	>2 days/week	Several times per day
	FEV_1 or peak flow	>80% predicted/personal best	60–80% predicted/personal best	<60% predicted/personal best
	Validated questionnaires: ATAQ			
	ACQ	0	1–2	3–4
	ACT	≤0.75	≥1.5	N/A
		≥20	16–19	≤15
Risk	Exacerbations requiring oral systemic corticosteroids	0–1/year	≥2/year	≥2/year
	Progressive loss of lung function	Evaluation requires long-term follow-up care		
	Treatment-related adverse effects	Medication side effects can vary in intensity from none to very troublesome and worrisome. The level of intensity does not correlate to specific levels of control but should be considered in the overall assessment of risk.		

Classification of asthma control[a]

[a]For patients ≥12 years.

ACQ, asthma control questionnaire; ACT, asthma control test; ATAQ, asthma therapy assessment questionnaire; EIB, exercise-induced bronchospasm; FEV_1, forced expiratory volume at 1 second; SABA, short-acting β_2-agonist.

Adapted from National Institutes of Health. National Heart, Lung, and Blood Institute. National Asthma Education and Prevention Program Expert Panel Report 3 (EPR-3): Guidelines for the Diagnosis and Management of Asthma. Summary Report 2007. NIH Publication 08-5846. Bethesda, MD. August 2007.

- **Airway hyperresponsiveness** results from exaggerated bronchoconstriction because of inflammation, neuroregulatory dysfunction, and structural changes.
- Bronchoconstriction can also be triggered in response to various stimuli, including tobacco smoke, weather changes, infections, and emotions.
- **Airway inflammation** is an important factor predisposing to bronchoconstriction.[10]
  - Even in the presence of well-controlled intermittent symptoms, airway inflammation persists.
  - Mast cells activated by allergen through cell-surface IgE receptors release **histamine, cysteinyl leukotrienes,** and **prostaglandin D2,** which cause bronchoconstriction.
  - Eosinophils release **major basic protein,** causing airway epithelial cell injury.
  - T_H2 cells release **interleukin (IL)-4, IL-5,** and **IL-13,** which potentiate eosinophilic inflammation and promote IgE production by B cells.
  - **Innate lymphocyte type 2 cells,** regulated by **IL-25** and **IL-33** secreted from airway epithelial cells, promote airway inflammation by secreting IL-5 and IL-13.
  - **Thymic stromal lymphopoietin (TSLP)** is an epithelial-derived cytokine that promotes T_H2 inflammation by modulating dendritic cell function, activating T_H2 cytokine production from T cells, and inhibiting regulatory T-cell function.[11]
- Multiple mediators are involved in asthma and mediate inflammatory responses.[12]
  - **Chemokines:** CCL11 or eotaxin recruits eosinophils. CCL17 and CCL22 recruit T_H2 cells.
  - **Cytokines:** IL-5 supports eosinophil differentiation and survival, IL-4 drives IgE expression and T_H2 cell differentiation, IL-13 promotes IgE expression, and IL-1β and tumor necrosis factor (TNF)-α amplify inflammatory response.
  - Deposition of collagen and proteoglycan causes subepithelial fibrosis. Smooth muscle cell hypertrophy and hyperplasia, under the influence of chitinase-like protein YKL-40 and vascular endothelial growth factors, lead to increased airway thickness.

Risk Factors

- **Atopy:** Epidemiologic studies consistently show an association between allergic sensitization and asthma.[5]
- **Genetics:** Asthma is often associated with gene-by-environment interactions, such that a combination of genetic susceptibility and an appropriate environmental stimulus increases asthma susceptibility. Genome-wide association studies have identified multiple genes associated with asthma. Studies suggest that a complex interaction of genes combined with environmental exposure(s) contributes to asthma risk.[13-15]
  - Parental diagnosis of asthma increases the risk of asthma in an offspring.
  - Twin studies show higher concordance rates in monozygotic twins.
- **Gender:** In early childhood, male children are at a higher risk for developing asthma, whereas in adolescents and adulthood, females are at higher risk.
- **Prematurity** and low birth weight have been associated with the development of symptoms consistent with asthma, both with and without a history of neonatal respiratory distress, but the mechanism and its involvement with other asthma risk factors are not known.
- **Passive tobacco smoke exposure:** In utero exposure to tobacco smoke affects airway responsiveness after birth. Children exposed to secondhand smoke have an increased frequency of wheezing and increased risk of more severe lower respiratory tract infections during the first year of life.[16]
- **Respiratory infections,** especially rhinovirus and respiratory syncytial virus, have been associated with recurrent childhood wheezing.[17] Respiratory infections are also associated with asthma exacerbations.
- The **hygiene hypothesis** suggests that the rising prevalence of asthma in developed countries is due to the overall decrease in viral and bacterial infections, which increase

activation of T_H2 lymphocytes. Also, the increased use of antibiotics in children may alter the normal gut flora in infants and increase the T_H2 immune response.[18]
- **Air pollutants** have been linked to asthma.[19]
  - Exposure to **nitrogen dioxide** in inner-city schoolchildren has been associated with an increase in airflow obstruction.[20]
  - Chronic exposure to nitrogen dioxide from indoor gas stoves may be associated with an increase in asthma symptoms in lower socioeconomic groups.[19]
  - **Diesel exhaust** particles may modulate immune response to a T_H2 phenotype.[21]
- **The Asthma Predictive Index** helps predict development of persistent asthma after 6 years of age.[22] The index is considered positive if there is
  - Recurrent wheezing in children aged 3 years or younger, *and*
  - One major criterion (parental asthma or physician-diagnosed eczema in patient) or
  - Two minor criteria (eosinophilia >4%, wheezing without colds, allergic rhinitis)
- **Risk factors for fatal asthma**
  - **Major risk** factors include
    - A recent history of poorly controlled asthma (e.g., increase in daily asthma symptoms and/or nocturnal awakening because of shortness of breath or wheezing, increased use of β_2-agonist, and variation in peak flow results).
    - A history of a near-fatal episode of asthma (intensive care unit admission and/or requirement of intubation previously).[23]
  - **Minor risk** factors include aeroallergen exposure, aspirin/NSAID exposure, cigarette smoke, illicit drug use, genetic factors, multiple ED visits or admissions for asthma, multiple oral corticosteroid requirements, psychosocial stress, depression, and poor medical adherence.

Prevention

- Identify **triggering factors** such as exposure to allergens, irritants, and viruses and **limit exposure** to these triggering factors.
- **Treatment of other comorbidities** that can worsen asthma should be optimized to reduce morbidity from asthma (e.g., conditions such as allergic rhinitis, sleep apnea, sinusitis, and gastroesophageal reflux disease).
- **Smoking cessation** must be a priority for any individual with asthma.

Associated Conditions

- Atopic diseases, including food allergy, atopic dermatitis, and allergic rhinitis, are frequently comorbid with asthma.
- The **atopic march** denotes the successive development of atopic dermatitis, allergic rhinitis, and asthma in childhood.[5]
- **Aspirin-exacerbated respiratory disease (AERD) (Samter triad)** is the co-occurrence of asthma, nasal polyps, and aspirin sensitivity.

DIAGNOSIS

Clinical Presentation

History
- Recurrent episodes of **reversible bronchoconstriction are the hallmark of asthma.**
- Four **classic symptoms** of asthma:
  - **Wheezing** (high-pitched whistling sound, usually upon exhalation) that may be audible without a stethoscope
  - **Cough (often worse at night)** that may be productive of secretions without being related to an infection cause

- Some patients rarely wheeze but cough instead, especially children. This is an important feature that should not be missed.
- **Curschmann spirals** are helical mucous plugs that may be observed in asthmatic sputum.
  ○ **Shortness of breath** or difficulty breathing
  ○ **Chest tightness**
- **Exercise-induced bronchospasm** can be the presenting symptom. Consider asthma if a patient cannot keep up with peers during athletic activity secondary to coughing, chest tightness, shortness of breath, or wheezing.
- **Nocturnal awakenings** with coughing or wheezing may be the presenting symptom. Nocturnal symptoms in a patient who has previously had only daytime symptoms may represent inadequate disease control or disease progression.
- **Family history** is frequently notable for the presence of atopic diseases.
- Asthma **triggers** such as exercise, viral infections, environmental triggers, and smoke should be identified during the history.
- **Environmental history** should be carefully reviewed for potential allergen and irritant exposures and should include
  ○ Details about the home/work/school environments
  ○ Whether the patient has a seasonal or perennial profile of symptoms
  ○ Animal exposure
  ○ Smoking history

Physical Examination
- Between acute exacerbations, patients with asthma may have a normal physical examination.
- Vital signs can be normal, even during an acute exacerbation. **Elevated heart rate and respiratory rate** are the most frequent abnormalities. Oxygen desaturation tends to be a late sign and may indicate impending respiratory failure.
- General appearance can be an important indicator of severity. **Inability to speak in complete sentences, agitation, and/or lethargy are alarming signs** and should prompt immediate intervention.
- Examination of the head, eyes, ears, nose, and throat may show signs of allergic disease or accessory muscle usage (especially in children). **Stridor or wheezing best heard in the neck suggests an alternative diagnosis,** such as vocal cord dysfunction (VCD) or upper airway obstruction.
- The lung examination frequently demonstrates high-pitched polyphonic end-expiratory wheezing with a prolonged expiratory phase. **In severe asthma exacerbations, wheezing may not be heard** ("silent chest") at all and may indicate impending respiratory failure.
  ○ Rhonchi or focal findings suggest a pulmonary infection that may have triggered the exacerbation or, in the absence of fever, may represent secretions commonly seen in asthmatics.
  ○ Respiratory muscle alternans is the paradoxical movement of the diaphragm with alternating abdominal and ribcage breathing. It represents a patient in extremis and is more commonly seen in children.
  ○ Retractions including suprasternal, intercostal, or subcostal retraction may be present during an exacerbation, particularly in children.

Differential Diagnosis
- The differential diagnosis of asthma in adults is presented in Table 5-3.
- **VCD** is voluntary or involuntary paradoxical adduction of the true or false vocal cords resulting in dyspnea that can mimic asthma.[24]

TABLE 5-3	DIFFERENTIAL DIAGNOSES OF ADULT ASTHMA
Chronic obstructive pulmonary disease (COPD)	Mechanical upper airway obstruction:
Congestive heart failure	Tumor
Pulmonary embolism	Epiglottitis
Tracheomalacia	Vocal cord dysfunction
Pulmonary eosinophilia	Foreign body
Allergic bronchopulmonary aspergillosis	Obstructive sleep apnea
Allergic rhinitis	

- In addition to dyspnea, patients often present with a choking sensation, dysphonia, and cough.
- Stridor (noisy breathing) may be inspiratory or expiratory or both and is heard best at the larynx.
- The flow-volume loops of pulmonary function test (PFT) may show flattening of the inspiratory curve.
- Definitive diagnosis of VCD is made by direct visualization of the vocal cords showing paradoxical movement during respiration.
- Treatment consists of speech therapy. Early diagnosis is important to avoid prolonged, unnecessary treatment, and some patients may also benefit from psychiatric counseling.

Diagnostic Testing

Laboratories
- Asthma is a clinical diagnosis. There are no blood tests that are diagnostic of asthma, although the presence of peripheral blood eosinophilia is often found.
- **Arterial blood gas measurement** may be indicated in the setting of an acute severe exacerbation in patients with signs of progressive respiratory failure.
  - Most patients will have an acute **respiratory alkalosis** from hyperventilation as the patient works to increase minute ventilation.
  - A patient whose CO_2 is normal or elevated during a severe exacerbation is in danger of respiratory failure. A "normal" or increasing value represents a patient who can no longer maintain a high minute ventilation and has begun to fatigue. Close monitoring is essential.

Imaging
- CXR is rarely necessary in the outpatient setting for an established asthmatic.
- A CXR of a pediatric patient who is wheezing for the first time may be helpful if history or physical examination suggests the possibility of aspiration of a foreign body or other atypical findings.
- In adults, CXR is particularly useful in patients who present with new-onset wheezing, have other comorbidities (e.g., congestive heart failure, chronic obstructive pulmonary disease [COPD], or pneumonia), or have focal findings on examination.
- CXR in asthma may demonstrate
  - Hyperinflation (flattening of the diaphragm)
  - Mucous plugging (linear atelectasis)
  - These findings may be indistinguishable from COPD.

Diagnostic Procedures

- **Spirometry** is a physiologic test that measures lung function. Measurement of forced expiratory volume in 1 second (FEV_1), forced vital capacity (FVC), and the ratio of FEV_1/FVC provides essential information for evaluation of asthma.[25]
  - **Reduced FEV_1/FVC ratio** indicates airflow obstruction.
  - The severity of airflow limitation is based on the **FEV_1% predicted**.
  - Assess the **reversibility** of the obstructive abnormality by repeating spirometry 15 minutes after administration of a bronchodilator. An **increase in FEV_1 of 12% and at least 200 mL** is considered a positive bronchodilator response.
- **Bronchoprovocation test:** Inhalation of **methacholine** induces bronchoconstriction by direct stimulation of airway smooth muscle receptors.[25] The provocative concentration 20 (PC20) is the dose of methacholine that provokes a 20% drop in FEV_1. **A methacholine PC20 of 8 mg/mL or less is considered a positive test.** This is a very sensitive test used to rule out asthma, although not all positive tests represent asthma.
- **Aeroallergen skin testing** may demonstrate positivity to aeroallergens in atopic asthma and is often useful in guiding therapy and counseling on allergen avoidance.
- **Peripheral blood eosinophilia** is often present and may be useful in phenotyping patients who are candidates for asthma biologics.

TREATMENT

- **Long-term goals** for the management of asthma include reduction of risk and impairment.
  - **Reduce risk** of morbidity and mortality by
    - Preventing exacerbations and minimizing ED visits/hospitalizations.
    - Preventing permanent loss of lung function.
    - Minimizing side effects of pharmacotherapy.
  - **Reduce functional impairment** by
    - Preventing day-to-day symptoms, including coughing, wheezing, or shortness of breath.
    - Minimizing use (≤ 2 days/week) of short-acting β_2-agonists (SABAs) for relief of symptoms (excluding pretreatment for exercise-induced asthma).
    - Maintaining normal activity levels to minimize interruption of exercise and attendance at work/school.

Medications

- **SABAs**, such as albuterol or levalbuterol, are inhaled medications that work through stimulation of airway β_2-adrenoreceptors to relax the airway smooth muscle.
  - Used in all types of asthma for relief of acute symptoms.
  - Also indicated for use as pretreatment in exercise-induced asthma.
- **Inhaled corticosteroids (ICSs) are the mainstay of persistent asthma therapy.**
  - They are anti-inflammatory, blocking late-phase reaction to allergen, reducing airway hyperresponsiveness, and inhibiting inflammatory cell migration and activation.
  - ICSs have an onset of action of several days, and their **maximal activity is seen 2–3 weeks after initiation of therapy**.
  - Local side effects include dysphonia, throat irritation, and oral candidiasis. Mouth rinsing after inhaler use may help prevent thrush.
  - Adrenal suppression is dose dependent, but the risk of symptomatic adrenal suppression is very low.
  - In children, ICSs are linked to a slight reduction in growth velocity. One study demonstrated a reduction of about 0.4 inches in final adult height.[26]

- **Leukotriene modifiers** are medications that alter the signaling or synthesis of leukotrienes, which are lipid inflammatory mediators.
  - **Leukotriene receptor antagonists** (LTRAs) (montelukast and zafirlukast) and a **5-lipoxygenase inhibitor** (zileuton) are commercially available.
  - They may be particularly effective in **aspirin-sensitive asthma** as well as **exercise-induced asthma**.[27]
- **Mast cell stabilizers** act by preventing degranulation of mast cells.
  - Generally, these are less effective medications and are considered alternative treatments for mild persistent asthma.
  - **Cromolyn sodium** and **nedocromil** are examples of mast cell stabilizers.
- **Anticholinergics** inhibit muscarinic cholinergic receptors and reduce intrinsic airway vagal tone, leading to bronchodilation.
  - Generally considered to be less effective in treating asthma symptoms than SABAs.
  - Most commonly used in combination with a SABA for moderate-to-severe asthma exacerbations and for those individuals who do not tolerate SABA (e.g., tachyarrhythmias).
- **Short-acting muscarinic antagonists (SAMAs)**
  - SAMAs such as ipratropium, when added to frequent SABA, may reduce the risk of hospitalization among children with severe exacerbations seen in the ED.[28]
- **Long-acting muscarinic antagonists (LAMAs)**
  - Adding tiotropium to ICS may benefit uncontrolled adult asthma patients already receiving ICS and adolescents receiving ICS with or without long-acting β_2-agonists (LABA), as it is associated with a lower risk of asthma exacerbation.[29]
  - Triple therapy with ICS, LABA, and LAMA is not associated with a lower risk of asthma exacerbation compared with ICS and LABA.[29]
- **LABAs** are long-acting inhaled medications providing bronchodilation for up to 12 (e.g., salmeterol and formoterol) or 24 (e.g., vilanterol) hours.
  - Early studies suggested increased mortality associated with LABA, though this seems to be associated with LABA monotherapy.[30] Four large Food and Drug Administration (FDA)-mandated studies concluded that LABA + ICS therapy did not result in a significantly higher risk of serious asthma-related events relative to ICS therapy alone, but did result in fewer severe exacerbations.[31]
  - **LABAs should not be used as monotherapy, but only as adjunctive therapy with ICSs for control of asthma.**[32]
- **Theophylline** is a methylxanthine drug that functions as both a phosphodiesterase inhibitor and an adenosine receptor antagonist to stimulate bronchodilation and reduce airway inflammation.
  - Serum levels of theophylline must be measured periodically because it has a relatively narrow therapeutic range. Target levels are 5–15 µg/mL.
  - Serious side effects include cardiac arrhythmia and seizure.
- **Systemic corticosteroids** are administered either parenterally or orally.
  - Primary indication in asthma is treatment of moderate-to-severe exacerbations.
  - Some patients with severe asthma may require chronic systemic corticosteroids to achieve and/or maintain asthma control.
  - Systemic corticosteroids should be reserved for asthma exacerbations with every effort made to transition to long-term controller medications.
  - The side effects of corticosteroids are multifold and include neuropsychiatric disturbances, weight gain, glucose intolerance, increased susceptibility to infections, avascular necrosis, growth stunting, and adrenal insufficiency when used chronically.
- **Magnesium sulfate** is administered via IV route. It has an effect on the smooth muscle, causing additional bronchodilation. Magnesium sulfate is safe and is used as an adjunct therapy in patients with severe exacerbations.[33]

- **Biologics**
  - **Omalizumab (anti-IgE)**[34]: Humanized monoclonal antibody against human IgE that is approved by the FDA for patients 6 years or older. Indicated as add-on therapy for allergic asthma with demonstrated sensitivity to perennial aeroallergens. Dose is based on IgE level and body weight. Administered every 2–4 weeks subcutaneously.
  - **Mepolizumab (anti-IL-5)**[35]: Humanized monoclonal antibody directed against the pro-eosinophil cytokine IL-5 and FDA approved as add-on therapy for asthma patients 6 years and older with an eosinophilic phenotype and for patients with eosinophilic granulomatosis with polyangiitis. It is a monthly subcutaneous injection in patients with severe asthma with eosinophil count ≥150 cells/μL at initiation or ≥300 cells/μL within the previous year.
  - **Reslizumab (anti-IL-5)**[36]: Humanized monoclonal antibody directed against the pro-eosinophil cytokine IL-5. This is an add-on maintenance treatment for patients 18 years and older with severe eosinophilic asthma. It is available as an IV preparation (dosed 3 mg/kg) administered every 4 weeks for patients with blood eosinophil counts ≥400 cells/μL.
  - **Benralizumab (anti-IL-5Rα)**[37]: Monoclonal antibody that binds to the α-subunit of the IL-5 receptor on eosinophils and basophils, which prevents IL-5 binding and enhances antibody-dependent cell-mediated cytotoxicity of these cells. It is indicated for the add-on management of severe asthma in patients 12 years and older with an eosinophilic phenotype. Benralizumab is subcutaneously administered 30 mg every 8 weeks (first three doses are every 4 weeks).
  - **Dupilumab (anti-IL-4Rα)**[38]: Humanized monoclonal antibody that binds to the IL-4Rα-subunit, which inhibits both IL-4 and IL-13 signaling and decreases IgE production. Dupilumab is indicated as add-on management for moderate-to-severe eosinophilic asthma and for atopic dermatitis in patients 12 years and older and is subcutaneously administered every 2 weeks.

Asthma Management

- **Acute exacerbation management** (see Table 5-4)
  - The focus of treatment is to immediately improve oxygenation, reduce airflow obstruction and inflammation, and alleviate symptoms.
  - **Antibiotics** are not routinely indicated for exacerbations unless there are signs or symptoms of coincident infection.
  - IV **magnesium sulfate** (2 g infused over 20 minutes) may provide some benefit for patients with severe exacerbations.[39]
- **Long-term management**
  - A stepwise approach to increasing therapy is recommended (Table 5-5).
  - Asthma control should be reassessed periodically while on therapy and treatment tailored to the level of control (Table 5-3).
  - Step-down therapy should be considered when asthma is well controlled for at least 3 months to determine the minimum amount of necessary medications.
- Frequent need for **oral corticosteroids** should prompt reevaluation of therapeutic management.
  - **Patient education** is key to long-term asthma control.
    - Home **peak flow monitoring** may be helpful in monitoring asthma control, especially in patients who have difficulty assessing their own symptoms.
    - **Asthma action plans** indicate a stepwise treatment plan tailored to each individual patient. Typically, they indicate warning signs of worsening symptoms, such as a decrease in peak flow, along with a therapeutic intervention.
    - **Identify and recognize triggers** so that patients are able to implement environmental controls to reduce exacerbations.
  - **Yearly influenza vaccination** is recommended because asthmatic patients are more susceptible to complications.

TABLE 5-4 ACUTE ASTHMA EXACERBATION MANAGEMENT

	Symptoms and signs	Initial PEF (or FEV$_1$)	Clinical course
Mild	Dyspnea only with activity (assess tachypnea in young children)	PEF ≥70% predicted or personal best	• Usually cared for at home • Prompt relief with inhaled SABA • Possible short course of oral systemic corticosteroids
Moderate	Dyspnea interferes with or limits usual activity	PEF 40–69% predicted or personal best	• Usually requires office or ED visit • Relief from frequent inhaled SABA • OSC; some symptoms last 1–2 days after treatment is begun
Severe	Dyspnea at rest; interferes with conversation	PEF <40% predicted or personal best	• Usually requires ED visit and likely hospitalization • Partial relief from frequent inhaled SABA • OSC; some symptoms last >3 days after treatment is begun • Adjunctive therapies may be helpful
Life-threatening	Too dyspneic to speak; perspiring	PEF <25% of predicted or personal best	• Requires ED/hospitalization; possible ICU • Minimal or no relief from frequent inhaled SABA • IV corticosteroids • Adjunctive therapies are helpful

ED, emergency department; FEV$_1$, forced expiratory volume at 1 second; ICU, intensive care unit; OSC, oral systemic corticosteroid; PEF, peak expiratory flow; SABA, short-acting β$_2$-agonist.

Adapted from National Institutes of Health. National Heart, Lung, and Blood Institute. National Asthma Education and Prevention Program. Expert Panel Report 3 (EPR-3): Guidelines for the Diagnosis and Management of Asthma. Summary Report 2007. NIH Publication 08-5846. Bethesda, MD. August 2007.

TABLE 5-5	STEPWISE ASTHMA MANAGEMENT FOR PATIENTS ≥12 YEARS					
	Step 1	Step 2	Step 3	Step 4	Step 5	Step 6
	Intermittent asthma	Persistent asthma: daily medication				
Preferred	SABA PRN	Low-dose ICS	Low-dose ICS + LABA or medium-dose ICS	Medium-dose ICS + LABA	High-dose ICS + LABA	High-dose ICS + LABA + oral corticosteroid Consider omalizumab for patients who have allergic asthma
Alternative		Cromolyn, LTRA Nedocromil or theophylline	Low-dose ICS + LTRA, theophylline, or zileuton	Medium-dose ICS + LTRA, theophylline, or zileuton	Consider omalizumab for patients who have allergic asthma	

Patient education and environmental control, and management of comorbidities at each step.

Steps 2–4: Consider SC allergen immunotherapy for patients who have allergic asthma.

Rescue medication
- SABA PRN for symptoms—up to three treatments at 20-minute intervals initially. Treatment intensity depends on symptom severity.
- Consider short course of oral corticosteroids.
- Increasing use of SABA or use >2 days/week for symptom relief (not prevention of EIB) generally indicates inadequate control and the need to step treatment.

Note
- If an alternative treatment is used and response is inadequate, discontinue it and use the preferred treatment before stepping up.
- Theophylline requires serum concentration levels monitoring; zileuton requires liver function monitoring.
- LABAs are not indicated for acute symptom relief and should be used in combination with an ICS.

EIB, exercise-induced bronchoconstriction; ICS, inhaled corticosteroid; LABA, long-acting β₂-agonist; LTRA, leukotriene receptor antagonist; SABA, short-acting β₂-agonist.

Adapted from National Institutes of Health. National Heart, Lung, and Blood Institute. National Asthma Education and Prevention Program. Expert Panel Report 3 (EPR-3): Guidelines for the Diagnosis and Management of Asthma. Summary Report 2007. NIH Publication 08-5846. Bethesda, MD. August 2007.

COMPLICATIONS

Status Asthmaticus

- Defined as a severe exacerbation unresponsive to repeated courses of β-agonist therapy, such as inhaled albuterol, levalbuterol, or SC epinephrine.[40]
- Patients at risk for status asthmaticus are those who are on oral corticosteroids, who smoke, who have previously been intubated, who have been admitted to an intensive care unit within the last year, and who frequently or recently visited the ED.

SPECIAL CONSIDERATIONS

Asthma during Pregnancy

- Asthma control during pregnancy is variable, with roughly one-third of women improving, one-third remaining stable, and one-third deteriorating.[41]
- Overall studies are reassuring that adverse effects on pregnancy are rare with albuterol and ICSs.
- The general goals and principles of asthma treatment are similar to those of nonpregnant patients.[42,43]
- The advantages of treating asthma in pregnancy markedly outweigh potential risks of controller and reliever medication.[42,43]
- Poorly controlled asthma increases the risk to the fetus because of maternal hypoxia.
- Careful reassessment of asthma control medications before pregnancy and discussion with the patient are necessary to minimize risk to the fetus.

Exercise-Induced Bronchoconstriction (EIB)

- Patients develop symptoms of asthma with bronchoconstriction during or after exercise.
- Pretreatment with SABAs before exercise is the preferred treatment.
- If SABA use is frequent, daily or pretreatment with LTRA is recommended.[44]
- Warm-up before exercise also reduces the occurrence of EIB.

REFERENCES

1. Boulet LP. Diagnosis of asthma in adults. In: Adkinson NF, Bochner B, Burks AW, et al., eds. *Middleton's Allergy: Principles and Practice.* 8th ed. Philadelphia, PA: Elsevier Saunders, 2014: 892–901.
2. National Institutes of Health. National Heart, Lung, and Blood Institute. National Asthma Education and Prevention Program. Expert Panel Report 3 (EPR-3): guidelines for the diagnosis and management of asthma. Summary Report 2007. NIH Publication 08-5846. Bethesda, MD. August 2007. https://www.nhlbi.nih.gov/sites/default/files/media/docs/EPR-3_Asthma_Full_Report_2007.pdf
3. de Nijs SB, Venekamp LN, Bel EH. Adult-onset asthma: is it really different? *Eur Resp J.* 2013;22(127):44–52.
4. Centers for Disease Control and Prevention. Most recent asthma data. 2019. Last Accessed 3/22/20. https://www.cdc.gov/asthma/most_recent_data.htm
5. Hill DA, Spergel JM. The atopic march: critical evidence and clinical relevance. *Ann Allergy Asthma Immunol.* 2018;120(2):131–7.
6. Masoli M, Fabian D, Holt S, et al. The global burden of asthma: executive summary of the GINA Dissemination Committee report. *Allergy.* 2004;59(5):469–78.
7. Moorman JE, Akinbami LJ, Bailey CM, et al. National surveillance of asthma: United States, 2001–2010. *Vital Health Stat 3.* 2012;(35):1–58.
8. To T, Simatovic J, Zhu J, et al. Asthma deaths in a large provincial health system. A 10-year population-based study. *Annals Am Thorac Soc.* 2014;11(8):1210–7.
9. Keet CA, Matsui EC, McCormack MC, et al. Urban residence, neighborhood poverty, race/ethnicity, and asthma morbidity among children on Medicaid. *J Allergy Clin Immunol.* 2017;140(3):822–7.
10. Holgate ST, Thomas M. Asthma. In: O'Hehir R, Holgate S, Sheikh A, eds. *Middleton's Allergy Essentials.* 1st ed. Philadelphia, PA: Elsevier, 2017.

11. Cianferoni A, Spergel J. The importance of TSLP in allergic disease and its role as a potential therapeutic target. *Expert Rev Clin Immunol.* 2014;10(11):1463–74.

12. Al Selahi EM, Cooke AJ, Kempe E, et al. Hypersensitivity disorders. In: Lee G, Stukus D, Yu J, eds. *ACAAI Review for the Allergy & Immunology Boards.* 3rd ed. Arlington Heights, IL: American College of Allergy, Asthma & Immunology, 2016.

13. Mathias RA. Introduction to genetics and genomics in asthma: genetics of asthma. *Adv Exp Med Biol.* 2014;795:125–55.

14. Ramasamy A, Kuokkanen M, Vedantam S, et al. Genome-wide association studies of asthma in population-based cohorts confirm known and suggested loci and identify an additional association near HLA. *PLoS One.* 2012;7(9):e44008.

15. Toncheva AA, Potaczek DP, Schedel M, et al. Childhood asthma is associated with mutations and gene expression differences of ORMDL genes that can interact. *Allergy.* 2015;70(10):1288–99.

16. Gaffin JM, Kanchongkittiphon W, Phipatanakul W. Perinatal and early childhood environmental factors influencing allergic asthma immunopathogenesis. *Int Immunopharmacol.* 2014;22(1):21–30.

17. Bacharier LB, Cohen R, Schweiger T, et al. Determinants of asthma after severe respiratory syncytial virus bronchiolitis. *J Allergy Clin Immunol.* 2012;130(1):91–100.e3.

18. von Mutius E, Vercelli D. Farm living: effects on childhood asthma and allergy. *Nat Rev Immunol.* 2010;10(12):861–8.

19. Kanchongkittiphon W, Mendell MJ, Gaffin JM, et al. Indoor environmental exposures and exacerbation of asthma: an update to the 2000 review by the Institute of Medicine. *Environ Health Perspect.* 2015;123(1):6–20.

20. Gaffin JM, Hauptman M, Petty CR, et al. Nitrogen dioxide exposure in school classrooms of inner-city children with asthma. *J Allergy Clin Immunol.* 2018;141(6):2249–55.e2.

21. Alexis NE, Carlsten C. Interplay of air pollution and asthma immunopathogenesis: a focused review of diesel exhaust and ozone. *Int Immunopharmacol.* 2014;23(1):347–55.

22. Castro-Rodriguez JA, Holberg CJ, Wright AL, et al. A clinical index to define risk of asthma in young children with recurrent wheezing. *Am J Respir Crit Care Med.* 2000;162(4 Pt 1):1403–6.

23. Alvarez GG, Schulzer M, Jung D, et al. A systematic review of risk factors associated with near-fatal and fatal asthma. *Can Respir J.* 2005;12(5):265–70.

24. Matrka L. Paradoxic vocal fold movement disorder. *Otolaryngol Clin North Am.* 2014;47(1):135–46.

25. Miller MR, Hankinson J, Brusasco V, et al. Standardisation of spirometry. *Eur Respir J.* 2005;26(2):319–38.

26. Loke YK, Blanco P, Thavarajah M, et al. Impact of inhaled corticosteroids on growth in children with asthma: systematic review and meta-analysis. *PLoS One.* 2015;10(7):e0133428.

27. de Benedictis FM, Vaccher S, de Benedictis D. Montelukast sodium for exercise-induced asthma. *Drugs Today (Barc).* 2008;44(11):845–55.

28. Griffiths B, Ducharme FM. Combined inhaled anticholinergics and short-acting β_2-agonists for initial treatment of acute asthma in children. *Cochrane Database Syst Rev.* 2013(8):CD000060.

29. Sobieraj DM, Baker WL, Nguyen E, et al. Association of inhaled corticosteroids and long-acting muscarinic antagonists with asthma control in patients with uncontrolled, persistent asthma: a systematic review and meta-analysis. *JAMA.* 2018;319(14):1473–84.

30. Cazzola M, Page CP, Rogliani P, et al. β_2-agonist therapy in lung disease. *Am J Respir Crit Care Med.* 2013;187(7):690–6.

31. Busse WW, Bateman ED, Caplan AL, et al. Combined analysis of asthma safety trials of long-acting β_2-agonists. *N Engl J Med.* 2018;378(26):2497–505.

32. Tovey D. Asthma challenges: the place of inhaled long-acting β-agonists. *Cochrane Database Syst Rev.* 2010;2011:ED000002.

33. Song WJ, Chang YS. Magnesium sulfate for acute asthma in adults: a systematic literature review. *Asia Pac Allergy.* 2012;2(1):76–85.

34. Humbert M, Busse W, Hanania NA, et al. Omalizumab in asthma: an update on recent developments. *J Allergy Clin Immunol Pract.* 2014;2(5):525–36.e1.

35. Bel EH, Wenzel SE, Thompson PJ, et al. Oral glucocorticoid-sparing effect of mepolizumab in eosinophilic asthma. *N Engl J Med.* 2014;371(13):1189–97.

36. Castro M, Zangrilli J, Wechsler ME, et al. Reslizumab for inadequately controlled asthma with elevated blood eosinophil counts: results from two multicentre, parallel, double-blind, randomised, placebo-controlled, phase 3 trials. *Lancet Respir Med.* 2015;3(5):355–66.

37. Bleecker ER, FitzGerald JM, Chanez P, et al. Efficacy and safety of benralizumab for patients with severe asthma uncontrolled with high-dosage inhaled corticosteroids and long-acting β_2-agonists (SIROCCO): a randomised, multicentre, placebo-controlled phase 3 trial. *Lancet.* 2016;388(10056):2115–27.

38. Wenzel S, Ford L, Pearlman D, et al. Dupilumab in persistent asthma with elevated eosinophil levels. *N Engl J Med.* 2013;368(26):2455–66.
39. Kew KM, Kirtchuk L, Michell CI. Intravenous magnesium sulfate for treating adults with acute asthma in the emergency department. *Cochrane Database Syst Rev.* 2014(5):CD010909.
40. Shah R, Saltoun CA. Chapter 14: acute severe asthma (status asthmaticus). *Allergy Asthma Proc.* 2012;33(suppl 1):47–50.
41. McCallister JW. Asthma in pregnancy: management strategies. *Curr Opin Pulm Med.* 2013; 19(1):13–17.
42. Murphy VE, Gibson PG. Asthma in pregnancy. *Clin Chest Med.* 2011;32(1):93–110, ix.
43. Alqalyoobi S, Zeki AA, Louie S. Asthma control during pregnancy: avoiding frequent pitfalls. *Consultant.* 2017;57(11):662–5.
44. Parsons JP, Hallstrand TS, Mastronarde JG, et al. An official American Thoracic Society clinical practice guideline: exercise-induced bronchoconstriction. *Am J Respir Crit Care Med.* 2013;187(9):1016–27.

Occupational Asthma

Kelsey Ann Childs Moon and Maya Jerath

6

GENERAL PRINCIPLES

Definition

- Occupational asthma (OA) is defined as variable airflow limitation and/or bronchial hyperresponsiveness caused by exposures in the workplace setting.
- OA also includes preexistent asthma that is worsened when exposed to the workplace.
- There are two types of OA.
  - **Sensitizer-induced OA,** previously known as latent OA
  - **Irritant-induced OA,** previously known as nonlatent OA

Classification

Sensitizer-Induced OA

- Symptoms of asthma occur after a **latency period** of months to years after initial exposure to a sensitizing substance in the workplace.
- After the patient has been sensitized, the reaction in the airway begins to develop at lower levels to the sensitizer than was previously tolerable. **Typically, this is an immunologically mediated reaction.**
- Different types of sensitizers are categorized by size.
  - **High molecular weight (HMW):** Agents >10 kD, **commonly inhaled proteins**
  - **Low molecular weight (LMW):** Agents <10 kD, **haptenated chemicals**

Irritant-Induced OA

- Exposure to high levels of an irritant agent can lead to **reactive airways dysfunction syndrome (RADS).**
- There is **no latent period,** and asthma symptoms occur within 24 hours of exposure to the irritant substance.
- Typical setting is an occupational accident that leads to exposure of unusually high levels of irritant.
- **Diagnosis cannot be made in patients with preexisting asthma.**

Epidemiology

- It is estimated that 15–25% of *de novo* adult asthma is due to work-related asthma.[1,2]
- In the United States, 2.7 million people might have asthma caused by or exacerbated by workplace conditions.[3]
- Up to 48% of adults with current asthma have work-related symptoms.[4]
- Prevalence of OA is difficult to assess as there are not many prospective studies. In addition, there are varying definitions of OA, making it difficult to gather data on the incidence of the disease.[1]
- Common occupations associated with OA
  - Animal handlers
  - Bakers and millers
  - Health care professionals

  ○ Hairdressers
  ○ Carpenters and cabinetmakers
  ○ Textile workers

Pathophysiology

There are more than 250 agents that have been identified to cause OA. Table 6-1 lists commonly associated allergens that cause OA.[5]

TABLE 6-1	AGENTS ASSOCIATED WITH OCCUPATIONAL ASTHMA		
Mechanism	**Type of agent**	**Causative agent**	**Occupations**
Immunologic IgE-dependent	HMW agents	Animal urine, dander, serum	Lab workers, veterinarians
		Cereal and soy flour	Bakers, millers
		Enzymes:	
		α-Amylase, cellulase	Bakers, pharmaceutical workers
		Papain, pepsin	Pharmaceutical and food workers
		Bacillus subtilis derived, *Aspergillus* derived	Detergent industry workers
		Gums (acacia, guar)	Printers, carpet manufacturers, hairdressers
		Psyllium	Pharmaceutical workers, nurses
		Egg proteins	Egg-processing workers
		Seeds— cottonseed, linseed, flaxseed	Bakers, oil producers
		Storage mites	Farmers, grain store workers
		Latex	Health care workers, manufacturers
Immunologic IgE dependent (often haptens)	LMW chemicals	Acid anhydrides: phthalic, trimellitic	Plastic, epoxy resin workers
		Platinum salts	Platinum refinery workers
		Reactive dyes	Textiles and dyeing workers
		Persulfate salts	Hairdressers

(*continued*)

TABLE 6-1	AGENTS ASSOCIATED WITH OCCUPATIONAL ASTHMA (continued)		
Mechanism	Type of agent	Causative agent	Occupations
Immunologic	LMW chemicals	Diisocyanates, toluene, methylene diphenyl, hexamethylene	Polyurethane, foundry workers, painters
		Western red cedar-plicatic acid	Sawmill workers, carpenters
		Amines	Photographers, shellac workers, chemist
		Colophony	Electronic workers, welders
Nonimmunologic (toxic effect)	LMW chemicals/ irritants	Chlorine	Pulp mill and chemical workers
		Sulfur dioxide	Pyrite workers, miners
		Ammonia	Spray painters, chemical workers
		Sodium fumes	Cleaners, chemical workers
		Smoke	Firefighters, police officers
		Diisocyanates	Spray painters, polyurethane workers

HMW, high molecular weight; LMW, low molecular weight.

Sensitizer-Induced OA

- HMW sensitizer
  - Proteins and/or glycoproteins act **as antigens in an IgE-mediated mechanism.** The allergen occasionally can be well characterized. However, several sensitizers are difficult to identify.[1]
  - This IgE-mediated response leads to **similar pathology seen in nonoccupational asthma** (see Chapter 5), with bronchial wall thickening, secondary eosinophilic infiltration, smooth muscle hypertrophy, fibroblast proliferation of subepithelium, and airway obstruction.
- LMW sensitizer
  - LMW sensitizers can cause OA by both **IgE and non–IgE-mediated mechanisms.**
  - LMW sensitizers can **haptenate to host proteins and drive IgE expression.**
  - Cell-mediated mechanisms may underlie some immunologic mechanisms to LMW sensitizers.

Irritant-Induced OA

- In contrast to sensitizer-induced OA, irritant-induced OA is caused by **direct toxic effects** of these agents on airway tissues (see Table 6-1 for a list of common irritant agents).
- Because these reactions are **not immunologically mediated,** prior exposure is not necessary to induce pathology.
- Exposure to high levels of irritant agents can lead to a cascade of events involving the nonadaptive immunologic response.
- Initially there is **injury to bronchial epithelial cells** causing release of inflammatory mediators and neurogenic inflammation. Nonspecific macrophage activation occurs with mast cell degranulation.

Risk Factors

- The most important risk factor is the **level and duration of exposure** to agents capable of causing OA. High levels and long duration of exposure lead to an increased likelihood of developing OA.
- **Atopy** is a risk factor for HMW allergens.
- Patients who develop **occupational rhinitis and/or conjunctivitis** are at increased risk of developing OA.
- There is geographic variation to the incidence of OA. Similar substances in different parts of the world are associated with different rates of OA. This may be due to the variation in exposure, coexposures, and recognition of disease.
- **Tobacco smoking**

Prevention

- Primary prevention efforts should focus on implementing **interventions that reduce exposure** to known OA-causing agents.[1]
- In a facility where there are known sensitizers, new cases of OA can be reduced by limiting ambient exposure to HMW sensitizers and by identifying patients with new occupational allergic symptoms.

DIAGNOSIS

Clinical Presentation

- Patients present with symptoms of asthma including dyspnea, wheezing, chest tightness, and cough.
- Symptoms of rhinitis and conjunctivitis will often precede the development of asthma.
- In OA, these **symptoms should be related to a workplace exposure** to a known OA-causing agent.
- History should include details about **occupational history** and all previous jobs held. The patient should also be asked about the use of **protective equipment.**
- Additional history will help differentiate OA from non–work-related asthma, vocal cord dysfunction, and hypersensitivity pneumonitis.

Differential Diagnosis

In addition to other diseases that can masquerade as asthma, other respiratory diseases should be considered along with OA.

- **Hypersensitivity pneumonitis** can usually be distinguished from OA by radiographic findings, which often show ground-glass nodularities, and pulmonary function testing (PFT) that typically shows restrictive disease.
- **Bronchiolitis obliterans** ("popcorn worker's lung") has been linked to diacetyl exposure in the workplace.

Diagnostic Testing

- Reversible airway limitation should be documented by spirometry and/or bronchial reactivity challenge with histamine, mannitol, or methacholine (described in Chapter 8).
  - Methacholine[6]
    - PC_{20} (methacholine concentration inducing a 20% fall in forced expiratory volume in 1 second [FEV_1]) <16 mg/mL at baseline—sensitivity 80%, specificity 47%, positive predictive value (PPV) 36%, negative predictive value (NPV) 86%
    - PC_{20} <16 mg/mL at work—sensitivity 98%, specificity 39%, PPV 44%, NPV 97%
  - Mannitol[7]
    - Patients experiencing wheezing, chest tightness, and dyspnea during the day and night—sensitivity 62%, specificity 90%, PPV 14%, NPV 99%
    - Any one symptom listed above—sensitivity 24%, specificity 95%, PPV 73%, NPV 71%
- In addition to establishing the presence of reversible airway obstruction, the diagnosis of OA must be confirmed by the evidence of **work-related symptom worsening.**
- Objective data that can be used to link workplace exposure to OA include spirometry, peak flow, and immunologic testing.
- **Serial spirometry or peak expiratory flow rates** (PEFRs) are often used to demonstrate a temporal worsening of airway obstruction after workplace exposures.
  - This approach is limited by patient compliance, but when used correctly has a high sensitivity and specificity.
  - Typically a patient with suspected OA will record serial flow rates for 2–4 weeks.
  - Ideally the patient will measure PEFR four times daily: morning, mid-shift, after work, and before sleeping.
  - One of those weeks includes a week away from work.
  - Patients with OA typically display the following pattern[1]:
    - Worsening of peak flow as the day progresses with improvement over the weekend
    - Progressively worsening peak flow as the work week progresses
    - Improvement in peak flows during a week away from work or during vacation
- **Specific inhalation challenge (SIC)** can be used to demonstrate reversible airway obstruction after exposure to a specific sensitizer.
  - During an SIC, the patient is exposed to a specific sensitizer in a controlled environment.
  - This allows the physician to identify a direct causal relationship between a sensitizer and airway obstruction.
  - OA is very unlikely if airway hyperresponsiveness is absent in the presence of continued exposure to the offending agent.[8]
  - Considered the **gold standard in the diagnosis of IgE-mediated OA**
  - Testing is limited by the necessity of trained personnel and emergency equipment.
  - **Sputum eosinophil counts** are helpful in the diagnosis of OA during SICs. Utility is limited by lack of widespread availability of sputum induction and processing.[8]
  - Blood eosinophil counts are not a reliable surrogate for sputum eosinophil counts.
  - Decrease in PC_{20} by at least threefold or >3% increase in sputum eosinophil counts achieved: sensitivity 84%, specificity 74%, NPV 91%.[8]
- **Immunologic testing** can establish sensitization to a particular sensitizer.
  - This has a **high negative predictive value,** indicating that if a patient has a negative test to a sensitizer that is a known work-related sensitizer, then the patient likely does not have OA.
  - Useful mostly for HMW sensitizers, because testing is dependent on IgE-mediated reaction.
  - Demonstration of sensitization does not necessarily establish that the tested agent is responsible for the patient's respiratory symptoms (SIC may be necessary).
- A simplified diagnostic workflow for OA is presented in Figure 6-1.

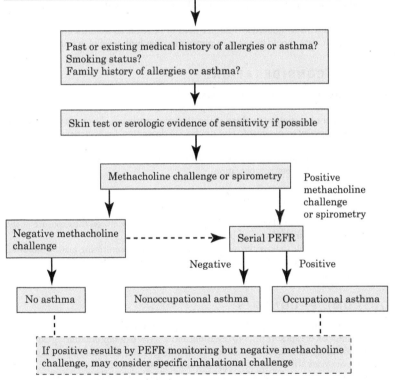

Clinical History

Cough? Wheeze? Sneezing? Rhinorrhea? Congestion? Itchy, watery eyes?
When during the day or week do you develop symptoms?
What jobs do you perform at work, and to what agents or materials are you exposed?
Have you had recurrent exposure with recurrent symptoms, or a single massive exposure?
Do your symptoms improve on your days off or on vacations?
Does anyone else at work have similar symptoms?
Describe your workplace in detail, including the type of ventilation.
Have there been any recent procedural changes in the workplace?
Do you wear protective gear? Is it always available, and does it fit?

Past or existing medical history of allergies or asthma?
Smoking status?
Family history of allergies or asthma?

Skin test or serologic evidence of sensitivity if possible

Methacholine challenge or spirometry

Positive methacholine challenge or spirometry

Negative methacholine challenge

Serial PEFR

Negative | Positive

No asthma | Nonoccupational asthma | Occupational asthma

If positive results by PEFR monitoring but negative methacholine challenge, may consider specific inhalational challenge

FIGURE 6-1 Algorithm for the diagnosis of occupational asthma. Mean peak expiratory flow rate (PEFR) consistently reduced by <20% with improvement away from work is diagnostic for occupational asthma.

TREATMENT

- The first-line and most important treatment for sensitizer-induced OA is **removal of the patient from the work environment.**
- Pharmacologic treatment of OA is the same as non–work-related asthma. The same treatment guidelines and symptomatic control are applied to the management of OA.
  - Pharmacologic treatment is second-line therapy after removal from the work environment.
  - **Patients who continue to be exposed to sensitizer despite optimal medications have poor outcomes because of chronic remodeling of the airways.**
  - Allergen immunotherapy is a treatment option for sensitized OA to a HMW agent that also has demonstrated an IgE-mediated reaction (i.e., laboratory animals, latex, and *Hymenoptera*). These are small studies and immunotherapy carries a risk of systemic reactions from immunotherapy.[9]
  - Use of omalizumab in a small cohort of 10 patients with sensitization to a LMW or a HMW agent showed improvement in asthma symptoms with decreased exposure to sensitizing agent.[10]
- Patients with irritant-induced OA do not need to be removed from their working environment, but steps should be taken to **prevent further high level of exposure.**

SPECIAL CONSIDERATIONS

- The socioeconomic consequences of being diagnosed with OA can have a lasting effect on the patient.
- Once a patient has stopped working at the offending workplace, he or she may have difficulty finding new employment. This can lead to depression, as the patient has financial obligations.
- In this setting, the specialty physician has a duty to be the patient's advocate in qualifying for disability or workers' compensation.

MONITORING/FOLLOW-UP

- Close monitoring should continue with patients who have removed the exposure of the sensitizing agent for resolution or persistence of symptoms.
- If patients are unable to leave the workplace, more frequent monitoring may be indicated and the patient should have an understanding that symptoms may worsen with continued exposure.

OUTCOME/PROGNOSIS

- Outcomes of patients with OA depend on the cessation of exposure to the offending agent, duration of exposure prior to cessation, and severity of symptoms during exposure.[1]
- If the patient is no longer exposed to the offending agent, asthma symptoms can still persist even years after exposure in approximately 70% of patients.[11]
- Continued exposure to the offending occupational agent can lead to a fatal asthma exacerbation.[12]

REFERENCES

1. Dykewicz M. Occupational asthma: current concepts in pathogenesis, diagnosis and management. *J Allergy Clin Immunol.* 2009;123:519–28.
2. Bernstein IL, Chang-Yeung M, Malo J-L, et al., eds. *Asthma in the Workplace.* New York, NY: Marcel Dekker, 1993.
3. *Sheehan* WJ, Gaffin JM, Peden DB, et al. Advances in environmental and occupational disorders in 2016. *J Allergy Clin Immunol.* 2017;140:1683–92.
4. Dodd KE, Mazurek JM. Asthma among employed adults, by industry and occupation—21 states, 2013. *MMWR Morb Mortal Wkly Rep.* 2016;65:1325–31.
5. Malo JL, Chang-Yeung M. Agents causing occupational asthma. *J Allergy Clin Immunol.* 2009;123:545–50.
6. Pralong JA, Lemiere C, Rochat T, et al. Predictive value of nonspecific bronchial responsiveness in occupational asthma. *J Allergy Clin Immunol.* 2015;137:412–6.
7. de Menezes MB, Ferraz E, Brannan JD, et al. The efficacy and safety of mannitol challenge in a workplace setting for assessing asthma prevalence. *J Asthma.* 2018;55:1278–85.
8. Racine G, Castano R, Cartier A, et al. Diagnostic accuracy of inflammatory markers for diagnosing occupational asthma. *J Allergy Clin Immunol Pract.* 2017;5:1371–7.
9. Moscato G, Pala G, Sastre J. Specific immunotherapy and biological treatments for occupational allergy. *Curr Opin Allergy Clin Immunol.* 2014;14(6):576–81.
10. Lavaud F, Bonniaud P, Dalphin JC, et al. Usefulness of omalizumab in ten patients with severe occupational asthma. *Allergy.* 2013;68:813–5.
11. Rachiotis G, Savani R, Brant A, et al. Outcome of occupational asthma after cessation of exposure: a systematic review. *Thorax.* 2007;62(2):147–52.
12. Ortega HG, Kreiss K, Schill DP, et al. Fatal asthma from powdering shark cartilage and review of fatal occupational asthma literature. *Am J Ind Med.* 2002;42(1):50–4.

Hypersensitivity Pneumonitis

7

Zhen Ren and Andrew L. Kau

GENERAL PRINCIPLES

Definition

- Hypersensitivity pneumonitis (HP), previously called **extrinsic allergic alveolitis,** is caused by an **inappropriate immunologic reaction to inhaled antigens,** resulting in respiratory and systemic symptoms.
- Diagnosis is based on a history of antigen exposure, clinical features, laboratory and radiologic findings, and, sometimes, histopathologic findings.
- HP is a complex syndrome whose clinical presentation and disease progression can vary significantly between patients. It may mimic other diffuse parenchymal lung diseases, such as sarcoidosis and idiopathic pulmonary fibrosis (IPF).

Classification

- HP is classically categorized as acute, subacute, and chronic based on the clinical presentation of each patient (see section Clinical Presentation).
- The three forms of the syndrome can be difficult to distinguish from one another and do not necessarily constitute stages of a single disease process, because patients with acute HP do not necessarily progress to chronic disease and those who present with the chronic form may not have had the acute presentation.[1]

Epidemiology

- HP is a rare disease, with an estimated 1-year prevalence of 1.67–2.71 and incidence of 1.28–1.94/100,000 people.[2]
- The greatest risk factor for developing HP is **exposure to inhaled organic particles and chemical compounds.** Contact with birds (e.g., pigeons, parakeets), humidifiers, moldy wood, and other environmental settings can also increase risk (see Table 7-1).[3] HP is more common among farmers ("farmer's lung").
- Sporadic outbreaks of HP are known to occur and are associated with workplace and seasonal exposures.
- **Genetic factors** have also been postulated to influence HP susceptibility.
- Cigarette smoking is associated with a decreased risk of developing HP. However, when HP occurs in smokers, it is associated with a more severe clinical course and a poorer survival rate.[4]

Etiology

- There are a wide range of antigens that can cause HP. These antigens are found in various settings, including the workplace, home, and recreational environments (see Table 7-1).[3] **Most antigens are organic,** but some low-molecular-weight chemical compounds can form haptens with serum albumin to create an antigenic particle.[5]
- Inhaled particles must be small enough (<5 μm) to reach the lung parenchyma and trigger an immune response.
- The causative agents for HP continue to increase as societal practices change.

TABLE 7-1	EXAMPLES OF ETIOLOGIC AGENTS IN HYPERSENSITIVITY PNEUMONITIS	
Disease	Environmental source	Antigen
Farmer's lung	Moldy hay and grain	Thermophilic actinomycetes, such as *Saccharopolyspora rectivirgula*
Bird fancier's lung	Pigeons, parakeets	Avian serum, droppings, and feather proteins
Bagassosis	Moldy sugarcane	*Thermoactinomyces sacchari, Tylenchorhynchus vulgaris*
Wine maker's lung	Moldy grapes	*Botrytis cinerea*
Coffee worker's lung	Coffee bean dust	Unknown
Tobacco grower's lung	Tobacco plants	*Aspergillus* spp.
Humidifier fever	Humidifier reservoirs, air conditioners, aquaria	Thermophilic actinomycetes, such as *Klebsiella oxytoca, Naegleria gruberi, Acanthamoeba* spp.
Hot tub lung	Mist, moldy ceilings, and tubs	*Mycobacterium avium* complex, *Cladosporium* spp.
Laboratory worker's lung	Laboratory rats	Rat serum, pelts, and urine proteins
Malt worker's disease	Moldy barley	*Aspergillus clavatus, Aspergillus fumigatus*
Wood dust pneumonitis	Oak, cedar, mahogany, pine dust	*Alternaria* spp., *Bacillus subtilis*
Chemical worker's lung		Diphenylmethane diisocyanate, toluene diisocyanate, and others

Adapted from Hirschmann JV, Pipavath SN, Godwin JD. Hypersensitivity pneumonitis: a historical, clinical, and radiologic review. *Radiographics.* 2009;29:1921–38.

Pathophysiology

- HP is an immune-mediated lung parenchymal inflammation disease with possible roles for both antibody and cellular immune responses.
  - The immune response to the inciting antigen can cause an **expression of antibodies**, resulting in an immune complex formation (type III hypersensitivity).
    - High-titer, antigen-specific, precipitating serum antibodies to the inciting antigen can result in complement fixation.
    - Presence of precipitating antibodies to a specific antigen is an important diagnostic marker of HP.
  - **Cell-mediated mechanisms** (type IV hypersensitivity) likely contribute as well.
    - Fixation of complement results in the recruitment of inflammatory cells, including lymphocytes and macrophages.
    - Once present in the lung tissue, these immune cells are thought to secrete Th1-skewed cytokines, including interferon-γ, which promote persistent inflammation and granuloma formation.

- Genetics also influence the development of HP. Major histocompatibility complex class II (MHC class II) alleles and polymorphisms in telomere-related genes, as well as other genes, have been implicated in the pathogenesis of HP.

Prevention

- HP can be prevented by reducing exposure to causative agents and using protective equipment.
- **Antigen reduction** focuses on ridding environments of antigenic particles.
  ○ Wetting compost before handling reduces dispersion of actinomycete spores.
  ○ Using antimicrobial agents while processing sugarcane reduces mold growth.
- **Facility design** can reduce the chances of contaminating the work environment.
  ○ Moisture plays a large role in indoor microbial overgrowth.
  ○ Humidity in buildings should be kept below 60%, carpeting should be avoided in moist areas, and water in ventilating systems should not be recirculated.
- **Protective devices:** In circumstances where it is impossible to completely eliminate environmental antigens, controls such as respirators should be used.[6]

DIAGNOSIS

- The diagnosis is based on exposure history, clinical presentation, as well as radiographic and physiologic findings. Bronchoalveolar lavage (BAL) and lung biopsy are helpful tools in supporting the diagnosis of HP or ruling out other potential diseases.
- Identifying the causative agent is particularly important to prevent ongoing exposure.

Clinical Presentation

Despite the diversity of inhaled agents that can cause HP, there are various diseases present with similar symptoms, suggesting that they may share pathogenic features.

- **Acute HP:** This form usually occurs within 4–6 hours of exposure. It is the most recognizable form of HP and presents with **fever, chills, cough, and dyspnea**. Symptoms last for hours to days and can be confused with a viral or bacterial illness. Physical examination often reveals tachypnea and fine inspiratory crackles, especially at the lung bases; wheezing is rarely heard.
- **Subacute HP:** This is characterized by a **more gradual onset of low-grade fever, cough, progressive dyspnea, fatigue, and, sometimes, anorexia and weight loss.** This may be superimposed with acute episodes. Examination reveals tachypnea, lung crackles, and sometimes cyanosis. This, like acute HP, is usually reversible with removal of the offending antigen.
- **Chronic HP:** This form often occurs after exposure to antigen for a long period. It presents with **insidious onset** over a period of months to years, with **progressive cough, dyspnea, fatigue, and weight loss**. Examination may reveal cyanosis and digital clubbing, which, if seen, suggests poor prognosis. This form is often disabling and is **usually irreversible**.[5] Patients with chronic HP may develop acute worsening of their symptoms and overlap with acute HP.

Differential Diagnosis

- There are many diseases apart from HP that are associated with inhalation of organic agents. Furthermore, other syndromes have clinical or histologic features similar to HP.
- **Inhalation fever** (e.g., metal fume fever): Occurs a few hours after inhaling the substance; characterized by fever, malaise, myalgias, and headache, without significant pulmonary symptoms. This is self-limited (usually within 24 hours) without long-term effects.[7]

- **Organic dust toxic syndrome** (ODTS): This is a reaction to inhaled antigens that occurs approximately 6 hours after exposure to **mycotoxins** or **endotoxins** produced by microorganisms found in moldy hay, grains, and contaminated textile materials. It is **more common in farmers than HP**. Symptoms and findings include fever, myalgias, cough, and dyspnea. Additional evaluation sometimes documents leukocytosis, diffuse opacities on CXR, and normal lung function or mild restriction with reduced diffusion capacity of the lungs for carbon monoxide (DLCO). Notably with ODTS, serum precipitins are negative, and there are no long-term sequelae.[8]
- **Obstructive lung disease**: Both asthma and chronic bronchitis are **much more common than HP** (see Chapter 5). Chronic bronchitis is thought to share some pathologic features with HP.
- **Sarcoidosis:** Both HP and sarcoidosis have lymphocytosis on BAL and may demonstrate noncaseating granulomas on lung biopsy. However, sarcoidosis is frequently associated with extrapulmonary organ involvement. In addition, granulomas in sarcoidosis are well formed and distributed in a lymphangitic pattern, whereas HP granulomas have a centrilobular distribution.
- **IPF**: The chronic form of HP can be difficult to distinguish from IPF, but can sometimes be differentiated by findings of centrilobular opacities and lack of lower lobe–predominant fibrosis in HP.[3]

Diagnostic Testing

Laboratories

- **Serum precipitins:** Patients with HP may have precipitating IgG antibodies specific to the inhaled antigen.
  - These antibodies are often present in asymptomatic exposed people. The **presence of serum precipitins simply indicates exposure** and not necessarily disease.
  - Absence of serum precipitins **does not rule out HP** because some HP-associated antigens may not be present in the routine precipitin panel and some antigens are still undiscovered.
  - There are several methods for detecting precipitins. The conventional Ouchterlony double immunodiffusion test is limited in both sensitivity and specificity. Enzyme-linked immunosorbent assay (ELISA) and ImmunoCAP testing are also available.
- Other laboratory tests
  - Nonspecific laboratories such as erythrocyte sedimentation rate (ESR), C-reactive protein (CRP), rheumatoid factor (RF), and lactate dehydrogenase (LDH) may be elevated in HP.
  - Serum IgE and eosinophils are not typically elevated.
  - **Skin testing is not useful** in the diagnosis of HP.

Imaging

- **CXR** in many patients with HP can be normal. Poorly defined infiltrates, diffuse airspace opacities, or nodules are seen in the acute or subacute form of the disease. Chronic HP may show reticulonodular infiltrates, fibrosis, or honeycombing.
- **High-resolution CT** (HRCT) is an important tool in the diagnosis of HP.
  - **Centrilobular ground-glass opacities or nodular opacities predominantly in upper and middle lobes with signs of air trapping are differentiating features of HP**.
  - In acute HP, HRCT can be normal or show diffuse ground-glass opacification.
  - In subacute HP, typical HRCT findings include poorly defined centrilobular nodules, ground-glass attenuation, focal air trapping or emphysema, and mild fibrotic changes.
  - In chronic HP, various changes can be seen, including honeycombing and fibrosis with upper and mid-lung zone predominance.
  - Findings not usually associated with HP are lung cavities, hilar adenopathy, and pleural thickening.[1]

Diagnostic Procedures
- Inhalation challenge
  - Inhalation challenge can be used to link HP symptoms to the suspected antigen.
  - A patient can be exposed to the offending environment, after which symptoms are observed.
  - Changes in clinical picture, pulmonary function tests (PFTs), and chest imaging are studied for 24 hours.
  - These tests are limited in utility as the **inhalation protocols lack standardization.**[5]
- Pulmonary function testing
  - PFTs cannot distinguish HP from other interstitial lung diseases.
  - PFTs are used to measure functional impairment and can help guide treatment (e.g., who should get corticosteroid treatment).
  - **Characteristically, PFTs show a restrictive pattern with decreased DLCO.**
  - An obstructive pattern can predominate in more insidious forms of HP, especially as emphysematous changes develop.
  - Mixed restrictive and obstructive defects can also occur.
- Bronchoalveolar lavage
  - BAL is an important tool in supporting the diagnosis of HP.
  - **Neutrophils in BAL fluid increase early after antigen exposure.**
  - **The BAL fluid in the subacute and chronic forms of HP has marked lymphocytosis >20%** (normal is 6–8%).
  - Eosinophils are not increased (except in some advanced cases), but mast cells and basophils can be increased.[1,5]
- Lung biopsy
  - Lung biopsy is sometimes needed to confirm the diagnosis of HP and can be obtained by transbronchial means or surgically.
  - Lung biopsy should be reserved for patients with a very unusual presentation or unexpected response to treatment, given the possible morbidity associated with surgical biopsy.
  - Histopathologic findings include **interstitial lymphocyte and plasma cell infiltrates, small, poorly formed noncaseating granulomas, and macrophages with foamy cytoplasm in the alveoli and interstitium.**
  - In chronic stages, peribronchiolar fibrosis can be seen. Schaumann bodies (calcium and protein inclusions) within isolated Langhans giant cells can also be seen.[5]

TREATMENT

- The principles of HP management are twofold: **avoidance of antigen exposure, and glucocorticoids.**
- Avoidance of the offending antigen through environmental control is the cornerstone of therapy in HP.
- If antigen exposure is related to the patient's job, avoidance can be difficult because of the potential loss of livelihood.
- Antigen can often persist at home despite removal of the primary offending agent (e.g., birds). In such cases, professional control measures and environmental modification may be sought.
- Medications
  - Some patients benefit from corticosteroids, the only drugs currently used for HP.
  - Indications for use are mainly in patients with subacute or chronic HP with persistent symptoms.
  - Glucocorticoids help control symptoms but do not improve long-term outcome.
  - The recommended regimen is 40–60 mg of prednisone or its equivalent corticosteroid. Treatment duration is 1–2 weeks followed by a taper over 2–4 weeks.[5,9,10]
  - Immune-modulating agents such as azathioprine and mycophenolate have been used in patients with refractory chronic HP.

OUTCOME/PROGNOSIS

- **The majority of patients with HP recover fully after they are removed from the offending environment,** and some recover despite continued exposure.
- Among the most well-studied types of HP, bird fancier's lung has a worse prognosis than farmer's lung.
- **Patients with chronic HP who have fibrosis or honeycombing on HRCT or lung biopsy have a worse prognosis,** and their disease may be irreversible despite environmental control or corticosteroid therapy.
- **Approximately 20% of patients with chronic HP develop pulmonary hypertension, which is associated with a greater mortality rate.**[11]

REFERENCES

1. Knutsen AP, Amin RS, Temprano J, et al. Hypersensitivity pneumonitis and eosinophilic pulmonary diseases. In: Victor C, Kendig E, eds. *Kendig's Disorders of the Respiratory Tract in Children.* 7th ed. Philadelphia, PA: Saunders/Elsevier, 2006:686–93.
2. Perez ERF, Kong AM, Raimundo K, et al. Epidemiology of hypersensitivity pneumonitis among an insured population in the United States: a claims-based cohort analysis. *Ann Am Thorac Soc.* 2018;15:460–9.
3. Hirschmann JV, Pipavath SN, Godwin JD. Hypersensitivity pneumonitis: a historical, clinical, and radiologic review. *Radiographics.* 2009;29:1921–38.
4. Ohtsuka Y, Munakata M, Tanimura K, et al. Smoking promotes insidious and chronic farmers lung-disease, and deteriorates the clinical outcome. *Intern Med.* 1995;34:966–71.
5. Girard M, Lacasse Y, Cormier Y. Hypersensitivity pneumonitis. *Allergy.* 2009;64:322–34.
6. Dion G, Duchaine A, Meriaux A, et al. Hypersensitivity pneumonitis (HP) prevention: benefits of industry and research community collaboration. *Am J Respir Crit Care Med.* 2008;177:A555.
7. Kaye P, Young H, O'Sullivan I. Metal fume fever: a case report and review of the literature. *Emerg Med J.* 2002;19:268–9.
8. Seifert SA, Von Essen S, Jacobitz K, et al. Organic dust toxic syndrome: a review. *J Toxicol Clin Toxicol.* 2003;41:185–93.
9. Mönkäre S. Influence of corticosteroid treatment on the course of farmer's lung. *Eur J Respir Dis.* 1983;64:283–93.
10. Kokkarinen JI, Tukiainen HO, Terho EO. Effect of corticosteroid treatment on the recovery of pulmonary function in farmer's lung. *Am Rev Respir Dis.* 1992;145:3–5.
11. Koschel DS, Cardoso C, Wiedemann B, et al. Pulmonary hypertension in chronic hypersensitivity pneumonitis. *Lung.* 2012;190:295–302.

Pulmonary Function Tests

Stacy Ejem and Aaron M. Ver Heul

8

GENERAL PRINCIPLES

Definition

- Pulmonary function tests (PFTs) include multiple methods of assessing the functional characteristics of an individual's lungs and are useful for the diagnosis of lung disease and monitoring response to treatment.
- Common PFTs utilized in clinical practice include spirometry, peak flow meter, lung volume measurement, and the diffusion capacity of the lung for carbon monoxide (DLCO).
- Acronyms and abbreviations used in this chapter are summarized in Table 8-1.

Classification

- **Spirometry** measures dynamic airflow during the respiratory cycle. Detailed guidelines have been published by the American Thoracic Society (ATS)/European Respiratory Society (ERS)[1] and were recently updated.[2]
  - Typically performed by one of two methods.
    - Open-circuit spirometry is generally less costly to implement.
    - Closed-circuit spirometry is generally more accurate, but hygiene is a concern because patients breathe directly from the instrument.
  - Normal baseline values for spirometry are dependent on various factors, including sex, age, weight, and height.
    - GLI-2012 multiethnic spirometry reference values are now recommended for use in North America.[2]
    - National Health and Nutrition Examination Survey (NHANES) III reference values (recommended for North America in 2005 ATS/ERS documents[1]) remain appropriate where maintaining continuity is important.
  - Spirometry depends on **patient effort**. Patients must have the mental and physical capacity to follow directions and perform the procedures for reliable results. **Criteria for acceptable spirometry** in patients >6 years of age include[1]
    - No hesitation or false start (defined as <5% forced vital capacity [FVC] or 0.150 L, whichever is greater)
    - A smooth continuous exhalation for >6 seconds demonstrating a plateau, with cessation of flow defined as <0.025 L in 1 second during expiration
      - In some patients, acceptable results can be obtained with forced expiratory time (FET) <6 seconds if they achieve a true plateau.
      - Instrument software may prematurely stop recording FET owing to meeting the low-flow criterion or because of artifacts, despite ongoing patient effort or flow.[2]
      - Accurate forced expiratory volume in 1 second (FEV_1) values require only high-quality data in the first second of the test.
- Lack of artifacts, such as coughing, glottic closure, early termination of exhalation, or obstructed mouthpiece
- Properly calibrated equipment without leaks

TABLE 8-1	ABBREVIATIONS USED IN PULMONARY FUNCTION TESTING

Measurement	Abbreviation	Description
Arterial blood gas	ABG	
Diffusion capacity of the lung for carbon monoxide (CO)	DLCO	The diffusion capacity between capillary and alveolar wall using CO
Expiratory reserve volume	ERV	The volume of gas that can be maximally exhaled from end-expiratory level during tidal breathing
Forced vital capacity	FVC	The volume of gas that can be forcefully expelled after maximal inhalation
Forced expiratory volume in 1 second	FEV_1	The volume measured in the first second of maximal forced exhalation
Forced expiratory flow during 25–75% of vital capacity	FEF 25–75%	The maximal mid-expiratory flow rate
Forced expiratory time	FET	The time taken to expire a given volume or a given fraction of VC during measurement of FVC
Functional residual capacity	FRC	The volume of gas present in the lungs after normal exhalation (TLC – IC)
Inspiratory capacity	IC	The maximum volume of gas that can be inspired after normal exhalation
Peak expiratory flow	PEF	The maximal airflow rate achieved during expiration
Total lung capacity	TLC	The volume of lungs after maximal inspiration
Slow vital capacity	SVC	It is the total volume of air expired slowly. It can be useful to diagnose airway obstruction when the FVC is reduced
Vital capacity	VC	The volume of gas measured with slow expiration after maximal inhalation

- Reproducibility is important for following longitudinal trends and to ensure that results can be compared between test centers. **Criteria for reproducibility** include[1]
  - A minimum of three respiratory loops. Making more than eight consecutive measurements has been shown to affect results owing to fatigue and is not recommended.
  - The best values for FEV_1 and FVC should be used for interpretation.
  - The largest values for FVC and FEV_1 should be within 0.15 L of their respective second largest values.
- A recent ATS/ERS update[2] notes that results not meeting ideal standards can still yield useful information and recommends applying a grading scale (Table 8-2) prior to interpretation. Grades A–C are considered clinically useful, D–E of limited use, and F not interpretable.
- ATS/ERS have modified criteria for children aged <5 years, but asthma guidelines, including Global Initiative for Asthma (GINA[3]) and Expert Panel Review (EPR3),[4] do not recommend PFTs in this age group because of issues with obtaining reliable results.

TABLE 8-2	ATS/ERS RECOMMENDED GRADING SCALE FOR QUALITY OF SPIROMETRY
Grade	Criteria for age ≥2
A	≥3 acceptable tests with repeatability within 0.150 L For ages 2–6, 0.100 L, or 10% of highest value, whichever is greater
B	≥2 acceptable tests with repeatability within 0.150 L For ages 2–6, 0.100 L, or 10% of highest value, whichever is greater
C	≥2 acceptable tests with repeatability within 0.200 L For ages 2–6, 0.150 L, or 10% of highest value, whichever is greater
D	≥2 acceptable tests with repeatability within 0.250 L For ages 2–6, 0.200 L, or 10% of highest value, whichever is greater
E	One acceptable test
F	No acceptable tests

ATS, American Thoracic Society; ERS, European Respiratory Society.

Adapted with permission of the American Thoracic Society. Copyright © 2020 American Thoracic Society. All rights reserved. Culver BH, Graham BL, Coates AL, et al. Recommendations for a standardized pulmonary function report. An official American Thoracic Society technical statement. *Am J Respir Crit Care Med.* 2017;196(11):1463–72. The American Journal of Respiratory and Critical Care Medicine is an official journal of the American Thoracic Society. Readers are encouraged to read the entire article for the correct context at https://www.atsjournals.org/doi/full/10.1164/rccm.201710-1981ST. The authors, editors, and the American Thoracic Society are not responsible for errors or omissions in adaptations.

- **Peak expiratory flow rates (PEFRs)** are calculated from a spirogram or measured with a handheld peak flow meter. Handheld devices are useful for **monitoring only**, not diagnosis.
  - Each measurement should be the highest value from three consecutive maneuvers.
  - Normal values of PEFR are based on age, gender, and height.
  - Peak flow values display a well-documented **diurnal variation**, with the lowest values in the early morning on awakening and the highest values during late afternoon.
    - GINA guidelines note that diurnal variations of >10% in adults or >13% in children warrant further evaluation or treatment.[3]
    - EPR3 guidelines no longer recommend twice-daily monitoring for diurnal variation.[4]
  - Handheld peak flow meters are useful for outpatient monitoring of
    - Response to therapy
    - Identification of provocative factors
    - Early detection of asthma exacerbations, in particular in patients with poor perception of worsening asthma symptoms
- **Lung volume measurement** determines the absolute capacity of a patient's lungs. Guidelines for measuring lung volumes were published by ATS/ERS.[5]
  - Lung volumes are related to body size. Standing height is the most important correlating variable.
  - **Total lung capacity (TLC)** is the most important lung volume measurement, along with spirometry, in interpretation of lung pathology.
  - **Functional residual capacity (FRC)** is a key component of lung volume measurements and is necessary to calculate TLC. Methods to determine FRC include body plethysmography, nitrogen washout, and helium dilution.
    - Plethysmography: includes ventilated and nonventilated lung compartments and yields higher results than gas dilation/washout methods. Gas dilation and washout

methods are more commonly used because they are less expensive and simpler to perform. Refer to Table 8-1 and Figure 8-1[5] for definitions and example test results.

- Nitrogen washout: The patient breathes 100% oxygen, and the initial alveolar N_2 concentration compared to the amount of N_2 washed out at 7 minutes is used to calculate lung volumes at the start of washout.

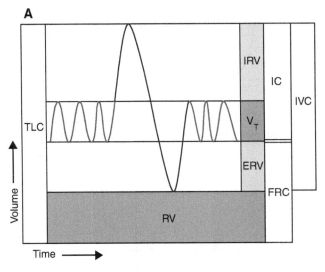

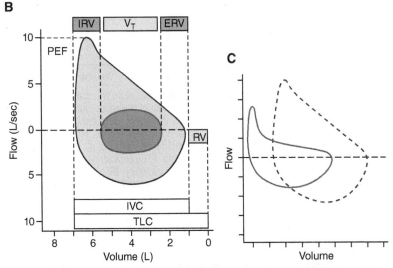

FIGURE 8-1 Example plethysmography and flow-volume loops. **A:** Static lung volumes and capacities based on a volume–time (V_T) spirogram of an inspiratory vital capacity (IVC). **B:** Normal flow-volume loop. Dark pink area represents tidal breathing loop, and light pink area represents maximal inspiratory and expiratory effort during the procedure. **C:** Obstructive ventilatory defect. Note the decreased PEF, "scooping" of the expiratory limb, and the left-shifted loop with increased TLC (air trapping).

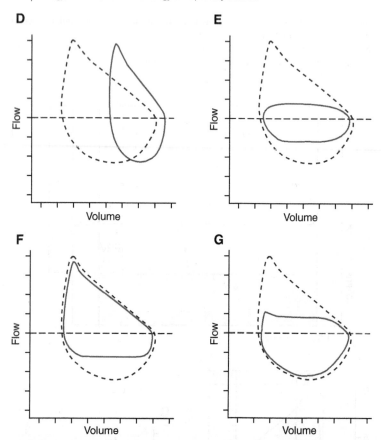

FIGURE 8-1 (*continued*) **D:** Restrictive lung disease. Note the narrowed and right-shifted flow-volume loop. **E:** Fixed obstruction of the upper airway (e.g., tracheal stenosis). Note the flattening of both the inspiratory and expiratory limbs. **F:** Variable extrathoracic obstruction (e.g., vocal cord dysfunction). Note the flattening of the inspiratory limb. **G:** Variable intrathoracic obstruction (e.g., tracheomalacia or goiter). Note the flattening of the expiratory limb. ERV, expiratory reserve volume; FRC, functional residual capacity; IC, inspiratory capacity; IRV, inspiratory reserve volume; PEF, peak expiratory flow; RV, residual volume; TLC, total lung capacity.

- ▪ Helium dilution: based on equilibration of gas in the lung with a known volume of gas containing helium[5]
- ○ The inspiratory capacity (IC) and expiratory reserve volume (ERV) must be measured in order to calculate the TLC and residual volume (RV).
  - ▪ The preferred method for determining ERV involves taking measurements immediately after obtaining FRC, followed by slow IC maneuvers.
  - ▪ A second method consists of performance of IC maneuvers immediately before acquiring the FRC to measure the TLC. This method may be performed in patients with severe obstruction and in those who are unable to follow the linked ERV maneuver due to dyspnea.

- The vital capacity (VC) can be derived from the IC maneuver or slow expiratory vital capacity (EVC) that follows an IC maneuver after the FRC determination.
- **DLCO** measurements assess the ability of the lung to transport gases by measuring diffusion of inspired gas across the alveolar capillary interface to red blood cells. ATS/ERS guidelines were recently updated.[6]
  - Many factors can affect gas exchange capacity, including lung volume, path length for diffusion, thickness and surface area of alveolar capillary membranes, volume of hemoglobin, absolute levels of ventilation and perfusion, composition of alveolar gas, and diffusion characteristics of the membrane.
  - In the **single-breath method**, the patient is connected to the test gas (0.3% CO, tracer gas, oxygen, and nitrogen), then inhales rapidly from RV to TLC in <4 seconds. Following a 10- to 12-second breath-hold, the patient exhales quickly and rapidly, and alveolar sample of exhaled gas is collected.
  - Criteria for acceptable DLCO include inspiratory volume >90% of the largest measurement of VC and at least 85% of the test gas inhaled in <4 seconds.
  - DLCO changes with anemia, carboxyhemoglobin levels, altitude, and lung volume, so adjustment for variance may be needed.
  - Isolated low DLCO can be due to pulmonary hypertension or pulmonary embolism. Asthmatic patients typically have normal or high DLCO. Restrictive lung disease coupled with low DLCO suggests interstitial lung disease, whereas normal DLCO with low lung volumes is suggestive of extrapulmonary cause of restriction, such as obesity or kyphoscoliosis.[6]
- **6-minute walk testing (6MWT)** assesses a patient's functional status, oxygen saturation, and heart rate in response to exertion.
  - 6MWT is a good index of physical function and therapeutic response and has prognostic value for chronic respiratory diseases.[7]
  - The walking path should be 30 m (100 feet) on level ground. Normal healthy subjects can walk 400–700 m in 6 minutes.
  - Although pulse oxygen saturation, heart rate, and perceived exertion (e.g., Borg scale) are measured at the beginning and end of the study, it is not designed to be an oxygen titration study.

DIAGNOSIS

- PFTs are obtained for various reasons.
- Diagnosis
  - Determine the presence of pulmonary disease.
  - Evaluate symptoms of dyspnea, cough, or wheezing.
  - Screen for high-risk individuals (e.g., smokers or those with occupational exposures).
  - Preoperative evaluation
  - **Flow-volume loops** can be invaluable in difficult diagnostic cases by providing insight into functional characteristics of the upper and lower airways as well as possible extrathoracic causes. Sample flow-volume loops are shown in Figure 8-1.
  - **Supine and sitting spirometry** can be used to diagnose respiratory muscle weakness. Diaphragmatic weakness is suggested by decrease in the supine VC by >10%. Unilateral diaphragmatic paralysis will have 15–25% decrease in VC, whereas bilateral paralysis is associated with 50% decrease.[8]
  - PFTs can identify **airway obstruction**.
  - Values of both FEV_1 and FVC can be reduced, but FEV_1 is disproportionately affected, thus giving a **low FEV_1/FVC**.
  - The primary criterion for the diagnosis of obstruction is FEV_1/FVC <0.7 of that predicted for age.[9]
  - There is some indication that a decrease in forced expiratory flow (FEF) 25–75% may detect early obstructive changes in the smaller and peripheral airways in the setting

of a normal FEV_1 and predict more severe symptoms in children[10,11] and adults.[12] However, the ATS/ERS do not find enough evidence to recommend routine use of this measurement at this time.[2]

- Monitoring
  - Assess response to therapy (e.g., inhaled corticosteroids, bronchodilators, biologics).
  - Follow progression of known pulmonary disease.
  - Monitor for adverse reactions to drugs that may have pulmonary side effects (e.g., amiodarone).
  - Characterize pulmonary dysfunction in response to environmental exposures.
- Other
  - Document disability for insurance.
  - Assess qualifications for rehabilitation programs.

Diagnostic Testing

- **Asthma**
  - EPR3 guidelines recommend an initial diagnostic PFT evaluation followed by repeated measures:
    - After treatment is initiated and lung function has stabilized (GINA guidelines specify 3–6 months)
    - During periods of progressive or prolonged loss of asthma control
    - At least every 1–2 years
  - Hallmark findings in asthma include **reversible airway obstruction** and **bronchial hyperresponsiveness (BHR)**.
  - **Reversible airway obstruction** can be demonstrated on spirometry by the measurement of FEV_1 and FVC before and after the administration of bronchodilators.
    - **An increase in FEV_1 >12% and 200 mL increase from baseline** supports a diagnosis of asthma.[3,4] There is even greater confidence if the increase is >400 mL.[3]
    - EPR3 guidelines utilize values of FEV_1 and FVC in schema to determine asthma severity at the time of diagnosis and also to determine the level of control. These classifications are given in Table 8-3 and compared to those of chronic obstructive pulmonary disease (COPD).
    - Table 8-4 lists sample PFT values of a patient with asthma.
    - The absence of improvement after bronchodilator treatment does not exclude reversible obstruction. Obstruction may be due to inflammation, which may only be reversible after prolonged anti-inflammatory therapy.
  - **BHR** can be documented via **bronchoprovocation** with agents known to cause bronchial constriction.[13,14]
    - BHR is demonstrable in nearly all patients with asthma.
    - Bronchoprovocation challenges are performed for
      □ Suspicion of asthma by history, but nondiagnostic PFTs
      □ Assessing the relative risk for developing occupational asthma
      □ Evaluation of severity of occupational asthma
    - **Absolute contraindications** for bronchoprovocation challenge are
      □ Severe airflow obstruction (FEV_1 <60% of predicted or <1.5 L)
      □ Myocardial infarction or stroke within 3 months
      □ Uncontrolled hypertension with systolic blood pressure >200 or diastolic blood pressure >100
      □ Known aortic aneurysm
      □ Recent eye surgery or intracranial pressure elevation risk
    - Relative contraindications are
      □ Inability to cooperate or follow directions for test
      □ Current use of cholinesterase inhibitor medication
      □ Pregnancy or breastfeeding (methacholine is considered category C in pregnancy)

TABLE 8-3 CLASSIFICATION OF COPD OR ASTHMA BASED ON PARAMETERS FROM SPIROMETRY

GOLD classifications—COPD		EPR3 classification—Asthma					
FEV_1/FVC <0.7			Severity (in patients not taking controller medication)			Control (in patients taking controller medication)	
Stage	FEV_1		Ages 5–11	Age >12		Ages 5–11	Age >12
GOLD 1	>80%	Intermittent	FEV_1 >80% FEV_1/FVC >0.85	FEV_1 >80% FEV_1/FVC normal	Well controlled	FEV_1 >80% FEV_1/FVC >0.8	FEV_1 >80%
GOLD 2	50–80%	Mild	FEV_1 >80% FEV_1/FVC >0.8	FEV_1 >80% FEV_1/FVC normal	Not well controlled	FEV_1 60–80% FEV_1/FVC 0.75–0.8	FEV_1 60–80%
GOLD 3	30–49%	Moderate	FEV_1 60–80%; FEV_1/FVC 0.75–0.8	FEV_1 60–80% FEV_1/FVC decr. 5%	Very poorly controlled	FEV_1 <60% FEV_1/FVC >0.75	FEV_1 <60%
GOLD 4	<30%	Severe	FEV_1 <60% FEV_1/FVC <0.75	FEV_1 60–80% FEV_1/FVC decr. >5%			

COPD, chronic obstructive pulmonary disease; EPR3, Expert Panel Review; FEV_1, forced expiratory volume in 1 second; FVC, forced vital capacity; GOLD, Global Initiative for Chronic Obstructive Lung Disease.

For asthma classification, normal values for FEV_1/FVC vary with age. Ages 8–19: 85%; ages 20–39: 80%; ages 40–59: 75%; ages 60–80: 70%. A decrease in FEV_1/FVC below the lower limit of normal should be calculated based on age in adult asthmatics.

Adapted from U.S. Department of Health and Human Services, National Institutes of Health. Expert Panel Report 3: Guidelines for the Diagnosis and Management of Asthma [EPR3]. Published July 2007. Last Accessed 7/31/18. http://www.nhlbi.nih.gov/health-pro/guidelines/current/asthma-guidelines; Global Initiative for Chronic Obstructive Lung Disease. Global strategy for the diagnosis, management, and prevention of chronic obstructive lung disease (2020 Report). https://goldcopd.org

| TABLE 8-4 | SAMPLE PULMONARY FUNCTION TEST OF PATIENTS WITH ASTHMA, COPD, AND RESTRICTIVE LUNG DISEASE |

	Asthma		COPD		Restrictive lung disease	
	Actual (L)	Percent predicted	Actual (L)	Percent predicted	Actual (L)	Percent predicted
FVC (L)	3.14	67	2.5	62	1.8	45
FEV$_1$ (L)	2.12	53	1.58	50	1.62	47
FEV$_1$/FVC	–	67	–	63	–	90
FEF 25–75% (L/sec)	0.63	14	1.3	33	1.4	41
TLC (L)	6.45	100	7.12	110	4.16	65
RV	–	–	4	160	–	–
DLCO (mL/min/mm Hg)	32	100	25	78	–	–

COPD, chronic obstructive pulmonary disease; DLCO, diffusion capacity of the lung for carbon monoxide; FEF, forced expiratory flow; FEV$_1$, forced expiratory volume in 1 second; FVC, forced vital capacity; RV, residual volume; TLC, total lung capacity.

| TABLE 8-5 | MEDICATIONS TO WITHHOLD BEFORE METHACHOLINE TESTING |

Medication	Minimum hold time (hours)
Short-acting β-agonists in conventional doses (e.g., albuterol)	6
Long-acting β-agonists (e.g., salmeterol, formoterol)	36
Ultra-long-acting β-agonists (e.g., indacaterol, olodaterol, vilanterol)	48
Ipratropium	12
Long-acting antimuscarinic agents (e.g., tiotropium)	≥168
Oral theophylline	12–24
The following agents have no effect on methacholine-induced BHR, but may affect other forms of provocation testing	
Leukotriene modifiers	24
Antihistamines	72
Caffeine (coffee, tea, chocolate)	Day of study

BHR, bronchial hyperresponsiveness.

Adapted from Coates AL, Wanger J, Cockcroft DW, et al. ERS technical standard on bronchial challenge testing: general considerations and performance of methacholine challenge tests. *Eur Respir J.* 2017;49:1–17; Crapo RO, Casaburi R, Coates AL, et al. Guidelines for methacholine and exercise challenge testing—1999. *Am J Respir Crit Care Med.* 2000;161:309–29.

- Medications that can decrease bronchial responsiveness are listed in Table 8-5.
- **Direct tests** use agents that act directly on bronchial smooth muscle to stimulate airway constriction. Examples include
  - **Methacholine: the agent of choice** among many clinicians because of extensive clinical experience and reduced side effects
  - Histamine: Challenges can have systemic side effects, such as headache, tachycardia, and flushing. Tachyphylaxis can also develop.
- **Indirect tests** utilize methods that stimulate bronchial smooth muscles through intermediate mechanisms. Examples include
  - Mannitol: a pharmacologic agent that induces BHR by changing the osmolarity of the bronchial epithelial surface, resulting in mast cell degranulation
  - Exercise: thought to induce BHR through changes in osmolarity related to increased ventilation rate
  - Eucapnic hyperventilation: for those unable to exercise, enables the osmotic changes due to hyperventilation without associated blood pH abnormalities
  - Adenosine monophosphate: causes bronchoconstriction by stimulation of inflammatory cell and mediators of the sensory nerves
- Methods for performing pharmacologic bronchoprovocation challenges
  - In the (recommended) **tidal breathing protocol**, the patient receives a dose of bronchoprovocation agent via continuous nebulizer or dosimeter while taking tidal breaths for at least 1 minute followed by FEV_1 measurement at 30 and 90 seconds postdosing. Initial doses are between 1 and 2 μg. In each subsequent cycle, doses are doubled or quadrupled until the FEV_1 changes by >20% from baseline or to the maximal recommended concentration.
  - In the **five-breath dosimeter protocol**, the patient uses a nebulizer with dosimeter attached to inhale the chosen bronchoprovocation agent after complete exhalation. The patient takes five slow (>5 seconds), deep breaths through the mouthpiece. FEV_1 is measured approximately 30 and 90 seconds after the fifth inhalation. As earlier, the cycle repeats with increasing doses until FEV_1 decreases by >20% from baseline or to the maximal recommended concentration.
- There are many ways to document bronchial challenge responses, including changes in FEV_1, airways resistance, maximum expiratory flow, or total respiratory resistance.
  - **Decrease in FEV_1** is the most common and is reported in conjunction with the **provocative dose 20 (PD20)**, which is defined as the delivered dose of constrictor agent at which FEV_1 falls by 20% from baseline. The PD20 end point is now favored because it allows for comparison between different devices or protocols.[13,14]
  - Prior ATS/ERS guidelines established a cutoff PC20 <8 mg/mL (equivalent to ~PD20 of 200 μg) for asthma,[15] but recent data show that this concentration is only suggestive of borderline airway hyperresponsiveness.[13,14]
  - Methacholine is a nonspecific bronchoconstrictor and can lead to a response in all people when given in high enough doses. A methacholine provocation test is more useful in excluding than confirming a diagnosis of asthma because its negative predictive value is much higher than its positive predictive valve. The utility of this test is highest for those patients with pretest probabilities of asthma between 30 and 70%. **A PD20 <25 μg (PC20 <1 mg/mL)** is highly specific for a diagnosis of asthma. A PD20 >400 μg (PC20 >16 mg/mL) is a negative test. **A negative test has a high predictive value and rules out the diagnosis of asthma.**
- **Chronic obstructive pulmonary disease**
  - The disease is characterized by persistent obstruction that is usually **not responsive to bronchodilator** administration.
  - In contrast to asthma, COPD often has reduced DLCO.

- ○ In advanced disease, air trapping becomes more evident—RV increases disproportionately to TLC, resulting in an elevated RV/TLC ratio.
- ○ Guidelines recommend repeating PFT evaluation for any changes in symptoms.[9,16]
- ○ Table 8-3 shows Global Initiative for Chronic Obstructive Lung Disease (GOLD) COPD severity classifications based on lung function in comparison to those of asthma. Table 8-4 lists sample PFT values for a patient with COPD.

- **Asthma–COPD Overlap**

GINA and GOLD guidelines both recognize clinical conditions in which patients have overlapping features of asthma and COPD. However, they also emphasize that this is no longer referred to as a separate entity. From the GINA guidelines,[3] "this is not a definition of a single disease entity, but a descriptive term for clinical use that includes several different clinical phenotypes reflecting different underlying mechanisms."

- **Features on PFTs suggestive of overlap include**
  - ▪ Persistent airflow obstruction with FEV_1/FVC below 0.7, a hallmark of COPD
  - ▪ A postbronchodilator increase in FEV_1 >12% and >400 mL, indicating significant reversibility (>200 mL is often found in COPD), which is both a hallmark of asthma and unusual in COPD alone
  - ○ Age, comorbid conditions such as smoking, and even asthma alone can predispose to development of overlapping COPD.[17,18]
  - ○ Routine monitoring with PFTs is crucial for early recognition and treatment, as studies show patients with overlapping features of asthma and COPD have higher morbidity and mortality than those with asthma or COPD alone.[19]

- **Vocal cord dysfunction (VCD),** also known as **paradoxical vocal fold motion (PVFM),** manifests as transient obstruction of the upper airway associated with inappropriate adduction of the vocal cords during inhalation and sometimes during exhalation.[20]
  - ○ It is underappreciated in clinical medicine and is often misdiagnosed as refractory asthma.[3,4,20]
  - ○ Symptoms can range from mild dyspnea to acute-onset respiratory distress.
  - ○ Its physiologic etiology is likely hyperresponsiveness and accentuation of the glottic closure reflex caused by intrinsic or extrinsic triggers, including psychogenic, exercise, or irritant (gastroesophageal reflux disease [GERD] or postnasal drip).
  - ○ **Characteristic flow-volume loops show flattening of the inspiratory limb.**
  - ○ Flow-volume loops have low negative predictive value and should not preclude rhinolaryngoscopy, which is the gold standard for diagnosis, if clinically suspected.

- **Restrictive lung disease** is characterized by a decreased **TLC <80% of predicted.**[13]
  - ○ FEV_1 and FVC are usually proportionately reduced and, therefore, will give a normal ratio of FEV_1/FVC.
  - ○ As the disease process progresses, FVC may decrease faster than FEV_1 and thus can increase the ratio of FEV_1/FVC. See Figure 8-1 and Table 8-4 for sample PFTs of a patient with restrictive lung disease.
  - ○ Restrictive defects are graded based on the severity of decrease in TLC or VC.

REFERENCES

1. Miller MR, Hankinson J, Brusasco V, et al. Standardisation of spirometry. *Eur Respir J.* 2005;26:319–38.
2. Culver BH, Graham BL, Coates AL, et al. Recommendations for a standardized pulmonary function report. An official American Thoracic Society technical statement. *Am J Respir Crit Care Med.* 2017;196:1463–72.
3. Global Initiative for Asthma. Global strategy for asthma management and prevention. 2020. www.ginasthma.org
4. U.S. Department of Health and Human Services, National Institutes of Health. Expert Panel Report 3: guidelines for the diagnosis and management of asthma [EPR3]. Published July 2007. Last Accessed 7/31/18. http://www.nhlbi.nih.gov/health-pro/guidelines/current/asthma-guidelines

5. Wanger J, Clausen JL, Coates A, et al. Standardisation of the measurement of lung volumes. *Eur Respir J.* 2005;26:511–22.

6. Graham BL, Brusasco V, Burgos F, et al. 2017 ERS/ATS standards for single-breath carbon monoxide uptake in the lung. *Eur Respir J.* 2017;49(1):1600016.

7. Holland AE, Spruit MA, Troosters T, et al. An official European Respiratory Society/American Thoracic Society technical standard: field walking tests in chronic respiratory disease. *Eur Respir J.* 2014;44:1428–46.

8. Dubé B-P, Dres M. Diaphragm dysfunction: diagnostic approaches and management strategies. *J Clin Med.* 2016;5(12):113.

9. Global Initiative for Chronic Obstructive Lung Disease. Global strategy for the diagnosis, management, and prevention of chronic obstructive lung disease (2020 Report). https://goldcopd.org/wp-content/uploads/2019/12/GOLD-2020-FINAL-ver1.2-03Dec19_WMV.pdf

10. Kanchongkittiphon W, Gaffin JM, Kopel L, et al. Association of FEF 25%–75% and bronchodilator reversibility with asthma control and asthma morbidity in inner-city children with asthma. *Ann Allergy Asthma Immunol.* 2016;117:97–9.

11. Rao DR, Gaffin JM, Baxi SN, et al. The utility of forced expiratory flow between 25% and 75% of vital capacity in predicting childhood asthma morbidity and severity. *J Asthma.* 2012;49:586–92.

12. Riley CM, Wenzel SE, Castro M, et al. Clinical implications of having reduced mid forced expiratory flow rates (FEF 25–75%), independently of FEV_1, in adult patients with asthma. *PLoS One.* 2015;10:e0145476.

13. Ranu H, Wilde M, Madden B. Pulmonary function tests. *Ulster Med J.* 2011;80(2):84–90. Last Accessed 7/31/18. http://www.ncbi.nlm.nih.gov/pubmed/22347750

14. Coates AL, Wanger J, Cockcroft DW, et al. ERS technical standard on bronchial challenge testing: general considerations and performance of methacholine challenge tests. *Eur Respir J.* 2017;49:1–17.

15. Crapo RO, Casaburi R, Coates AL, et al. Guidelines for methacholine and exercise challenge testing—1999. *Am J Respir Crit Care Med.* 2000;161:309–29.

16. Qaseem A, Wilt TJ, Weinberger SE, et al. Diagnosis and management of stable chronic obstructive pulmonary disease: a clinical practice guideline update from the American College of Physicians, American College of Chest Physicians, American Thoracic Society, and European Respiratory Society. *Ann Intern Med.* 2011;155:179–91.

17. Lange P, Celli B, Agustí A, et al. Lung-function trajectories leading to chronic obstructive pulmonary disease. *N Engl J Med.* 2015;373:111–22.

18. McGeachie MJ, Yates KP, Zhou X, et al. Patterns of growth and decline in lung function in persistent childhood asthma. *N Engl J Med.* 2016;374:1842–52.

19. Alshabanat A, Zafari Z, Albanyan O, et al. Asthma and COPD overlap syndrome (ACOS): a systematic review and meta analysis. *PLoS One.* 2015;10:e0136065.

20. Dunn NM, Katial RK, Hoyte FCL. Vocal cord dysfunction: a review. *Asthma Res Pract.* 2015;1:9.

Allergic Rhinitis and Sinusitis

Niharika Thota and Jennifer Marie Monroy

9

RHINITIS

GENERAL PRINCIPLES

- One of the most common chronic diseases, allergic rhinitis (AR) is characterized by rhinorrhea, nasal congestion, postnasal drainage, nasopharyngeal itching, and sneezing.
- AR symptoms are a result of a hypersensitivity reaction to environmental allergens.
- The prevalence of AR is increasing.[1]
- Rhinitis can be broadly classified as allergic, nonallergic (NAR), or infectious.

Definition

- AR is allergen-driven mucosal inflammation.
- AR must contain one or more of the following symptoms[1]:
  - Nasal congestion
  - Sneezing
  - Itching
  - Rhinorrhea
  - Postnasal drainage
- For rhinitis to be classified as allergic, the patient must have evidence of IgE sensitization to an allergen by skin testing or ImmunoCAP testing.

Classification

- Rhinitis can be classified into
  - AR
  - NAR: vasomotor, gustatory, infectious
  - NAR with eosinophilia syndrome (NARES)
  - Atrophic
- AR can be further classified as
  - **Seasonal:** Patients have signs and symptoms of AR occurring in one or more seasons, but not year-round. They are sensitized to seasonal allergens, such as trees, grasses, or weeds.
  - **Perennial:** Patients have signs and symptoms of AR throughout the year, and they may also have seasonal exacerbations if they are sensitized to seasonal allergens.
    - Allergens typically include dust mites, molds, pet dander, or cockroaches.
    - Symptoms must be present >2 hours/day, >9 months out of the year.
  - **Episodic:** Patients have signs and symptoms of AR, but the aeroallergens to which they are sensitized are not present regularly in their environment. An example would be a patient who has symptoms only when visiting a friend who has a cat and is otherwise asymptomatic.[1]
  - **Local:** Patients have signs and symptoms of AR but no evidence of atopy on conventional testing. However, patients have a positive response to nasal allergen challenge. It is characterized by the production of specific IgE, eosinophils, and mast cells in the nasal mucosa.
  - **Mixed:** Patients have a combination of AR and NAR.

Epidemiology

- AR affects 10–30% of people worldwide, and the prevalence in the United States is 19.9%.[2,3]
- 43% of patients have AR, 34% have mixed rhinitis, and 23% have NAR.[4]
- In 2010, approximately $17.5 billion was attributable to AR-related care.[5]
- Most individuals develop symptoms before 20 years of age, with 40% of patients becoming symptomatic by 6 years of age. AR is more common in males in the pediatric population but more common in females in the adult population.[6]
- Adults have a higher prevalence of perennial AR, and children have a higher prevalence of seasonal AR.

Etiology

- AR is an **IgE-mediated** disease that is provoked by either seasonal or perennial inhalant allergens. Sensitization to aeroallergens may occur even in the first 2 years of life.[1]
- Anatomic causes of rhinitis include septal deviation, foreign bodies, adenoid hypertrophy, choanal atresia, and tumors.

Pathophysiology

- Mast cells and basophils located on the superficial mucosa of the respiratory tract have specific IgE bound to cell membranes. When allergens bind and cross-link the IgE, cellular degranulation occurs.
  - Mast cells degranulate and release both preformed and newly synthesized mediators that cause the allergic reaction.[7]
  - Preformed mediators include histamine, tryptase, chymase, kininogenase, heparin, and other enzymes. Newly formed mediators include prostaglandins, leukotriene (LT)C4, LTD4, and LTE4.
- AR may be characterized by a dual-phase reaction.
  - **Early phase:** occurs within a few minutes of exposure to an inhaled allergen. Characterized by sneezing, rhinorrhea, and postnasal drip. These symptoms abate in about 1 hour.
  - **Late phase:** recurrence of symptoms a few hours later with predominantly nasal obstruction. Eosinophils release mediators, causing tissue damage in the late-phase response.[1]
- **Priming** occurs with prolonged allergen exposure, resulting in repeated late-phase responses even with very small exposures such that inflammatory mediators continue to be released and symptom resolution may lag behind the decrease in pollen.[1]
- NAR causes include hormones, gustatory, vasomotor, and medications.

Risk Factors

- Family history of atopy
- Atopic march: Atopic dermatitis and food allergies in infancy and early childhood are associated with an increased risk of AR.[8]
- A serum IgE >100 IU/mL before age 6
- Higher socioeconomic status
- Presence of a positive percutaneous skin test[1]
- First-born children are more likely to have AR.
- Smoke exposure
- Exposure to pets in early life was found to be inversely associated with rhinitis incidence in adolescence.[9]
- Protective factors include exposure to a farm environment in early life and increased number of siblings.

DIAGNOSIS

Clinical Presentation

- Patients typically present with sneezing, rhinorrhea, postnasal drip, nasal itching, and congestion.[1]
- Other symptoms include itching of palate, conjunctiva, throat, Eustachian tubes, and middle ear.
- Ear fullness and popping, as well as pressure over cheeks and forehead may be reported.
- Occasionally, chronic cough may be the presenting symptom.
- Often patients can associate the onset of symptoms to a particular trigger.

History
- History is vital in making the diagnosis.
- Important elements to ask
  - Symptom frequency
  - Symptom severity both past and present
  - Seasonal variation in symptoms
  - Temporal association of symptoms to potential allergens (indoor and outdoor)
  - Relationship of symptoms when at home and/or in the workplace
- Assessment of **home environmental conditions**
  - Water damage or mold
  - Pets
  - Carpet
  - Indoor plants
  - Cockroach and/or mouse infestation
  - Age of mattress and pillows as well as the type of filling (e.g., synthetic or feather)
  - Presence of irritants nearby (e.g., factories, farms, woods, vacant lots)
  - Type of heat and air-conditioning (central, window unit). Presence of air filters and how often they are changed
  - Use of fireplace, wood burning stove, or humidifiers
  - Exacerbation of symptoms from activities like dusting or vacuuming the home
- Medications
  - Aspirin, NSAIDs, oral contraceptives, angiotensin-converting enzyme (ACE) inhibitors, or β-blockers
  - Current and past medications used to treat symptoms
- Other associated medical conditions
  - Asthma: found in 19–38% of patients with AR, and approximately 85–95% of asthmatics have AR.[10]
  - Allergic conjunctivitis
  - Food allergies
  - Atopic dermatitis
  - Oral allergy syndrome
  - Recurrent otitis media or effusions
  - Obstructive sleep apnea
  - Nasal obstruction from severe nasal septal deviation
  - Refractory sinusitis
- Family history of atopic disease
- Quality-of-life assessment
  - Presence of fatigue, learning and attention problems, sleep disturbances
  - Time missed from work or school
  - The effect on quality of life is often underrecognized and inadequately treated.[1]

- Timing of exacerbations
  - Worse upon awakening?
  - Are particular seasons worse and are there seasons where symptoms are absent?
- Assess symptom severity
  - Mild: normal sleep, daily activities and work/school not affected, no bothersome symptoms
  - Moderate or severe: sleep disturbance, impairment of daily activities, school/work performance, and having bothersome symptoms.
- Assess duration of symptoms
  - Intermittent: Symptoms occur fewer than 4 days a week or for <4 weeks.[11]
  - Persistent: Symptoms occur >4 days a week or >4 weeks.[11]

Physical Examination
- A thorough examination of the head, eyes, ears, nose, and throat should be performed.
- Note if findings are unilateral or bilateral.
- Common findings in AR include
  - **Allergic salute** is a crease across the bridge of the nose and is a result of rubbing the nose.
  - **Dennie lines** are infraorbital creases.
  - **Conjunctivitis** may be present in those with ocular symptoms.
  - **Allergic shiners** are infraorbital hyperpigmentation secondary to nasal congestion.
  - The interior of each nostril should be carefully examined using a handheld otoscope with nasal adapter. A pneumatic otoscope can be used to assess the mobility of the tympanic membrane.
  - Turbinates are often edematous and pale. They may sometimes appear blue.
  - **Cobblestoning** in the posterior oropharynx indicates postnasal drainage.
  - Ears should be evaluated for otitis or Eustachian tube dysfunction.
  - The presence of **septal deviation** or **nasal polyps** should be noted.
  - Assess for concomitant sinusitis, wheezing, and eczema.
- If **septal perforation** is present, the differential diagnosis includes
  - Inappropriate intranasal steroid technique or adverse effects of nasal medications
  - Intranasal narcotic abuse
  - Prior surgery
  - Systemic disease such as granulomatosis with polyangiitis

Differential Diagnosis

- **NAR** is characterized by periodic or perennial symptoms of rhinitis without evidence of sensitization to allergens. There is inflammation of the nasal mucosa and symptoms are similar to AR, but pruritus is often absent.
- **Vasomotor rhinitis** is a type of NAR in which excessive vasomotor activity causes chronic nasal congestion.
  - The underlying mechanism is unknown.
  - Etiologies include **odors, chlorine, tobacco smoke, alcohol, spicy foods, emotions, temperature change, cold dry air, and sexual and emotional states**.
  - When associated with eating, it is called **gustatory rhinitis**. Anticholinergics are the preferred treatment.
- **NARES** causes similar symptoms to AR, and large numbers of eosinophils are present on nasal smear.
  - Patients tend to be middle aged and often have paroxysmal exacerbations.
  - There is an increased risk for developing obstructive sleep apnea.[1]
- **Drug-induced rhinitis:** Common offenders include ACE inhibitors, β-blockers, aspirin, NSAIDs, oral contraceptives, phosphodiesterase-5-selective inhibitors, α-receptor antagonists, and cocaine.

- **Rhinitis medicamentosa:** occurs from prolonged use of **intranasal α-adrenergic decongestants**
  - Rebound congestion occurs followed by nasal mucosal hypertrophy that appears as red, beefy mucosa.
  - Once the medication is discontinued and intranasal corticosteroids are used, resolution occurs.
- **Hormonal rhinitis:** Hormone-altering events induce nasal obstruction and hypersecretion.
  - Events include **hypothyroidism, oral contraceptive use, menstruation, and pregnancy.**
  - For pregnant women, symptoms usually appear during the second trimester, but disappear 2 weeks after delivery.
- **Occupational rhinitis**
  - Can be separated into IgE-mediated (bakers, farmers, lab workers) or irritant-mediated (anhydrides, ammonia, diisocyanates)
  - Differentiated from work-exacerbated AR where preexisting rhinitis symptoms are worse in the workplace
- **Nasal polyposis**
  - Outgrowths from the nasal passages that typically start along the lateral walls and appear smooth, round, pale, and gelatinous
  - Growth likely occurs from eosinophil-associated growth factors found in the contained eosinophils and immunoglobulins.
  - Persistent nasal congestion, anosmia, and dysgeusia should prompt consideration.
  - When seen in children, must rule out cystic fibrosis.
- **Anatomic abnormalities** should be considered, particularly in difficult-to-treat rhinitis.
- If **cerebrospinal fluid (CSF) rhinorrhea** is suspected, test for the presence of β-transferrin in nasal secretions.
- **Inflammatory disorders** such as granulomatosis with polyangiitis, eosinophilic granulomatosis with polyangiitis, sarcoidosis, amyloidosis, relapsing polychondritis, and other granulomatous infections are associated with rhinitis.

Diagnostic Testing

- **Skin testing and ImmunoCAP testing** are used to determine allergen sensitization and are discussed in detail in Chapter 3.
- The purpose of testing is to determine evidence of an allergic basis by confirming or denying suspected allergens so as to implement avoidance measures, symptom control, and/or immunotherapy.
- Epicutaneous skin testing is the preferred initial test, whereas intradermal testing could be considered subsequently given its higher sensitivity.
- The allergens tested include local trees, weeds, and grasses, while molds and other perennial allergens are usually included as well.

Laboratory Testing/Imaging

- **ImmunoCAP** (specific IgE) **testing** is used when skin testing is unable to be performed, such as the continued use of antihistamines, extensive skin disease, a history of anaphylaxis to skin testing, or the inability to remain still for the 15–20 minutes it takes for the testing to be performed.
- The average sensitivity of serum-specific IgE assays is only 70–75%.[1]
- Serum IgE and IgG subclasses **are not** used as diagnostic tools for AR.
- If anatomic abnormalities or chronic sinusitis is suspected, a CT scan may be helpful.

Diagnostic Procedures

- **Rhinoscopy** can be used to assess the structure of the nasal passages, search for nasal polyps and sinusitis, and evaluate the vocal cords.

- **Nasal provocation testing** is not routinely used in clinical practice but is used in research to confirm an allergen sensitivity. It is the test of choice in local AR.[1]
- **Nasal cytology** to look for eosinophils can be used to diagnose NARES.
- **Saccharin test/ciliary biopsy** can be used as a screening test for primary and secondary mucociliary dysfunction but have limited value and are not diagnostic.
- **Other diagnostics** include pulmonary function testing in asthmatics, sleep study evaluation for obstructive sleep apnea, and sweat chloride testing for cystic fibrosis.

TREATMENT

- Options include environmental control, pharmacologic therapy to treat symptoms, and allergen immunotherapy.[12]
- If AR is mild, single-agent therapy or combination therapy may be used in addition to avoidance measures.
- For all intranasal preparations, patients should be instructed to spray medication **away from the septum** to avoid irritation and perforation.

Medications

First Line

- **Intranasal steroids** are the mainstay of therapy because they help prevent both the early- and late-phase response.
  - Intranasal steroids significantly lower mediator and cytokine release, thereby reducing recruitment of basophils, eosinophils, neutrophils, and mononuclear cells to nasal secretions.[12]
  - Options include beclomethasone, budesonide, flunisolide, fluticasone furoate, fluticasone propionate, mometasone, triamcinolone, and ciclesonide.
  - Typical adult dosing is two sprays in each nostril once daily. Daily use is more effective than PRN use.
  - Also improves conjunctivitis symptoms like itching, redness, and watery eyes
  - For seasonal AR, intranasal steroids should be started 1–2 weeks before the onset of the pollen season.
- **Oral antihistamines** are also commonly used.
  - They reduce symptoms of rhinorrhea, nasal pruritus, sneezing, ocular pruritus, and tearing but are less effective at reducing nasal congestion.
  - Nonsedating second-generation antihistamines include loratadine, desloratadine, fexofenadine, cetirizine, and levocetirizine.
  - First-generation antihistamines, such as chlorpheniramine, diphenhydramine, doxepin, and hydroxyzine, are not generally used for AR because of their sedating properties.
    - Cumulative use of first-generation antihistamines with strong anticholinergic properties has been associated with a higher risk of dementia.
    - Second-generation antihistamines are more specific for peripheral H_1-receptors and have limited penetration of the blood–brain barrier.
- **Intranasal antihistamines** may be as effective or superior to oral second-generation antihistamines.[1]
  - They have a rapid onset of action and help reduce nasal congestion but are generally less effective than intranasal steroids.
  - Examples include azelastine and olopatadine.
  - These are combined with intranasal steroids in preparations, such as azelastine/fluticasone propionate.
- **Nasal saline irrigations** are beneficial in treating symptoms of chronic rhinorrhea and rhinosinusitis both as a sole modality and for adjunctive treatment.

Second Line
- **Montelukast** is approved for seasonal and perennial AR.
  - Can consider for patients with both AR and asthma
  - Side effects include headache, abnormal dreams, aggression, and depression.
- **Intranasal cromolyn** inhibits mast cell degranulation.[1,11]
  - The onset of action is 4–7 days, and it is effective for episodic AR.
  - It must be used qid for maximum effect and is not as effective as intranasal steroids or antihistamines.
- **Intranasal anticholinergics (ipratropium)** reduce rhinorrhea.
  - Not useful for nasal congestion and side effects include epistaxis and nasal xerosis
  - Should be used with caution in patients with glaucoma or prostate hypertrophy
- **Nasal decongestants (oxymetazoline, phenylephrine)**
  - Causes vasoconstriction to improve edema but does not affect the antigen-provoked nasal response[1]
  - Should not be used as a single agent and continuous use should be limited to 5 days to prevent rhinitis medicamentosa[11]
- **Oral decongestants (pseudoephedrine, phenylephrine)**
  - May play a role in select patients during acute flares, but chronic use is not recommended[11]
  - Not recommended in children, the elderly, and patients with a history of arrhythmia, coronary artery disease, cerebrovascular disease, hypertension, glaucoma, bladder neck dysfunction, and hyperthyroidism[12]
- **Oral steroids** are rarely indicated because of side effects, but a 5- to 7-day course may be considered for severe, intractable symptoms.

Immunotherapy
- The only treatment known to modify the natural course of AR and is successful approximately 80% of the time[12]
- May be used for the treatment of perennial and seasonal AR when a specific allergen has been identified
- Treatment is for 3–5 years and is considered unsuccessful if there is no symptom relief after 1 year of maintenance therapy.
- Is delivered either subcutaneously (SCIT) or sublingually (SLIT). See Chapter 11 for further details.
- Food and Drug Administration (FDA)-approved SLIT options
  - Timothy grass (Grastek)
  - Ragweed (Ragwitek)
  - Sweet vernal, orchard, perennial rye, timothy, and Kentucky blue grass (Oralair)
  - Dust mite (Odactra)

Lifestyle/Risk Modification
- Dust mite avoidance[1]
  - Dust mite proof covers for mattresses and pillows are designed to help decrease exposure.
  - Vacuum with a high-efficiency particulate air (HEPA) filter.
  - Wash linens in hot water.
  - Keep indoor humidity <50% to avoid growth of dust mites as well as fungi.
  - Hard surface flooring is preferable over carpet.
  - A multifaceted approach is more effective than any single intervention.
  - Acaricides are not recommended.
- Furry animals[1,13]
  - Remove the pet from the environment or keep out of the bedroom.
  - Bathing cats or dogs at least twice a week has been shown to reduce the level of allergens.

- Pollen
  - Counts are highest on sunny, windy days with lower humidity.
  - Keep windows and doors closed during pollen seasons.
  - Outdoor activities should be done in the evening when counts are lower.
- Mold
  - Sources of water damage or moisture should be eliminated, and porous surfaces should be replaced.
  - A dilute bleach solution will denature mold allergens on nonporous surfaces.
- Eliminate cockroaches (much easier said than done).

SPECIAL CONSIDERATIONS

Pregnancy
- Symptoms of AR increase in one-third of pregnant patients.[1]
- First- and second-generation antihistamines may be used.
- Oral decongestants should be avoided, particularly in the first trimester.
- Other medications that may be used include intranasal steroids, montelukast, and sodium cromolyn.
- Immunotherapy may be continued without dose escalation, but not initiated during pregnancy.

Elderly Patients
- Age-related changes such as cholinergic hyperactivity, anatomic changes, or concomitant medication use may affect rhinitis.
- Allergy is not a common cause of new-onset rhinitis in people aged >65 years.[7]
- Gustatory rhinitis is more commonly seen.
- Intranasal steroids and ipratropium may be used safely.
- If antihistamines are used, nonsedating agents are preferred.[7]

Rhinitis in Athletes
- Performance can be affected by rhinorrhea and chronic or rebound nasal congestion.
- Special consideration should be taken when prescribing treatment so as to avoid prescribing medications on the list of doping agents.

COMPLICATIONS

- Psychological impact of untreated AR can include depression, anxiety, and low self-esteem.
- Improperly or untreated AR can result in rhinosinusitis, otitis media, and rhinitis medicamentosa.[1]

REFERRAL

- Indications for referral to an allergist and immunology specialist
  - Consultation with an allergist-immunologist has been shown to improve outcomes such as adherence, quality of life, and patient satisfaction.[1]
  - Patients considering allergen immunotherapy to prevent progression of disease
- Indications for referral to an otolaryngologist
  - Nasal obstruction from severe nasal septal deviation
  - Inferior turbinate hypertrophy requiring reduction in those who have failed medical therapy
  - Nasal polyposis (NP) requiring polypectomy
  - Complications from refractory rhinosinusitis

MONITORING/FOLLOW-UP

- Clinical improvement is a better measure of appropriate environmental control rather than the amount of allergen concentration.[1]
- Patients should be assessed 2–4 weeks after initiation of therapy.
- If one medication regimen does not seem to be effective, addition of an agent or changing to a different class may be warranted.

SINUSITIS

GENERAL PRINCIPLES

Normal sinus function requires patient sinus ostia normal mucociliary function, and normal local and systemic immune function.[7]

Definition

- **Sinusitis** is defined as inflammation of one or more of the paranasal sinuses.
- Characterized by two or more symptoms, one of which should be either nasal blockage/obstruction/congestion or nasal discharge[14]
  - +/− Facial pain
  - +/− Anosmia
- Plus endoscopic signs of
  - Nasal polyps
  - Mucopurulent discharge
  - Edema/mucosal obstruction
- And/or CT revealing mucosal changes within the ostiomeatal complex and/or sinuses
- Rhinosinusitis is the preferred term because inflammation of the sinus cavities is almost always accompanied by inflammation of the nasal cavities.[15]

Classification

- Sinusitis can be **acute, chronic,** or **recurrent.**
- No consensus for defining chronic rhinosinusitis (CRS) vs. acute rhinosinusitis (ARS)
- ARS usually lasts for <4 weeks with complete symptom resolution.[14]
- CRS consists of inflammation of the nasal passages lasting a minimum of 12 weeks despite medical management.[7]
- CRS is characterized by abnormal findings on nasal endoscopy or sinus CT.[15]
- Recurrent sinusitis is characterized by three episodes of acute sinusitis per year.[16] Patients may need evaluation for underlying AR, primary immunodeficiency, NP, or neoplastic lesions.

Epidemiology

- About 90–98% of episodes of sinusitis are preceded by an acute viral upper respiratory infection.[1]
- About 31 million people in the United States have rhinosinusitis annually.[7]
- Viral upper respiratory infections evolve into bacterial rhinosinusitis in 0.5–2% of the population.[7]
- CRS is associated with AR in 60% of adults.[7]
- Increasing resistance to first-line therapies is well known and includes β-lactamase production (gram-negative organisms) and alterations in penicillin-binding proteins (gram-positive organisms).
  - More than one-third of *Haemophilus influenzae* strains and virtually all *Moraxella catarrhalis* strains are penicillin resistant.

Etiology

- ARS is usually infectious, viral, bacterial, or fungal.
- **Viruses** are the most common cause of ARS, and symptoms usually last for fewer than 10 days. **Acute postviral rhinosinusitis** is defined as an increase in symptoms after 5 days or persistent symptoms after 10 days with a <12 weeks duration.[14]
- The most common **bacterial** etiologies include *Streptococcus pneumoniae*, *H. influenzae*, and *Staphylococcus aureus*.
- *S. aureus*, coagulase-negative *staphylococcus*, and anaerobic bacteria are more common in CRS, but CRS is more often inflammatory.[7]
- *S. aureus* is increased in prevalence in CRS with NP.[7]
- *Pseudomonas aeruginosa* is frequently found in patients with cystic fibrosis.
- **Fungal** rhinosinusitis is classified into three forms.
  - **Allergic fungal rhinosinusitis (AFRS)**
    - Seen in patients with asthma and nasal polyps
    - CT imaging demonstrates hyperattenuated areas within opacified sinuses corresponding to eosinophilic mucin deposits.
  - **Fungal ball**
    - Typically occurs in the maxillary or sphenoid sinuses and is usually unilateral
    - Causes chronic nasal congestion and headache
- **Invasive fungal sinusitis**
    - Seen in immunocompromised patients and the acute presentation is an aggressive, fulminant disease
    - *Aspergillus fumigatus* is most commonly associated.

Pathophysiology

- Acute sinusitis often develops when the sinus ostia are obstructed, leading to infection.
- Conditions that **disrupt mucociliary clearance** of secretions and **promote ostial obstruction** predispose patients to sinusitis, including:
  - Rhinitis
  - Nasal polyps
  - Anatomic abnormalities
  - Foreign bodies
  - Impaired mucociliary transport
    - Cystic fibrosis
    - Primary ciliary dyskinesia
    - Viral infections and other causes of inflammation may result in ciliary dysfunction themselves.
- Obstruction of the ostia can lead to mucous impaction and decrease oxygenation in the sinus cavities, resulting in bacterial growth.

DIAGNOSIS

Clinical Presentation

- The diagnosis of rhinosinusitis is usually entirely clinical, and the differentiation between viral and bacterial infections can be difficult.
- Investigation into the utility of symptoms and signs for diagnosing acute sinusitis has resulted in differing conclusions. Not all studies have used the true gold standard (i.e., sinus puncture and culture) but instead have used a surrogate standard (e.g., sinus plain films and CT). Radiography cannot differentiate viral from bacterial sinusitis.

- ARS symptoms lasting 7–10 days typically indicate a viral rhinosinusitis, whereas symptoms lasting longer suggest a bacterial infection.[7]
- Acute bacterial rhinosinusitis (ABRS) symptoms include nasal congestion, purulent rhinorrhea, facial and dental pain, postnasal drainage, headache, and cough.
- Signs include sinus tenderness, purulent nasal discharge, erythematous mucosa, pharyngeal secretions, and periorbital edema.
- Fever may or may not be present. ABRS is mostly a clinical diagnosis, and radiologic confirmation is not essential, except in complicated cases.
- CRS can be differentiated into CRS with NP and CRS without NP. Nasal congestion, sinus pressure, and hyposmia/anosmia are prominent in CRS with NP, whereas facial pain is more prominent in CRS without NP.[15]

Diagnostic Testing

Laboratories
If **immunodeficiency** is suspected, obtain a complete blood count (CBC) with differential, quantitative immunoglobulin levels, and vaccine titers. Otherwise, lab tests are of little use.

Imaging
- Imaging to confirm the diagnosis of acute uncomplicated rhinosinusitis is usually not necessary.[17–19]
- Standard radiography cannot readily differentiate viral from bacterial acute sinusitis.
- The limited sinus CT has become the most widely used radiographic study for the diagnosis of sinusitis.
  - It is obtained in the coronal projection with cuts through the frontal sinuses, anterior ethmoid/maxillary sinuses, and posterior ethmoid and sphenoid sinuses.
  - Allows for assessment of patency of the ostiomeatal unit and the critical confluence of drainage from the maxillary and anterior ethmoid sinuses
  - In CRS, imaging will reveal mucosal thickening and ostial plugging.
  - Can also evaluate for variants (infraorbital ethmoid, Haller cells, mucoceles)[15]
- MRI is useful for evaluating allergic or infectious fungal sinusitis to rule out soft-tissue extension into the orbital or intracranial space.

Diagnostic Procedures
- Skin-prick testing to evaluate for underlying AR
- Endoscopically directed middle meatus cultures may be helpful in adults.[1]
- Rhinoscopy can help determine nasal and sinus anatomy.
- Biopsy is indicated if there is suspicion for a tumor or vasculitis. May also be necessary to confirm the presence of an invasive fungal infection.
- Ciliary function testing is indicated in the setting of recurrent otitis, sinusitis, and pneumonia with bronchiectasis (primary ciliary dyskinesia or Kartagener syndrome).
- Electron microscopy of nasal mucosal biopsy is the only way to document abnormal cilia structure.
- Nasal cytology
  - Eosinophils may indicate AR, NARES, and nasal polyps.
  - Neutrophils are more indicative of an infection.

TREATMENT

- Most cases of ARS are caused by viruses and are expected to significantly improve without antibiotic treatment within 10–14 days. Treatment should, therefore, be symptomatic for those without clinical signs suggestive of a bacterial infection.[19]

- Uncomplicated ABRS may be treated with or without antibiotics.[7,17,18] Those without severe or prolonged symptoms may be treated for symptoms alone and followed for resolution. Worsening symptoms should prompt reconsideration of antibiotic therapy.
- Patients with severe initial symptoms, symptoms that persist for >10 days after diagnosis, or recrudescence of symptoms after improvement are typically treated with antibiotics.
  - Amoxicillin–clavulanate is recommended as a first-line therapy, although the optimal duration of therapy is unclear.[19,20]
  - Penicillin allergy should be clarified to prevent antibiotic resistance.
- Alternative antibiotic therapy should be considered in patients who worsen or do not improve during the initial 7 days of therapy.[19,20]
- Although evidence is somewhat limited, the addition of intranasal steroids may have a modest positive benefit in the treatment of ARS.[7,17,21]
- There are no controlled trials of systemic steroids, and these are not routinely recommended.
- Analgesics should be used for those with significant pain.[17]
- Data to support the use of decongestants, antihistamines, mucolytics/expectorants, and sinus irrigation are lacking, but they are at least theoretically beneficial and often recommended.[7,19]
  - Intranasal steroids, either as monotherapy or in combination with antibiotics, are used in uncomplicated rhinosinusitis.[7]
  - Systemic antibiotics and a short course of oral steroids can be considered in the treatment of CRS, with greater benefit in those with CRS without NP than CRS with NP.[15]
  - Nasal irrigation is frequently recommended.[22]
- AR should be maximally treated.
- Aspirin desensitization can be considered in patients with aspirin-exacerbated respiratory disease (AERD).[23]
- The exhalation delivery system with fluticasone propionate (Xhance®) is approved for treating CRS with NP.[24]
- The monoclonal antibody dupilumab inhibits interleukin (IL)-4 and IL-13 signaling and can be used in patients with CRS with NP as well as those with moderate-to-severe atopic dermatitis and moderate-to-severe asthma.[25]

COMPLICATIONS

- Rare but dangerous complications may occur when sinus disease extends outside the sinus cavity, including orbital cellulitis, cavernous vein thrombosis, brain abscess, meningitis, osteomyelitis, oroantral fistula, and mucoceles.[1,7,16]
- It should be remembered that *Clostridium difficile* colitis and candidiasis can be a complication of prolonged antibiotic therapy.

REFERRAL

Indications for referral to an otolaryngologist[1,7,16]

- Evidence of anatomic defects by CT or physical examination, including foreign bodies, and tumors
- Nasal polyps that obstruct sinus drainage despite medical treatment
- Persistent sinusitis despite aggressive medical management
- Sinus condition requiring biopsy (granulomatous disease, neoplasm, ciliary dyskinesia, or fungal ball)

- Sinusitis complicated by extension into local structures
- When anatomic defects obstruct the sinus outflow tract, particularly the ostiomeatal complex (and adenoidal tissues in children)

MONITORING/FOLLOW-UP

- Symptoms are expected to resolve between episodes of ARS.
- If symptoms persist after one course of antibiotics for ARS, an alternative antibiotic may be considered.
- If symptoms have not resolved after multiple antibiotic courses, a CT scan should be performed and further workup for underlying conditions should be performed.

REFERENCES

1. Wallace DV, Dykewicz MS, Bernstein DI, et al. The diagnosis and management of rhinitis: an updated practice parameter. *J Allergy Clin Immunol.* 2008;122:S1–84
2. Pawanker R, Canonica G, Holgate S, et al. *White Book on Allergy 2011–2012 Executive Summary.* Milwaukee, WI: World Health Organization, 2011.
3. Wallace DV, Dykewicz MS. Seasonal allergic rhinitis: a focused systematic review and practice parameter update. *Curr Opin Allergy Clin Immunol.* 2017;17:286–94.
4. Bernstein JA. Allergic and mixed rhinitis: epidemiology and natural history. *Allergy Asthma Proc.* 2010;31:365–9.
5. Blaiss MS, Hammerby E, Robinson S, et al. The burden of allergic rhinitis and allergic rhinoconjunctivitis on adolescents: a literature reviews. *Ann Allergy Asthma Immunol.* 2018;121:43–52.
6. Meltzer EO, Blaiss MS, Derebery MJ, et al. Burden of allergic rhinitis: results from the Pediatric Allergies in America survey. *J Allergy Clin Immunol.* 2009;124:S43–70.
7. Dykewicz MS, Hamilos DL. Rhinitis and sinusitis. *J Allergy Clin Immunol.* 2010;125:S103–15.
8. Berger WE. Overview of allergic rhinitis. *Ann Allergy Asthma Immunol.* 2003;90:7–12.
9. Matheson MC, Dharmage SC, Abramson MJ, et al. Early-life risk factors and incidence of rhinitis: results from the European Community Respiratory Health Study—an international population-based cohort study. *J Allergy Clin Immunol.* 2011;128:816–23
10. Khan DA. Allergic rhinitis and asthma: epidemiology and common pathophysiology. *Allergy Asthma Proc.* 2014;25:357–61.
11. Brozek JL, Bousquet J, Agache I, et al. Allergic rhinitis and its impact on asthma (ARIA) guidelines: 2016 revision. *J Allergy Clin Immunol.* 2017;140:950–8.
12. Dykewicz MS, Wallace DV, Baroody F, et al. Treatment of seasonal allergic rhinitis: an evidence-based focused 2017 guideline update. *Ann Allergy Asthma Immunol.* 2017;119(6):489–511.
13. Portnoy J, Kennedy K, Sublett J, et al. Environmental assessment and exposure control: a practice parameter—furry animals. *Ann Allergy Asthma Immunol.* 2012;108(4):223.e1–15.
14. Fokkens WJ, Lund VJ, Mullol J, et al. EPOS 2012: European position paper on rhinosinusitis and nasal polyps 2012. A summary for otorhinolaryngologists. *Rhinology.* 2012;23:S1–229.
15. Peters AT, Spector S, Hsu J, et al. Diagnosis and management of rhinosinusitis: a practice parameter update. *Ann Allergy Asthma Immunol.* 2014;113:347–85.
16. Bachert C, Gevaert P, Cauwenberge P. Nasal polyps and rhinosinusitis. In: Adkinson NF, Holgate ST, Bochner BS, et al., eds. *Middleton's Allergy: Principles and Practice.* 7th ed. Philadelphia, PA: Mosby/Elsevier, 2009:995–1004.
17. Rosenfeld RM. Clinical practice guideline on adult sinusitis. *Otolaryngol Head Neck Surg.* 2007;137:365–77.
18. Hickner JM, Bartlett JG, Besser RE, et al. Principles of appropriate antibiotic use for acute rhinosinusitis in adults: background. *Ann Intern Med.* 2001;134:498–505.
19. Slavin RG, Spector SL, Bernstein IL, et al. The diagnosis and management of sinusitis: a practice parameter update. *J Allergy Clin Immunol.* 2005;116:S13–47.
20. Piccirillo JF. Acute bacterial sinusitis. *N Engl J Med.* 2004;351:902–10.
21. Snidvongs K, Kalish L, Sacks R, et al. Topical steroid for chronic rhinosinusitis without polyps. *Cochrane Database Syst Rev.* 2011;(8):CD009274.

22. Harvey R, Hannan SA, Badia L, et al. Nasal saline irrigations for the symptoms of chronic rhinosinusitis. *Cochrane Database Syst Rev.* 2007;(3):CD006394.

23. Stevenson DD. Aspirin desensitization in patients with AERD. *Clin Rev Allergy Immunol.* 2003;24(2):159–68.

24. Leopold DA, Elkayam D, Messina JC, et al. NAVIGATE II: randomized, double-blind trial of the exhalation delivery system with fluticasone for nasal polyposis. *J Allergy Clin Immunol.* 2019;143:126–34.

25. Bachert C, Hellings PW, Mullol J, et al. Dupilumab improves patient-reported outcomes in patients with chronic rhinosinusitis with nasal polyps and comorbid asthma. *J Allergy Clin Immunol Pract.* 2019;7(7):2447–9.e2.

Ocular Allergic Diseases

Xiaowen Wang and Brooke Ivan Polk

10

GENERAL PRINCIPLES

Ocular allergic diseases can be considered a spectrum of diseases ranging from mild itching and redness associated with seasonal allergic conjunctivitis (AC) to severe, sight-threatening sequelae secondary to atopic keratoconjunctivitis (AKC).

Definition

IgE-mediated inflammation of the conjunctivae, the clear membrane that covers the sclera and lines the eyelids

Classification

Ocular allergic conditions may be classified as follows[1]:
- **AC, seasonal or perennial**: a self-limited, generally bilateral conjunctivitis in individuals sensitized to environmental allergens
- **Vernal keratoconjunctivitis (VKC)**: a sight-threatening condition consisting of severe photophobia, pruritus, and thick, ropy discharge predominantly affecting young males living in warm, arid climates
- **AKC**: a chronic, bilateral, sight-threatening condition with severe ocular pruritus, flaking periocular skin, and mucoid discharge generally in adults with atopic dermatitis
- **Giant papillary conjunctivitis (GPC)**: a benign condition with mild ocular pruritus, foreign-body intolerance, and giant papillae generally caused by contact lenses that does not require aeroallergen sensitization

Epidemiology

Approximately 20–30% of the population of the United States (60–90 million people) have ocular allergic diseases.[2]

Etiology

Genetic predisposition for atopy and formation of specific IgE after exposure to environmental allergens

Pathophysiology

- AC is the prototype of the group of diseases that begin as an **antigen–IgE antibody interaction on the surface of the conjunctival mast cells** (also see Chapter 2).[3]
- The allergen binds two separate IgE molecules, creating a dimer formation (cross-linking) that initiates the chain of reactions on the mast cell plasma membrane.
- Cross-linking of the IgE causes the release of preformed mediators (e.g., histamine) and newly formed mediators produced via metabolism of arachidonic acid (AA).
- Metabolism of AA produces **prostaglandins** via the cyclooxygenase pathway and **leukotrienes** via the lipoxygenase pathway.
- Conjunctival surface contains both H1 and H2 histamine receptors.
  - Histamine binding to the H1 receptor results in symptoms of ocular **itching**.
  - Histamine binding to the H2 receptors produces **vasodilation of conjunctival vessels**.

- Other mediators
  - Eosinophils release **major basic protein** (MBP) that has been demonstrated to cause epithelial toxicity.
  - Lymphocytes release **interleukins** that are involved in further recruitment of inflammatory cells and their release of inflammatory mediators.

Risk Factors

- AC (seasonal and perennial)
  - Family history of atopy
  - Atopic disease, such as allergic rhinitis, asthma, or atopic dermatitis
  - Aeroallergen sensitization
- VKC
  - Male gender (3:1 M:F ratio)
  - Warm, dry climate
  - Strong family history of atopic disease
  - Aeroallergen sensitization
- AKC
  - Age 20–60 years
  - No gender predilection
  - Long history of atopic dermatitis
  - Aeroallergen sensitization
- GPC
  - Exogenous materials causing chronic inflammation of the upper tarsal conjunctival surface
  - Most cases are secondary to **contact lens wear,** but ocular prostheses and nylon sutures used in ophthalmic surgical procedures may be an etiologic agent.

DIAGNOSIS

- Diagnosis is usually made through an appropriate clinical history in combination with epicutaneous skin-prick testing to environmental allergens to demonstrate the presence of allergic sensitization.
- Physical examination of the eyes, including assessment of the eyelids, conjunctiva, and quality of tears that are formed, and slit-lamp examination can aid in the diagnosis, but findings may not always be apparent (especially if the patient is currently asymptomatic).

Clinical Presentation

History
- AC
  - Bilateral, red, itching eyes associated with tearing and burning
  - Occasionally unilateral response may occur when there has been hand-to-eye contact with allergen (e.g., animal dander).
  - Generally associated with rhinitis
- VKC
  - Typically a young boy (age 3–20 years) will present with marked itching associated with stringy, ropy mucus discharge.
  - Severe cases may be associated with photophobia, pain, and decreased visual acuity.
- AKC
  - Chronic year-round itching; associated with burning, light sensitivity, tearing, and chronic redness of the eyes
  - Red or flaking periocular skin
  - Rubbing may cause corneal erosions and scarring.

- GPC
  - Chronic irritation, redness, discharge, and mild itching
  - Decreased wearing time of contact lenses, foreign-body sensation

Physical Examination
- AC
  - Edematous and erythematous periocular tissues
  - Conjunctiva with mild-to-moderate chemosis with mucus discharge in the tear film, with **limbal sparing**
  - Cornea is rarely involved.
  - May have **allergic shiners,** owing to decreased venous return to overlying skin
- VKC
  - Edematous and ptotic upper eyelid
  - Corneal examination may reveal superficial infiltrates and, in severe cases, **shield ulcers,** which are epithelial defects with plaque-like deposition of material at the base, centrally located just above the visual axis.
  - Upper tarsal surface develops large raised **cobblestone papillae,** which are pathognomonic of the disease.
  - Papillae appear injected and commonly have mucus strands running in the crevices.
  - **Horner–Trantas dots** caused by aggregation of eosinophils, grossly appearing as gelatinous elevations with whitish inclusions located at the limbus
- AKC
  - Eczematous changes of the upper and lower eyelids, induration, erythema, and scaling.
  - Slit-lamp examination reveals marked plugging of the Meibomian gland orifices with purulent secretions and a concurrent poor precorneal tear film.
  - Bulbar conjunctiva may show mild-to-moderate injection and changes consistent with keratoconjunctivitis sicca (KCS) (dry eye).
  - Severe cases may result in conjunctival subepithelial fibrosis and **symblepharon** formation.
  - Tarsal conjunctival surfaces usually reveal mild-to-moderate injection.
  - Corneal involvement in AKC may vary according to the severity of disease.
    - In mild forms, the cornea may show minimal punctate staining with fluorescein dye.
    - Severe cases demonstrate marked surface irregularity with epithelial desiccation associated with corneal neovascularization, keratinization, and scarring.
- GPC
  - Examination may reveal minimal pathology.
  - Hyperemia and **giant papillae** may develop with chronic trauma to the upper tarsal conjunctival surfaces.
  - Papillae are the result of chronic collagen deposition and tend to be more uniformly distributed, smaller, and flatter in appearance than those seen in the cobblestone appearance of patients with VKC.
  - With disease progression, cornea may show diffuse punctate keratitis or even corneal epithelial abrasions.

Differential Diagnosis

- Viral conjunctivitis[4]
  - Usually characterized by an acute onset of a unilateral red eye associated with preauricular lymph node swelling
  - Patients complain of matting of the eyelids with clear to mucopurulent discharge.
  - Examination of the tarsal conjunctivae reveals a follicular appearance.
  - Infection often spreads to the opposite eye 3–9 days later.
  - May have concurrent upper respiratory infection

- Bacterial conjunctivitis
  - Usually characterized by an acute onset of a unilateral or bilateral red eye associated with eyelid erythema
  - Patients complain of matting of the eyelashes with yellow to green purulent discharge.
  - Examination of the tarsal conjunctivae reveals a papillary appearance.
- Chlamydial conjunctivitis
  - Usually characterized by an indolent, chronic onset of at least 6 weeks of a unilateral or bilateral mildly red eye
  - Examination of the tarsal conjunctivae reveals a mixed follicular and papillary appearance.
- Noninfectious
  - Irritant contact dermatitis
  - Drug-induced allergic contact dermatitis
  - KCS (dry eye syndrome)
  - Meibomian gland dysfunction (MGD), blepharitis

Diagnostic Testing

- For AC, VKC, and AKC, the offending allergen can be identified by either epicutaneous skin-prick testing (preferred) or specific IgE testing of the serum (also see Chapter 3). Serum IgE testing may be performed if the patient is not able to discontinue antihistamine medications, if he/she is uncooperative, or if he/she has extensive skin disease precluding skin testing.
- No testing is generally needed for GPC.

TREATMENT

- Identify and remove the offending allergen, if present.
- Prevent circulating allergens from interacting with conjunctival mast cells with refrigerated artificial tears.
- Basic eye care includes avoiding rubbing and use of cool compresses.
- Suppress cellular and extracellular inflammation with concomitant redness (vascular dilation) and chemosis (edema) using vasoconstrictor agents, NSAIDs, and steroidal agents.
- Decrease and prevent itching-associated redness by using mast cell stabilizer/antihistamine dual-acting agents (see Table 10-1).[5]
- Decrease itching by using H1-receptor antihistamines.
- **For GPC specifically, discontinue the use of contact lens for 4 weeks.**
- Consider the use of allergen immunotherapy for AC, VKC, and AKC.
- **Seasonal AC**
  - For mild-to-moderate disease, topical mast cell stabilizers/antihistamine dual-acting agents are first-line therapy.
    - Greatest benefit achieved if started prior to peak symptom severity
    - Most products dosed once to bid
  - Severe disease requires combination therapy, generally consisting of
    - Topical mast cell stabilizers/antihistamine dual-acting agents
    - Oral second-generation anti-H1 medications
  - Extreme cases may require short courses of topical steroids.
  - Treat accompanying nasal symptoms with steroid nasal spray.
  - Avoid first-generation systemic antihistamines as they decrease tear production.
  - Topical medications containing vasoconstrictor medications are generally not recommended.
  - Consider SC or sublingual aeroallergen immunotherapy.

TABLE 10-1 MEDICATIONS FOR OCULAR ALLERGIC DISEASES

Combined mast cell stabilizer/H1-receptor antagonist

Olopatadine (Patanol®, Pataday®, Pazeo®, or generic)
Bepotastine (Bepreve®)
Alcaftadine (Lastacaft®)
Azelastine (Optivar®)
Epinastine (Elestat®)
Ketotifen (Alaway®, Zaditor®, or generic OTC)

Selective H1-receptor antagonists

Emedastine (Emadine®)
Pheniramine (available in combination with naphazoline as Naphcon-A®, Opcon-A®, Visine-A®)

Mast cell stabilizers

Lodoxamide tromethamine (Alomide®)
Nedocromil (Alocril®)
Pemirolast (Alamast®)
Cromolyn (Opticrom®)

NSAIDs

Ketorolac (Acular®)

"Soft" topical steroids

Prednisolone acetate 0.12% (Pred Mild®)
Fluorometholone 0.1% (FML®, Flarex®, or generic)
Loteprednol etabonate 0.2% (Alrex®) or 0.5% (Lotemax®)
Rimexolone 1% (Vexol®)

OTC, over the counter.

- **Vernal keratoconjunctivitis**
  - In addition to basic eye care and aeroallergen avoidance, first-line therapy includes topical mast cell stabilizers/antihistamine dual-acting agents, with oral antihistamines if frequent itch/irritation or visual deficits.
    - Topical antihistamines alone are not effective.
    - Topical mast cell stabilizers are effective but not first line for acute symptoms.
  - If not responsive to 2–3 weeks of initial therapy, refer to ophthalmology for initiation of topical steroids.[6]
    - Seasonal exacerbations may require topical pulse steroids such as dexamethasone 0.1% or prednisolone phosphate 1%, often dosed eight times daily for 1 week with taper.
    - Less severe cases can be treated with "soft" steroids such as prednisolone acetate 0.12%, fluorometholone, loteprednol etabonate 0.5 or 0.2%, or rimexolone 1% dosed bid to qid for 2 weeks.
  - Topical calcineurin inhibitors (cyclosporine, tacrolimus) may be started if unable to reduce topical steroids, or if the cornea is compromised.
  - Consider aeroallergen immunotherapy.
  - Shield ulcers are sight-threatening and should be treated with topical cyclosporine and broad-spectrum topical antibiotics.

- **Atopic keratoconjunctivitis**
  - In addition to environmental control, first-line therapy includes topical mast cell stabilizer/antihistamine dual-acting agents.
  - If no response to 2–3 weeks of consistent mast cell stabilizer/antihistamine, a transient course of steroids may be required for 1–2 weeks, with referral to ophthalmology.
  - Topical vasoconstrictor–antihistamine combination medications may bring transient relief, but prolonged use is not recommended.
  - Topical cyclosporine A and tacrolimus are effective second-line, steroid-sparing agents.
  - Severe, refractory cases are managed with systemic immunosuppressive agents, with case reports of amniotic membrane transplantation.[7]
  - Topical antibiotic drops or ointments if corneal abrasion or keratitis is present
  - Treat comorbid eyelid dermatitis with topical calcineurin inhibitors.
  - Concurrent bacterial or viral infections must be treated appropriately.
  - May need to correct trichiasis or lid position abnormalities
- **GPC**
  - In addition to initial contact lens holiday followed by reduction in the wearing time of contacts, first-line therapy includes frequent use of artificial tears.
  - Topical antihistamines, mast cell stabilizers, and dual-acting agents can provide relief from symptoms.
  - Severe cases may require short courses of "soft" steroids.

SPECIAL CONSIDERATIONS

- Patients being treated with topical steroid drops should have close ophthalmology monitoring to watch for increased intraocular pressure, corneal ulcers, and cataracts.
- The most important aspects of treating ocular allergic disease are careful history taking and making a differential diagnosis.

REFERRAL

- Allergy/immunology evaluation to confirm or exclude IgE-mediated disease
- Ophthalmology should evaluate any patient requiring topical steroids.

REFERENCES

1. Berdy GJ, Berdy SS. Ocular allergic disorders: disease entities and differential diagnoses. *Curr Allergy Asthma Rep.* 2009;9:297–303.
2. Leonardi A, Castegnaro A, Valerio AL, et al. Epidemiology of allergic conjunctivitis: clinical appearance and treatment patterns in a population-based study. *Curr Opin Allergy Clin Immunol.* 2015;15(5):482–8.
3. Ono SJ, Abelson MB. Allergic conjunctivitis: update on pathophysiology and prospects for future treatment. *J Allergy Clin Immunol.* 2005;115:118–22.
4. Bielory L. Differential diagnoses of conjunctivitis for clinical allergist immunologists. *Ann Allergy Asthma Immunol.* 2007;98:105–15.
5. Berdy GJ, Spangler DL, Bensch G, et al. A comparison of the relative efficacy and clinical performance of olopatadine hydrochloride 0.1% ophthalmic solution and ketotifen fumarate 0.025% ophthalmic solution in the conjunctival antigen challenge model. *Clin Ther.* 2000;22:826–33.
6. Vichyanond P, Pacharm P, Pleyer U, et al. Vernal keratoconjunctivitis: a severe allergic eye disease with remodeling changes. *Pediatr Allergy Immunol.* 2014;25(4):314–22.
7. Li J, Luo X, Ke H, et al. Recalcitrant atopic keratoconjunctivitis in children: a case report and literature review. *Pediatrics.* 2018;141(suppl 5):S470–4.

Allergen Immunotherapy

Christopher J. Rigell and Jeffrey R. Stokes

11

GENERAL PRINCIPLES

- Noon and Freeman established allergen immunotherapy (AIT) >100 years ago when they treated grass pollen allergic patients with pollen extracts.[1,2]
- AIT is the only therapy that has a disease-modifying effect on allergic disease.[3-5]
- AIT is used in the treatment of allergic rhinitis, allergic conjunctivitis, allergic asthma, stinging insect hypersensitivity, and atopic dermatitis if associated with aeroallergen sensitivity.[6]

Definition

- AIT consists of administering increasing doses of allergen extract to patients with IgE-mediated conditions to alleviate symptoms associated with the specific allergens.[6]
- SC immunotherapy (SCIT) consists of SC injections that build up to an effective maintenance dose.
- Sublingual immunotherapy (SLIT) consists of daily tablets or liquid placed under the tongue.

Mechanism

- The mechanism of action of AIT is complex and not yet completely understood.
- Allergic disease that is targeted by immunotherapy involves IgE-based reactions under the influence of a subset of T lymphocytes (T_H2).
- One current paradigm is that high-dose allergen exposure results in suppression of T_H2 immunity through induction of regulatory T cells (Tregs), leading to immune deviation from T_H2 to T_H1, or deletion or anergy of antigen-specific T cells.[7,8]
- Studies have shown that AIT leads to
  - Transient increase in specific IgE followed by blunting of the usual seasonal rise with prolonged treatment
  - 10- to 100-fold increase in IgG (specifically IgG4 and IgG1) as well as increases in serum IgA
  - IgG4 may compete with IgE for allergen, preventing cross-linking of high-affinity IgE receptors on basophils and mast cells.
  - IgG4 also blocks binding of allergen–IgE complexes to low-affinity IgE receptor (Fcε RII) on B cells, downregulating T_H2 responses.
  - Downregulation of the cellular and inflammatory mediators of allergic response
  - Decrease in platelet-activating factor and histamine-releasing factor levels
  - Decrease in number of mast cells, basophils, and eosinophils in secretions
  - Increase in natural Tregs (nTregs) expressing FOXP3 and CD25
  - Increase in inducible Tregs (iTregs) that produce interleukin (IL)-10, IL-35, and transforming growth factor (TGF)-β.
  - Increase in regulatory B cells that also produce IL-10, IL-35, and TGF-β
  - Upregulation of the counterregulatory cytokines expressed by T_H1 phenotype

TREATMENT

Subcutaneous Immunotherapy

Indications
- SCIT is indicated for allergic rhinitis/conjunctivitis, allergic reactions to stinging insects, allergic asthma, and atopic dermatitis resulting from sensitivity to aeroallergens.
- It is **not indicated for food or drug allergy, urticaria, or angioedema.**[6]
- Prior to initiating, patients should have
  - Clinical signs and symptoms based on history and physical examination
  - Evidence of IgE sensitization preferably by epicutaneous skin testing. In vitro testing with specific allergen IgE is an alternative.
- **Allergic rhinitis/allergic conjunctivitis**: Reasons for initiating AIT in allergic rhinitis[9]
  - To prevent symptoms and improve quality of life
  - To reduce ongoing expenses for symptomatic medications
  - To reduce side effects of antihistamines and decongestants
  - To reduce development/aggravation of allergic asthma
  - To reduce comorbidity due to recurrent sinusitis/otitis
  - To improve the limited efficacy of allergen avoidance
  - Potentially preventing the development of allergic asthma[10]
  - Potentially preventing the development of new aeroallergen sensitizations[10]
- **Allergic asthma**: In the past, the role of AIT in allergic asthma had been controversial, but two large meta-analyses confirmed the effectiveness of AIT in treating mild-to-moderate allergic asthma compared to placebo.[11,12]
  - These studies demonstrated that patients treated with AIT had reductions in allergen-specific bronchial hyperresponsiveness, medication requirements, and overall symptoms.
  - Therefore, AIT has been endorsed by the World Health Organization (WHO) for the treatment of mild-to-moderate allergic asthma.[9]
- **Hymenoptera and fire ant allergy**
  - Effectiveness of immunotherapy for venom hypersensitivity has been well established.[13,14]
  - Venom immunotherapy (VIT) is indicated for patients with a history of systemic reactions from venom.[15] VIT is usually not required for patients who have experienced only cutaneous systemic reactions after an insect sting, whereas patients >16 years old with large local reactions can receive VIT when considering high-risk factors and quality-of-life concerns.[16]
- **Atopic dermatitis**
  - Has been controversial as to whether AIT is helpful, but studies have demonstrated improvement in patients when there is sensitization to house dust mites, grass, and tree pollen[17,18]
  - AIT has shown improvement in atopic dermatitis symptoms and in quality of life.[17,18]

Relative Contraindications
- **AIT should not be initiated in allergic asthma patients whose asthma is unstable or poorly controlled.** The risk of fatal or near-fatal events is much higher in this group.[19]
- Patients receiving β-blockers may be at increased risk for severe systemic reactions that may be resistant to epinephrine administration. Although most evidence demonstrates treatment with a **β-blocker** does not cause more anaphylaxis, it is a relative contraindication for receiving AIT to inhalant allergens, but not for VIT. When feasible, β-blocker should be substituted with an alternative.[20]

- There are conflicting data regarding whether **angiotensin-converting enzyme (ACE) inhibitors** lead to more severe anaphylaxis. In theory, the renin–angiotensin system (RAS) is part of the compensatory physiologic response to anaphylaxis.[20] It is a possibility that those on ACE inhibitors have a higher risk of VIT failure and that substitution should be considered before initiating VIT.[16]
- Tryptase levels should be measured in all patients before initiating VIT. **A higher baseline tryptase correlates with an increased risk of systemic reactions.**[16,21]
- Serious immunodeficiency (i.e., AIDS), active malignancy or autoimmune disease, significant cardiovascular disease, or the inability to communicate clearly, such as very young children, are all contraindications.[20]
- Patients with a fever, asthmatics with an upper respiratory infection (URI), patients with wheezing, or patients with significantly reduced pulmonary function tests (peak expiratory flow rate [PEFR] <70% of predicted) should wait for resolution of these symptoms to receive scheduled AIT.
- Strenuous exercise should be avoided immediately after an injection.
- Women who become pregnant can continue their scheduled AIT at lower doses than normal, but AIT is not initiated in pregnant patients. This is due to the potential harmful effects of allergic reactions to AIT, not due to effectiveness.[6]

Dosing
- Standardized extracts (cat, dust mite, grasses, short ragweed, and Hymenoptera venoms) should be used when available.[9]
- Allergen SCIT needs to be individualized to the patient, and only clinically relevant allergens should be included.[6]
- When writing immunotherapy, consideration has to be given to cross-reactive allergens as well as potential degradation from mold and cockroach extracts that contain proteolytic enzymes.[6]
- The use of glycerin can help prevent degradation from proteolytic enzymes.[6]
- SCIT is traditionally given in two phases
  ○ Buildup: weekly injections starting at 1,000- to 10,000-fold less than maintenance dose and increasing until maintenance dose is achieved
  ○ Maintenance: final effective dose
- Vials are color coded: red = maintenance 1:1 (no dilution), yellow = 10-fold dilution, blue = 100-fold dilution, green = 1,000-fold dilution, silver = 10,000-fold dilution[6]
- Rush protocols (injections given daily) and cluster protocols (multiple injections/day) are alternative dosing regimens used to achieve maintenance dosing in a shorter period of time. Typically associated with increased reactions to build up doses
- Maintenance dosages for aeroallergens are usually given every 2–4 weeks.
- VIT may be given every 8–12 weeks.[16]
- Table 11-1 provides recommended maintenance doses set forth by the Joint Task Force for AIT practice parameters.[6]
- Allergen extract concentrations can be expressed as a weight per volume ratio (wt/vol), protein nitrogen unit (PNU) or, the biologically active measure, in allergen units (BAU).
- The goal is to attain the highest tolerated dose; usually 5–20 μg of the major allergen per 0.5 mL maintenance dose is required.
- **A physician needs to be immediately available with proper equipment on hand in case a severe reaction occurs.**
- When extracts are administered SC, the recommended injection site is the outer aspect of the upper arm between the deltoid and triceps muscles.
- Oral antihistamines and leukotriene antagonists may be given to reduce local reactions.
- The patient should be **observed for at least 20–30 minutes after each injection** because life-threatening anaphylactic reactions are rare after the initial 30 minutes.[9,22]

TABLE 11-1 PROBABLE EFFECTIVE DOSE RANGES

Allergenic extract	Labeled potency or concentration	Probably effective dose range	Range of estimated major allergen content in U.S.-licensed extracts
Dust mites: *Dermatophagoides pteronyssinus* and *Dermatophagoides farinae*	3,000, 5,000, 10,000, and 30,000 AU/mL	500–2,000 AU	10,000 AU/mL
Cat hair	5,000 and 10,000 BAU/mL	1,000–4,000 BAU	10,000 BAU/mL 20–50 µg/mL Fel d 1 30–100 µg/mL cat albumin
Cat pelt	5,000–10,000 BAU/mL	1,000–4,000 BAU	10,000 BAU/mL 20–50 µg/mL Fel d 1 400–2,000 µg/mL cat albumin
Grass, standardized	100,000 BAU/mL	1,000–4,000 BAU	100,000 BAU/mL 425–1,100 µg/mL Phl p 5 506–2,346 µg/mL group 1
Bermuda	10,000 BAU/mL	300–1,500 BAU	10,000 BAU/mL 141–422 Cyn d 1 425–1,100 µg/mL
Short ragweed	1:10, 1:20 wt/vol, 100,000 AU/mL	6–12 µg of Amb a 1 or 1,000–4,000 AU	1:10 wt/vol 300 µg/mL Amb a 1

(continued)

TABLE 11-1 PROBABLE EFFECTIVE DOSE RANGES (*continued*)

Allergenic extract	Labeled potency or concentration	Probably effective dose range	Range of estimated major allergen content in U.S.-licensed extracts
Nonstandardized acetone precipitated (AP) dog	1:100 wt/vol	15 µg Can f 1	80–400 µg/mL Can f 1 10–20 µg/mL dog albumin
Nonstandardized extract: dog	1:10 and 1:20 wt/vol	15 µg Can f 1	0.5–10 µg/mL Can f 1 <12–1,500 µg/mL dog albumin
Nonstandardized extracts: pollen	1:10 to 1:40 wt/vol or 10,000–40,000 PNU/mL	0.5 mL of 1:100 or 1:200 wt/vol	NA
Nonstandardized extracts: mold/fungi, cockroach	1:10 to 1:40 wt/vol or 10,000–40,000 PNU/mL	Highest tolerated dose	NA
Hymenoptera venom	100 µg/mL single venom, 300 µg/mL in mixed vespid extract	50–200 µg of each venom	100–300 µg/mL of venom protein
Imported fire ant	1:10 to 1:20 wt/vol whole-body extract	0.5 mL of a 1:100 wt/vol to 0.5 mL of a 1:10 wt/vol extract	NA

AU, allergy unit; BAU, bioequivalent allergy unit; NA, not applicable; PNU, protein nitrogen unit.

Based on a maintenance injection of 0.5 mL.

Reprinted with permission from: Cox L, Nelson H, Lockey R, et al. Allergen immunotherapy: a practice parameter third update. *J Allergy Clin Immunol.* 2011;127(suppl):S1–55.

Duration of Treatment
- Clinical improvement is usually observed within 6–12 months after reaching maintenance dosing. If clinical benefit is not apparent at this point, consideration for discontinuing AIT should be given.
- Therapy is generally given for 3–5 years; however, the actual length of time for treatment is unclear, and the decision to continue or stop should be individualized.
- The recommendation of 3–5 years duration is based on data from venom hypersensitivity and only one study of a single seasonal allergen (grass); clearly, further studies need to be performed.[23]
- There are no markers to distinguish who will remain in remission and who will worsen after discontinuation of SCIT to inhalant allergens.
- Some patients experience return of symptoms within 1–2 years after cessation of AIT; if desired, it may be restarted, but needs to be incrementally increased to the maintenance dose.
- For VIT, an elevated baseline tryptase level, history of a severe reaction to a sting or VIT, honeybee venom allergy, and treatment duration <5 years are associated with a higher risk of relapse.[16]

Side Effects and Risks
- **Local reactions to AIT are common.**
  - Significant local reactions are identified as erythema, pruritus, and swelling, with wheal >2 cm in diameter or wheal lasting >24 hours.
  - Local reactions should be treated with cold compresses and topical corticosteroids.
  - Premedication with antihistamines may help reduce local reactions.
  - Large local reactions do not seem to predict systemic reactions.[6]
  - Montelukast may reduce local reactions in VIT.
- **Systemic reactions and anaphylaxis are rare but can occur.**
  - A physician needs to be available to treat potentially serious reactions to AIT.[9]
  - Contributing factors to severe systemic reactions include dosing errors, symptomatic asthma, β-blocker use, the first injection from new vials, or injections when symptoms are active during the allergy season.
  - Historically, fatalities were estimated to occur in 1 out of every 2.5 million injections (3.4 events/year).[19] According to the American Academy of Allergy, Asthma & Immunology (AAAAI)/American College of Allergy, Asthma & Immunology (ACAAI) surveillance study, there were 3 fatalities out of 54.4 million injections (1 per 18 million injections) from 2008 to 2016.[24,25]
  - Signs/symptoms of systemic reaction include one or more of the following: generalized erythema and/or urticaria, pruritus, angioedema, sneezing, nasal congestion, oropharyngeal pruritus, bronchospasm, laryngeal edema, and shock/cardiac arrest.
  - **Systemic/anaphylaxis reactions should be treated with IM aqueous epinephrine (0.3–0.5 mL of 1:1,000) every 5 minutes PRN** (see Chapter 4).
  - To limit systemic absorption of the antigen, a tourniquet should be placed above the injection site and released every 15 minutes.
  - Proper emergency resuscitation protocol should be followed to ensure patent airway and maintenance of adequate blood pressure.
  - If patient is on a β-blocker, IV glucagon 1–5 mg can be used for refractory hypotension.[6]
  - Antihistamines are used as adjunctive therapy with cetirizine or diphenhydramine most commonly used.
  - IV hydrocortisone (5 mg/kg) is another adjunctive agent; however, **corticosteroids have limited effect on the immediate response**. Additional data suggest that corticosteroids may not be effective in preventing late phase (biphasic) anaphylaxis.[26]

Efficacy
- VIT reduces large local reactions to stings, and 80–98% individuals will be protected from systemic reactions with subsequent stings.[13]
- The clinical efficacy of SCIT in allergic rhinitis has been well documented, and AIT has been shown to improve symptoms, reduce medications, and provide long-term benefits even after cessation of therapy.[23,27,28]
- Allergen-specific SCIT has the potential to alter the natural course of allergic disease.[3-5]
- SCIT improves asthma symptoms, decreases use of asthma medications, and reduces bronchial hyperreactivity.[29]
- Long-term benefits >12 years after discontinuation of therapy in patients with allergic rhinitis have been documented.[4,5]
- When comparing the cost of immunotherapy to the savings from the decrease in medications, outpatient and inpatient visits, immunotherapy is cost-effective.

Potential Reasons for Failure of Immunotherapy
- Environmental modifications to control allergens are inadequate or insufficient.
- Significant or contributing allergen not recognized and omitted in AIT regimen
- Inadequate doses of major allergen in preparation (normally need 5–20 μg of the major allergen to be successful)
- Poor quality of extracts
- Inability to achieve optimal dosing
- New allergies develop during treatment course.
- Exposure to nonallergen triggers like cigarette smoke
- Original causative allergen is misdiagnosed.

Sublingual Immunotherapy

Worldwide, SLIT is administered as either a liquid formulation or tablet. In the United States, only the tablets are Food and Drug Administration (FDA) approved.

FDA-Approved Extracts
- Oralair = five grass combination (sweet vernal, orchard, perennial, rye, timothy, Kentucky blue)
- Grastek = timothy grass
- Ragwitek = short ragweed
- Odactra = house dust mite allergen

Indications
- Allergic rhinitis and allergic conjunctivitis[30,31]
- Can be used for add-on therapy for allergic asthma[32,33]
- Similar to SCIT, studies have shown benefit for atopic dermatitis, but this indication is not FDA approved.[34]

Contraindications
- Contraindications include eosinophilic esophagitis, severe or uncontrolled asthma, severe systemic reaction to SLIT or SCIT, and severe local reaction to SLIT[30,31]
- SLIT should be used with caution in pregnancy and breastfeeding.
  - Ragwitek is category C.
  - Oralair and Grastek are category B.
  - Odactra does not have sufficient data to inform associated risks in pregnancy.

Efficacy
- Improvement is seen within 1 year of treatment.
- Duration of therapy seems to be at least 3 years.[35]

- Effective doses, which include amount of major allergen in the tablet:
  - Single grass tablet: 2,800 BAU daily, which has 15 μg Phl p 5.[36]
  - 5-Grass tablet: 300 IR daily, which has 25 μg group 5 major allergens from five grasses[37]
  - Ragweed tablet: 12 Amb a 1-U daily, which has 12 μg Amb a 1[38]
  - House dust mite tablet: 12 SQ-HDM daily, which has 15 μg Der p 1 and Der f 1, 15 μg Der p 2 and Der f 2[39]
- One study has shown that for patients who need treatment with grass and weed extracts, overlapping treatment was tolerated.[40]
- It remains to be seen if adequate doses can be achieved with more than two extracts delivered at the same time.

Safety and Side Effects
- Common side effects include pruritus (oral, ear, tongue), sore throat, and mouth edema. Most common during the first week of treatment
- Oral H1 and H2 antihistamines can help with mild symptoms.
- Systemic allergic reactions are rare: symptoms include rhinitis, asthma, urticarial, angioedema, and/or hypotension. IM epinephrine is the treatment.

Dosing and Practical Considerations
- Pollen extract tablets should be started 12–16 weeks prior to the relevant season.
- The first dose should be given in a physician's office, and the patient should be observed for 30 minutes.
- The tablet is placed under the tongue for at least 1 minute until it dissolves. Afterward, the patient must ensure to wash their hands and to avoid eating or drinking for 5 minutes.
- Adherence is poor but can be improved with 3-month follow-up and repeat prescriptions.
- The single grass tablet, ragweed tablet, and house dust mite tablet do not require buildup.
- The 5-grass tablet has a buildup for ages 10–17 years, with 100 IR on day 1, 200 IR on day 2, 300 IR on day 3 and beyond.
- When to hold dose: increased asthma symptoms in the last 24 hours, worsening dysphagia or gastroesophageal reflux disease (GERD), recent oral surgery/dental work or oral lesions, increased viral URI symptoms, any episode of urticaria or angioedema, and fever[31]
- If patient misses one dose, do not double dose the next day. If >1 day is missed, it is recommended that the patients call their physician.[31]
- The duration of missing doses has not been extensively studied, but if it has been <7 days, then there is no dose reduction; if it has been between 7 and 14 days, the patient should restart at day 1; if it has been >14 days, then the patient should return to clinic to restart at day 1.
- Although severe systemic reactions are rare and there are no known fatalities associated with SLIT, all patients should be prescribed epinephrine to have with them.[31]

Sublingual Immunotherapy vs. Subcutaneous Immunotherapy
- SLIT was approved in Europe based on two trials that separately demonstrated SCIT and SLIT led to similar symptom improvement in patients with severe grass pollen seasonal allergic rhinitis.[41,42]
- SCIT vs. SLIT is not well studied because there is significant heterogeneity in the studies.[43]
- Few direct head to head trials: Two demonstrated more improvement with SCIT that was not statistically significant, and one showed equal effect.[44-46]
- Indirect evidence suggests SLIT is safer than SCIT, whereas SCIT seems more effective.
- SLIT requires larger doses of allergen compared to SCIT.
- More studies are required assessing the safety and efficacy of taking multiple tablets in patients who are polysensitized, thus limiting the role of SLIT.

PATIENT EDUCATION

- Patients should be educated regarding the possible signs and symptoms of systemic reactions.
- Before AIT is started, patients should be educated about the benefits and risks of AIT, as well as the methods for minimizing risks.
- Realistic outcomes from AIT should also be discussed with patients.

MONITORING/FOLLOW-UP

Patients should be seen for a follow-up visit with the physician at least every 6–12 months. More frequent visits may be needed depending on response to therapy, adverse reactions, modifications in dosage needed, or alteration in underlying allergic diseases.

REFERENCES

1. Noon L. Prophylactic inoculation against hay fever. *Lancet.* 1911;1:1572–3.
2. Freeman J. Further observations of the treatment of hay fever by hypodermic inoculations of pollen vaccine. *Lancet.* 1911;2:814–7.
3. Bousquet J, Demoly P, Michel FB. Specific immunotherapy in rhinitis and asthma. *Ann Allergy Asthma Immunol.* 2001;87:38–42.
4. Eng PA, Borer-Reinhold M, Heijnen IA, et al. Twelve-year follow-up after discontinuation of preseasonal grass pollen immunotherapy in childhood. *Allergy.* 2006;61:198–201.
5. Jacobsen L, Niggemann B, Dreborg S, et al. Specific immunotherapy has long-term preventive effect of seasonal and perennial asthma: 10-year follow-up on the PAT study. *Allergy.* 2007;62:943–8.
6. Cox L, Nelson H, Lockey R, et al. Allergen immunotherapy: a practice parameter third update. *J Allergy Clin Immunol.* 2011;127(suppl):S1–55.
7. Shamji MH, Durham SR. Mechanisms of allergen immunotherapy for inhaled allergens and predictive biomarkers. *J Allergy Clin Immunol.* 2017;140:1485–98.
8. Zhang W, Lin C, Sampath V, et al. Impact of allergen immunotherapy in allergic asthma. *Immunotherapy.* 2018;10:579–93.
9. Theodoropoulos DS, Lockey RF. Allergen immunotherapy: guidelines, update, and recommendations of the World Health Organization. *Allergy Asthma Proc.* 2000;21:159–66.
10. Moller C, Dreborg S, Ferdousi HA, et al. Pollen immunotherapy reduces the development of asthma in children with seasonal rhinoconjunctivitis (the PAT-Study). *J Allergy Clin Immunol.* 2002;109:251–6.
11. Abramson M, Puy R, Weiner J. Immunotherapy in asthma: an updated systematic review. *Allergy.* 1999;54:1022–41.
12. Abramson MJ, Puy RM, Weiner JM. Is allergen immunotherapy effective in asthma? A meta-analysis of randomized controlled trials. *Am J Respir Crit Care Med.* 1995;151:969–74.
13. Golden DB, Kagey-Sobotka A, Normal PS, et al. Outcomes of allergy to insect stings in children, with and without venom immunotherapy. *N Engl J Med.* 2004;351:668–74.
14. Golden DB, Kelly D, Hamilton RG, et al. Venom immunotherapy reduces large local reactions to insect stings. *J Allergy Clin Immunol.* 2009;123:1371–5.
15. Hunt KJ, Valentine MD, Sobotka AK, et al. A controlled trial of immunotherapy in insect hypersensitivity. *N Engl J Med.* 1978;299:157–61.
16. Golden DB, Demain J, Freeman T, et al. Stinging insect hypersensitivity: a practice parameter update 2016. *Ann Allergy Asthma Immunol.* 2017;118:28–54.
17. Nahm DH, Kim ME, Kwon B, et al. Clinical efficacy of subcutaneous allergen immunotherapy in patients with atopic dermatitis. *Yonsei Med J.* 2016;57:1420–6.
18. Slavyanakaya TA, Derkach VV, Sepiashvili RI. Debates in allergy medicine: specific immunotherapy efficiency in children with atopic dermatitis. *World Allergy Organ J.* 2016;9:15.
19. Bernstein DI, Wanner M, Borish L, et al. Twelve-year survey of fatal reactions to allergen injections and skin testing: 1990–2001. *J Allergy Clin Immunol.* 2004;113:1129–36.
20. Pitsios C, Demoly P, Bilo MB, et al. Clinical contraindications to allergen immunotherapy: an EAACI position paper. *Allergy.* 2015;70:897–909.

21. Rueff F, Przybilla B, Bilo MB, et al. Predictors of side effects during the buildup phase of venom immunotherapy for hymenoptera venom allergy: the importance of baseline serum tryptase. *J Allergy Clin Immunol.* 2010;126:105–11.

22. Lockey RF, Nicoara-Kasti GL, Theodoropoulos DS, et al. Systemic reactions and fatalities associated with allergen immunotherapy. *Ann Allergy Asthma Immunol.* 2001;87(suppl 1):47–55.

23. Durham SR, Walker SM, Varga EM, et al. Long-term clinical efficacy of grass-pollen immunotherapy. *N Engl J Med.* 1999;341:468–75.

24. Epstein TG, Liss GM, Murphy-Berendts K, et al. AAAAI/ACAAI surveillance study of subcutaneous immunotherapy, years 2008–2012: an update on fatal and nonfatal systemic allergic reactions. *J Allergy Clin Immunol Pract.* 2014;2:161–7.

25. Epstein TG, Liss GM, Murphy-Berendts K, et al. Recent trends in fatalities, waiting times, and use of epinephrine auto-injectors for subcutaneous allergen immunotherapy (SCIT): AAAAI/ACAAI national surveillance study 2008–2016. *J Allergy Clin Immunol.* 2018;141(suppl 2):AB401.

26. Shaker MS, Wallace DV, Golden DBK, et al. Anaphylaxis-a 2020 practice parameter update, systematic review, and Grading of Recommendations, Assessment, Development and Evaluation (GRADE) analysis. *J Allergy Clin Immunol.* 2020;145:1082–123.

27. Lowell FC, Franklin WF, Williams M. A double-blind study of the effectiveness and specificity of injection therapy in ragweed hay fever. *N Engl J Med.* 1965;273:675–9.

28. Varney VA, Gaga M, Frew AJ, et al. Usefulness of immunotherapy in patients with severe summer hay fever uncontrolled by antiallergic drugs. *BMJ.* 1991;302:265–9.

29. Abramson MJ, Puy RM, Weiner JM. Injection allergen immunotherapy for asthma. *Cochrane Database Syst Rev.* 2010;(8):CD001186.

30. Greenhawt M, Oppenheimer J, Nelson M, et al. Sublingual immunotherapy: a focused allergen immunotherapy practice parameter update. *Ann Allergy Asthma Immunol.* 2017;118:276–82

31. Epstein TG, Calabria C, Cox LS, et al. Current evidence on safety and practical considerations for administration of sublingual allergen immunotherapy (SLIT) in the United States. *J Allergy Clin Immunol Pract.* 2017;5:34–40

32. Mosbech H, Deckelmann R, de Blay F, et al. Standardized quality (SQ) house dust mite sublingual immunotherapy tablet (ALK) reduces inhaled corticosteroid use while maintaining asthma control: a randomized, double-blind, placebo-controlled trial. *J Allergy Clin Immunol.* 2014;134:568–75.

33. Virchow JC, Backer V, Kuna P, et al. Efficacy of a house dust mite sublingual allergen immunotherapy tablet in adults with allergic asthma: a randomized clinical trial. *JAMA.* 2016;315:1715–25.

34. You HS, Yang MY, Kim GW, et al. Effectiveness of specific sublingual immunotherapy in Korean patients with atopic dermatitis. *Ann Dermatol.* 2017;29:1–5.

35. Didier A, Malling HJ, Worm M, et al. Post-treatment efficacy of discontinuous treatment with 300IR 5-grass pollen sublingual tablet in adults with grass pollen-induced allergic rhinoconjunctivitis. *Clin Exp Allergy.* 2013;43:568–77.

36. Durham SR, Yang WH, Pedersen MR, et al. Sublingual immunotherapy with once-daily grass allergen tablets: a randomized controlled trial in seasonal allergic rhinoconjunctivitis. *J Allergy Clin Immunol* 2006;117:802–9.

37. Didier A, Malling HJ, Worm M, et al. Optimal dose, efficacy, and safety of once-daily sublingual immunotherapy with a 5-grass pollen tablet for seasonal allergic rhinitis. *J Allergy Clin Immunol.* 2007;120:1338–45.

38. Nolte H, Hebert J, Berman G, et al. Randomized controlled trial of ragweed allergy immunotherapy tablet efficacy and safety in North American adults. *Ann Allergy Asthma Immunol.* 2013;110:450–6.

39. Nolte H, Bernstein DI, Nelson HS, et al. Efficacy of house dust mite sublingual immunotherapy tablet in North American adolescents and adults in a randomized, placebo-controlled trial. *J Allergy Clin Immunol.* 2016;138:1631–8.

40. Maloney J, Berman G, Gagnon R, et al. Sequential treatment initiation with timothy grass and ragweed sublingual immunotherapy tablets followed by simultaneous treatment is well tolerated. *J Allergy Clin Immunol Pract.* 2016;4:301–9.

41. Dahl R, Kapp A, Colombo G, et al. Efficacy and safety of sublingual immunotherapy with grass allergen tablets for seasonal allergic rhinoconjunctivitis. *J Allergy Clin Immunol.* 2006;118:434–40.

42. Frew AJ, Powell RJ, Corrigan CJ, et al. Efficacy and safety of specific immunotherapy with SQ allergen extract in treatment-resistant seasonal allergic rhinoconjunctivitis. *J Allergy Clin Immunol.* 2006;117:319–25.

43. Durham SR, Penagos M. Sublingual or subcutaneous immunotherapy for allergic rhinitis? *J Allergy Clin Immunol.* 2016;137:339–49.

44. Khinchi MS, Poulsen LK, Carat F, et al. Clinical efficacy of sublingual and subcutaneous birch pollen allergen-specific immunotherapy: a randomized, placebo-controlled, double-blind, double-dummy study. *Allergy.* 2004;59:45–53.

45. Quirino T, Iemoli E, Siciliani E, et al. Sublingual versus injective immunotherapy in grass pollen allergic patients: a double blind (double dummy) study. *Clin Exp Allergy.* 1996;26:1253–61.

46. Ventura MT, Carretta A, Tummolo RA, et al. Clinical data and inflammation parameters in patients with cypress allergy treated with sublingual swallow therapy and subcutaneous immunotherapy. *Int J Immunopathol Pharmacol.* 2009;22:403–13.

Urticaria and Angioedema   12

Jeffrey A. Kepes and Maya Jerath

GENERAL PRINCIPLES

- Urticaria and angioedema are common conditions with heterogeneous origins.
- A detailed history and physical examination are the most important factors in determining the etiology.
- Urticaria and angioedema are a spectrum disorder that can occur concurrently or independently of each other.
- Urticaria is mediated by mast cell degranulation.
- Angioedema can be **mast cell mediated** (histaminergic) or **bradykinin mediated.**
- Urticaria is defined as a raised, round area of edema (wheal) surrounded by reflex erythema (flare) that involves only the superficial dermis of the skin.
- The lesions are usually pruritic and may develop rapidly. Any single lesion does not ordinarily last >24 hours.
- Urticaria is defined as **acute** if the episode lasts <6 weeks and **chronic** if it goes on for longer.[1]
- Angioedema extends into the deep dermis or subcutaneous tissue and often affects areas of loose connective tissue, such as the face.
- Angioedema may be uncomfortable or painful rather than pruritic, especially when the viscera are involved.
- Angioedema involving a patient's larynx can threaten the airway and lead to asphyxiation.
- Resolution is slower for angioedema and can take up to 72 hours.

MAST CELL–MEDIATED URTICARIA AND ANGIOEDEMA

- Mediated by **histamine and cytokine release** by mast cell degranulation in tissues
- The mechanism of mast cell degranulation can be allergic or nonallergic in nature.
- Urticaria is often a symptom of another allergic disorder such as anaphylaxis or food allergy, in which case it is generally considered a secondary diagnosis.
- Most cases of isolated urticaria are mild and self-limited.
- Chronic spontaneous urticaria (CSU) is nonallergic and often idiopathic.

Epidemiology

- Between 15 and 24% of the U.S. population will experience acute urticaria or angioedema at some time in their life.[1]
- CSU is common, affecting about 3% of the population with an economic and social burden comparable to that seen with severe coronary artery disease.[2] The syndrome lasts an average of 3–5 years, with 20% of patients still symptomatic at 20 years after diagnosis.[3]

- Angioedema occurs in approximately 50% of cases of chronic urticaria, whereas about 10% of individuals experience angioedema alone.[4]
- Chronic urticaria is more common in adults and women.

Allergic Urticaria and Angioedema

Etiology
- Food: Peanuts, tree nuts, and shellfish are the most common causes in adults.
- Drugs
  ○ The most common drugs causing urticaria are antibiotics and opiate analgesics.
  ○ Penicillin and cephalosporins cause IgE-mediated allergic reactions.
  ○ Platinum-based chemotherapy (e.g., oxaliplatin) and monoclonal antibodies can cause IgE-mediated reactions.
  ○ Nonsteroidal anti-inflammatory drugs (NSAIDs) are the most common cause of non–IgE-mediated ("pseudoallergic") reactions.
- Latex
- Stinging insects
- Aeroallergens

Diagnosis
- Skin testing can identify a potential allergic trigger.
  ○ Contraindications include the presence of wheezing, poorly controlled asthma, and a history of severe reactions to skin testing.
  ○ Dermatographism can make skin testing uninterpretable.
- Allergen-specific IgE (blood testing) can be used in patients unable to undergo skin prick testing.
- **No routine laboratory tests are indicated for most patients**.

Treatment
- Therapy is focused on avoiding triggers.
- In the event of an exposure to allergen with reaction, therapy is aimed at mitigating the effects of mast cell degranulation by blocking histamine with fast-acting agents such as cetirizine.
- Urticaria that progresses to anaphylaxis is treated with epinephrine.
- Steroids may be used to potentially help prevent a late-phase reoccurrence of symptoms.

Nonallergic Urticaria and Angioedema

- Sometimes has an underlying etiology/association
  ○ Postviral urticaria
  ○ Autoimmune (e.g., related to an antibody directed against the IgE receptor [FcεRI] on the mast cell)
  ○ Hypo- or hyperthyroidism, including Graves' disease or Hashimoto thyroiditis
- Chronic or undiagnosed infections
- Malignancy
- CSU is a diagnosis of exclusion if no etiology is found.
  ○ Can be associated with significant morbidity
  ○ Patients with CSU are more prone to physical urticaria in addition to spontaneous lesions.

Physical Urticarias
- **Cold urticaria**
  ○ Seen in cold, exposed areas of the skin
  ○ Fatalities have been reported from hypotension occurring while swimming in cold water.

- Secondary acquired cold urticaria is related to cryoglobulins resulting from systemic disease (hepatitis B or C) or lymphoreticular malignancy.
- **Cholinergic urticaria**
  - Related to elevated core temperature from exercise, a hot shower, or emotional stress
  - Lesions are typically tiny and diffuse.
  - Occurs in approximately 15% of the population
  - Severe forms may progress to anaphylaxis although lesions usually resolve with normalization of body temperature.
- **Dermatographism**
  - Literally means "skin writing" and is another common form of physical urticaria
  - Affects approximately 4% of the population
  - Can be elicited on examination by briskly stroking skin with tongue blade or fingernail
  - May confound ability to read allergen skin tests
  - Lesions are transitory and respond to suppression with antihistamines.
- **Delayed pressure urticaria/angioedema**
  - Unlike other physical urticarias, lesions appear 4–6 hours after the stimulus of pressure.
  - Mediators are thought to be similar to late-phase reactants rather than histamine.
  - Poorly responsive to antihistamines; systemic steroids may be needed to control severely afflicted patients.
- **Exercise-induced urticaria**
  - Different from cholinergic urticaria in that it is not related to core body temperature.
  - Lesions are typically urticarial and can progress to anaphylaxis.
  - In some patients, the ingestion of a specific food before exercise is necessary (e.g., celery) to trigger the reaction, although eating before exercise in general will worsen symptoms in most patients.[1]

Urticarial Vasculitis
- A form of vasculitis that affects the skin and presents with urticaria.
- Examination usually reveals large lesions and ecchymoses at sites of resolved ones.
- Other signs of vasculitis, such as petechiae and palpable purpura, are often evident.
- Lesions tend to last >**24 hours** and be more painful than pruritic.
- A punch biopsy is necessary to make the diagnosis and will show **leukocytoclastic vasculitis**.
- Management is similar to that of CSU, but the condition may evolve into a hypocomplementemic form, which is on the spectrum with lupus.

Diagnosis
- As stated earlier, conducting a **thorough history** and review of systems is key.
- In addition, some testing may be selected to help rule out underlying associated conditions based on the history or review of systems, such as:
  - Complete blood count with differential
  - Complete metabolic panel
  - Thyroid-stimulating hormone (TSH) and free thyroxine (FT4) to evaluate thyroid function
  - Erythrocyte sedimentation rate (ESR) and C-reactive protein (CRP) to evaluate systemic inflammation
  - Chest X-ray to evaluate for potential infection or malignancy (e.g., non-Hodgkin lymphoma)
  - Antinuclear antibody (ANA) to screen for autoimmune disorders
  - Autologous serum skin testing and chronic urticaria index/anti-FcεRI antibody are tests that can be used to demonstrate the presence of autoantibodies that may be the cause of chronic urticaria.

Treatment

- If a cause is identified, treatment of the underlying malignancy and autoimmune or thyroid disorder can help ameliorate symptoms.
- Pharmacologic therapy as recommended by the 2014 Practice Parameters published by the American Academy of Allergy, Asthma and Immunology (AAAAI)[1]
  - Goal of therapy is to block end-effects of both histamine and leukotrienes.
  - Step 1: **Daily monotherapy with second-generation antihistamines**[1]
    - Cetirizine, loratadine, fexofenadine, levocetirizine, or desloratadine
    - About 44% of patients benefit from H1-antagonist monotherapy.
    - Daily monotherapy rather than as-needed dosing is more efficacious for reducing symptom burden.[5]
  - Step 2: **Increasing dose of H1-antihistamine, addition of a H2-anthistamine and/or a leukotriene receptor blocker**[1]
    - May increase H1-antihistamine dosing to up to fourfold Food and Drug Administration (FDA)-approved dose.
    - H2-antihistamines may have synergistic effect with H1-antihistamines, but data are conflicting.[6]
    - Potential benefit may be due to cytochrome P450 inhibition by many H2-antihistamines, yielding an increased serum levels of H1-antihistamines.[7]
    - Leukotriene antagonists like montelukast (Singulair®) have also been shown to be beneficial in combination with H1-anthistamines in some studies.[8]
  - Step 3: **Addition of a potent first-generation H1-antihistamine**
    - Doxepin or hydroxyzine
    - This step has been removed in the most recent 2018 World Allergy Organization guidelines.[9]
  - Step 4: **Addition of a biologic agent or immunomodulator**
    Omalizumab (Xolair®), a recombinant humanized monoclonal antibody that binds to free IgE and inhibits binding to high-affinity IgE receptors, is indicated in patients who fail to respond to high-dose H1-antihistamines.[1,10]
  - Other immunomodulators like **hydroxychloroquine**,[11] **cyclosporine**,[12] and **dapsone**[13] also have some benefit in patients resistant to antihistamine therapy.
  - Topical corticosteroids may have a role in patients with localized delayed pressure urticaria (DPU).[14]
  - NSAIDs can exacerbate urticaria in up to 30% of patients with chronic urticaria, and in these patients they should be avoided.[15,16]

BRADYKININ-MEDIATED ANGIOEDEMA

Angioedema occurs **without** urticaria.

Angiotensin-Converting Enzyme Inhibitor and Angiotensin II Receptor Blocker–Mediated Angioedema

Pathophysiology

- Vasodilation and increased vascular permeability because of angiotensin-converting enzyme inhibitor (ACEi)-induced inhibition of bradykinin degradation
- Angiotensin II receptor blocker (ARB) does not directly affect bradykinin metabolism and mechanism of induction of angioedema is not well understood.
  - Rate of angioedema with ARBs is significantly lower than with ACEi.
  - Risk of ARB-induced angioedema in patients who had angioedema on an ACEi is <1%.[17]
- Lesions are typically not pruritic and often involve the tongue and the airway.

Diagnosis
- Suggested by history of being on an ACEi or ARB. Implicated in 11% of angioedema without urticaria[18]
- No testing is available.

Treatment
- Discontinuation of ARB or ACEi.
- Monitoring of airway and, if necessary, prophylactic intubation until resolution of swelling.
- Epinephrine, antihistamines, and glucocorticoids have no therapeutic benefit.
- Patients may develop recurrent angioedema for up to 6 weeks after discontinuation of ACEi or ARB.

Hereditary Angioedema

Pathophysiology
- Hereditary angioedema (HAE) is caused by **lack of** (Type I) or **dysfunctional** (Type II) **C1 esterase inhibitor (C1-INH)**.
- Majority of patients possess an autosomal dominant mutation in the gene encoding C1-INH.
- Lack of C1-INH quantity or function results in accumulation of bradykinin, which is the main mediator responsible for the symptoms in HAE.

Epidemiology
- Incidence is roughly 1:30,000–1:80,000 without any significant differences in distribution based on race or sex.[1]
- Type I HAE accounts for 85% of cases, with type II HAE accounting for almost 15% of cases.[19]
- Autosomal dominant pattern of inheritance; however, 25% of patients have a *de novo* mutation of C1INH gene and so have no family history.[20]
- Type III HAE is very rare and the mechanism is unknown; it is believed to involve a mutation in factor XII in some patients.

Clinical Presentation
- Episodic swelling that peaks within 24 hours and resolves over 48–72 hours
- Usually presents within first two decades of life
- May be preceded by a prodromal rash (**erythema marginatum**) or localized tingling of the skin
- Episodes are never associated with urticaria.
- Characterized by periodic attacks of angioedema that are often, but not always, triggered by trauma (i.e., dental surgery) or stress
- **Frequently involves abdominal viscera; may involve extremities, face, oropharynx, and larynx**.
- When involving the viscera, HAE can present similarly to a small bowel obstruction.
- Laryngeal angioedema is a significant cause of mortality.

Diagnosis
- Often a **family history of angioedema**
- C4 (complement) level is a sensitive and inexpensive screening test and should be low.
- Other tests can be ordered to distinguish type of angioedema. See Table 12-1.
  - C1-INH level
  - C1-INH functional level
  - C1q level

TABLE 12-1	TESTING TO DISTINGUISH FORMS OF BRADYKININ-MEDIATED ANGIOEDEMA			
	C1-INH level	C1-INH function	C4	C1q level
Type I HAE	Low	Low	Low	Normal
Type II HAE	Normal or high	Low	Low	Normal
Type III HAE	Normal	Normal	Normal	Normal
Acquired angioedema	Low	Low	Low or normal	Low
ACEi/ARB-induced angioedema	Normal	Normal	Normal	Normal

ACEi, angiotensin-converting enzyme inhibitor; ARB, angiotensin II receptor blocker; C1-INH, C1 esterase inhibitor HAE, hereditary angioedema.

Treatment

- Acute management of HAE is directed at stabilizing the patient and reducing the extent of swelling.
  - Fluid resuscitation may be necessary due to third spacing.
  - Elective intubation may be necessary for laryngeal attacks.
  - Medications for acute HAE attacks:
    - **Human C1-INH** (Berinert®), which is a plasma-derived concentrate of C1-INH, is an FDA-approved treatment for acute abdominal or facial attacks of HAE.[21] Administered intravenously and may be done either at home by the patient or in a medical facility
    - **Recombinant C1 inhibitor** (Ruconest®) is a short half-life product collected from the milk of transgenic rabbits. Higher dosing is required than for human-derived products. Patients must be monitored for allergic reactions during administration, especially if they have known rabbit allergies.
    - Bradykinin B2-receptor antagonist **Icatibant** (Firazyr®) is a synthetic B2-receptor antagonist given by SC injection and can be administered by the patient at home. Dose can be repeated every 6 hours for a total of three doses.
    - **Ecallantide (Kalbitor®)** is a reversible inhibitor of plasma kallikrein that has been shown to be effective for acute attacks of swelling in HAE.[22] Should be administered in a medical facility as there is a significant risk of anaphylaxis (2–3%).
  - **Second-line therapy:** Fresh-frozen plasma (FFP) seeks to replace C1-INH; however, no controlled trials have been performed to assess efficacy.
  - Epinephrine has often been used for attacks, but there are no studies to support its efficacy and mechanistically it has no role.
  - The use of antihistamines and corticosteroids is of little value.
- Chronic prophylactic therapy seeks to prevent or lessen severity of angioedema attacks.
  - **Human C1-INH** (Cinryze®) is also approved to help prevent angioedema attacks in teenagers and adults with HAE.[23] It is administered intravenously twice weekly for prophylaxis.
  - **Recombinant C1 inhibitor** (Ruconest®) can also be given intravenously once or twice weekly for prophylaxis.
  - **Human monoclonal antibody IgG1/κ light chain** (Lanadelumab®) binds plasma kallikrein and inhibits proteolysis, preventing excess bradykinin accumulation. It can be given every 2–4 weeks for prophylaxis.

○ **Second-line agents**
  ▪ **Synthetic androgenic steroids** (danazol or stanozolol) increase the synthesis of C1 inhibitor and can prevent angioedema episodes. Despite having attenuated virilizing effects, these agents do have significant side effects and should not be used in pregnant women. Patients should also be monitored for hyperlipidemia, liver dysfunction, and hepatic neoplasms with routine liver function tests, lipid profiles, and abdominal ultrasounds every 6 months.
  ▪ **Fibrinolytic agents** (such as tranexamic acid or ε-aminocaproic acid) have also been shown to ameliorate symptoms. Unfortunately, this therapy also carries the risk of numerous side effects including retinal damage and increased risk of thromboembolic events.

Acquired Angioedema

- Unlike HAE, acquired angioedema (AAE) usually presents after the fourth decade of life and in patients **without a family history of angioedema.**
- Most commonly due to **autoantibodies** directed against C1-INH or other **inhibitors** of its function
- May also be due to inappropriate activation of the classical complement pathway leading to consumption of C1-INH

Etiology
- B-cell lymphoproliferative disease
- T-cell lymphoma
- Multiple myeloma
- Myelofibrosis
- Autoimmune disorders (systemic lupus erythematosus, cryoglobulinemia, and autoimmune hemolytic anemia)

Diagnosis
- Evaluation of C1-INH function and quantity
- Demonstration of activation of complement by reduced levels of C3, C4
- **Differentiated from HAE by decreased levels of C1q**
- After diagnosis is made, evaluation for an underlying cause should be undertaken.

Treatment
- **Treatment of underlying condition**
- Like in HAE, corticosteroids, epinephrine, and antihistamines have no therapeutic benefit.
- Ecallantide and icatibant have both been shown to be efficacious in acute attacks.
- Androgens and antifibrinolytics (tranexamic acid and ε-aminocaproic acid) may be more efficacious in AAE than in HAE, although they should be used with great caution.

REFERENCES

1. Bernstein J, Lang D, Khan D, et al. The diagnosis and management of acute and chronic urticaria: 2014 update. *J Allergy Clin Immunol.* 2014;133:1270–7.
2. Fox RW. Chronic urticaria and/or angioedema. *Clin Rev Allergy Immunol.* 2002;23:143–5.
3. Najib U, Sheikh J. An update on acute and chronic urticaria for the primary care provider. *Postgrad Med.* 2009;121:141–51.
4. O'Donnell BF, Lawlor F, Simpson J, et al. The impact of chronic urticaria on the quality of life. *Br J Dermatol.* 1997;136:197–201.

5. Grob JJ, Auquier P, Dreyfus I, et al. How to prescribe antihistamines for chronic idiopathic urticaria: desloratadine daily vs PRN and quality of life. *Allergy.* 2009;64:605–12.

6. Salo OP, Kauppinen K, Mannisto PT. Cimetidine increases the plasma concentration of hydroxyzine. *Acta Derm Venereol.* 1986;66:349–50.

7. Sharpe GR, Shuster S. In dermographic urticaria H2 receptor antagonists have a small but therapeutically irrelevant additional effect compared with H1 antagonists alone. *Br J Dermatol.* 1993;129:575–9.

8. Pacor ML, Di Lorenzo G, Corrocher R. Efficacy of leukotriene receptor antagonist in chronic urticaria. A double-blind, placebo-controlled comparison of treatment with montelukast and cetirizine in patients with chronic urticaria with intolerance to food additive and/or acetylsalicylic acid. *Clin Exp Allergy.* 2001;31:1607–14.

9. Zuberbier T, Aberer W, Asero R, et al. The EAACI/GA²LEN/EDF/WAO guideline for the definition, classification, diagnosis and management of urticaria. *Allergy.* 2018;73:1393–414.

10. Saini S, Rosen KE, Hsieh HJ, et al. A randomized, placebo-controlled, dose-ranging study of single-dose omalizumab in patients with H1-antihistamine-refractory chronic idiopathic urticaria. *J Allergy Clin Immunol.* 2011;128:567–73.

11. Reeves GE, Boyle MJ, Bonfield J, et al. Impact of hydroxychloroquine therapy on chronic urticaria: chronic autoimmune urticaria study and evaluation. *Intern Med J.* 2004;34:182–6.

12. Vena GA, Cassano N, Colombo D, et al. Cyclosporine in chronic idiopathic urticaria: a double-blind, randomized, placebo-controlled trial. *J Am Acad Dermatol.* 2006;55:705–9.

13. Cassano N, D'Argento V, Filotico R, et al. Low-dose dapsone in chronic idiopathic urticaria: preliminary results of an open study. *Acta Derm Venereol.* 2005;85:254–5.

14. Barlow RJ, Macdonald DM, Black AK, et al. The effects of topical corticosteroids on delayed pressure urticaria. *Arch Dermatol Res.* 1995;287:285–8

15. Doeglas HM. Reactions to aspirin and food additives in patients with chronic urticaria, including the physical urticarias. *Br J Dermatol.* 1975;93:135–44.

16. Moore-Robinson M, Warin RP. Effect of salicylates in urticaria. *BMJ.* 1967;4:262–4.

17. Haymore BR, Yoon J, Mikita CP, et al. Risk of angioedema with angiotensin receptor blockers in patients with prior angioedema associated with angiotensin-converting enzyme inhibitors: a meta-analysis. *Ann Allergy Asthma Immunol.* 2008;101:495–9.

18. Zingale LC, Beltrami L, Zanichelli A, et al. Angioedema without urticaria: a large clinical survey. *CMAJ.* 2006;175:1065–70.

19. Frank MM, Gelfand JA, Atkinson JP. Hereditary angioedema: the clinical syndrome and its management. *Ann Intern Med.* 1976;84:580–93.

20. Pappalardo E, Cicardi M, Duponchel C, et al. Frequent de novo mutations and exon deletions in the C1inhibitor gene of patients with angioedema. *J Allergy Clin Immunol.* 2000;106:1147–54.

21. Craig TJ, Lew RJ, Wasserman RL, et al. Efficacy of human C1 esterase inhibitor concentrate compared with placebo in acute hereditary angioedema attacks. *J Allergy Clin Immunol.* 2009;124:801–8.

22. Sheffer AL, Campion M, Lew RJ, et al. Ecallantide (DX-88) for acute hereditary angioedema attacks: integrated analysis of 2 double-blind, phase 3 studies. *J Allergy Clin Immunol.* 2011;128:153–9.

23. Zuraw BL, Busse PJ, White M, et al. Nanofiltered C1 inhibitor concentrate for treatment of hereditary angioedema. *N Engl J Med.* 2010;363:513–22.

Atopic Dermatitis

13

Watcharoot Kanchongkittiphon and Tiffany Dy

GENERAL PRINCIPLES

- Atopic dermatitis (AD) is the most common chronic skin disease of young children, affecting 17% of U.S. schoolchildren and a significant number of adults.[1]
- Skin barrier abnormalities, innate immune system defects, T_H2-skewed adaptive immune responses (see Chapter 2), and altered resident skin microbial flora play a key role in the manifestations of AD.

Definition

- AD is a **chronically relapsing skin disease** characterized by pruritic skin lesions, disrupted skin barrier function, dysregulation of the immune system, and a personal or family history of atopy or sensitization to food and environmental allergens. It involves the local infiltration of T_H2 cells, which is the same type of inflammatory response seen in asthma and allergic rhinitis.
- The cause remains unknown, although it is understood to involve a complex relationship of genetic, environmental, immunologic, and epidermal mechanisms.

Epidemiology

- AD affects a **higher proportion of children than adults.**
  - AD affects 20–30% of children and 7–10% of adults. Patients with AD usually have other atopic diseases such as asthma, allergic rhinitis, and food allergy.[2]
  - 90% of patients with AD develop symptoms before the age of 5.[1]
  - The majority of children affected by AD appear to outgrow this inflammatory skin disease.
- Multiple studies suggest that the prevalence of AD is on the rise.
  - A recent systematic review of epidemiological studies of AD showed an increase in the prevalence of atopic eczema in Africa, eastern Asia, western Europe, and parts of northern Europe.[3] The prevalence of AD increased from 9.9% to 20.9% within a 7-year period in Moroccan children aged 13–14 years.[4]
  - This increased frequency is not unique to AD and is paralleled by increases in the prevalence of other atopic diseases, such as allergic rhinitis and asthma.

Etiology

- Compromise of the epidermal barrier, which can occur through various mechanisms, is thought to lead to increased water loss and facilitates entry of allergens and microbes.
  - **Mutations in filaggrin, a protein involved in keratinization of the skin and in barrier function maintenance, have been demonstrated to be a major predisposing factor for a significant subset of patients with AD.**[5] Mutations in the *FLG* gene, specifically *R501X* and *2282del4*, can induce a reduction of natural moisturizing factors, including sodium pyrrolidone carboxylic acid, urocanic acid, and lipoprotein components, especially ceramides.[6,7]
  - Mutations in *SPINK5*, which encodes the serine protease inhibitor Kazal-type 5, can increase cleavage of intercellular attachments in the stratum corneum and can compromise barrier function.[8]

- **Thymic stromal lymphopoietin (TSLP) causes dysregulation of the cutaneous immune response.**
  ○ TSLP expression in keratinocytes is induced by mechanical injury, such as scratching.
  ○ TSLP activates dendritic cells, which leads to T_H2 upregulation.[9]
  ○ TSLP also stimulates mast cells, basophils, and eosinophils, which play a crucial role in cutaneous inflammation.[8]
- Most patients with AD have an **atopic predisposition** and develop an IgE response to common environmental allergens.
  ○ Elevated IgE and detectable reactions to allergens upon skin testing are seen in up to 85% of patients with AD.[1]
  ○ Allergic inflammation causes intrinsic hyperreactivity of inflammatory cells, resulting in lower threshold for irritation.
  ○ Exposure to food allergens and aeroallergens can cause exacerbations in some patients with AD.

Pathophysiology

- Inflammation in AD is characterized by
  ○ Increased secretion of prostaglandin E2 and interleukin (IL)-10 by monocytes, both of which inhibit interferon (IFN)-γ (a T_H1 cytokine)
  ○ Infiltration of **Langerhans cells and macrophages** with surface-bound IgE. These cells do not typically have surface-bound IgE in patients without AD.
  ○ **Activated eosinophils**, particularly in chronic AD lesions
  ○ Absent neutrophils in skin biopsies of AD, which is a result of defective chemotactic activity. This partially explains the increased frequency of cutaneous infections.
- Keratinocytes secrete proinflammatory cytokines such as TSLP, which induces the secretion of the inflammatory cytokines IL-4, IL-5, and IL-13 by T_H2 upregulation.
- IL-4, IL-13, and IL-31 signaling occurs through the JAK-STAT pathway. This can lead to transcriptions of genes, causing decreased keratinocyte differentiation, increased T_H2 differentiation, and increased pruritus.[10]
- IL-22, a major cytokine of T_H22, can cause epidermal hyperplasia and abnormal keratinocyte differentiation.[10] Reduced production of antimicrobial peptides, such as β-defensins and cathelicidins, predisposes patients to greater infection and colonization with *Staphylococcus aureus*, viruses, and fungi.[11]
- IL-22, in synergy with the T_H17 cytokine IL-17, drives an increase in a subset of terminal differentiation proteins, such as S100A7 and S100A8, leading to disruption of the skin barrier.[12]
- Increased levels of IL-4, IL-5, and IL-13 result in **increased IgE** synthesis by B cells.
  ○ Immediate response of pruritus and erythema after allergen exposure is a result of degranulation of mast cells bearing allergen-specific IgE.
  ○ Antigen presentation is potentiated by epidermal Langerhans cells expressing IgE on their surface.
- Chronic inflammation in AD is the result of multiple factors.
  ○ Repeated exposure to allergens which leads to T_H2-type cell expansion.
  ○ Monocytes in patients with AD have a lower incidence of apoptosis, which results in increased production of factors promoting a T_H2-type inflammatory response.
  ○ Allergen-induced inflammation alters corticosteroid receptor binding affinity, which blunts the anti-inflammatory effects of corticosteroids.
  ○ Scratching injures keratinocytes, which can lead to cytokine release and attraction of cells to the inflammatory site.

Risk Factors

- A family history of atopy (AD, allergic rhinitis, or asthma) and a loss-of-function mutation in the *FLG* gene are associated with the development of AD.[13]

- Children with atopic parents have up to a fivefold increased risk of developing AD.[14]
- Environmental exposures such as allergens, irritants, and changes in humidity and temperature may cause flares of AD, particularly in older children and adults.[15]
- Hygiene hypothesis: Exposure to bacterial endotoxins, farm animals, dogs, unpasteurized milk, and early day care has been demonstrated to have protective effects from development of AD.[16]

Prevention

- Skin barrier enhancement with regular application of emollients can decrease the incidence of AD. Three randomized trials have shown that AD can be prevented using regular application of emollients from birth to 6 or 8 months of age.[17]
- There is controversy regarding a preventive effect of probiotics.[18,19]

Associated Conditions

AD is an early manifestation of the atopic march, which describes the progressive development of food allergy, allergic rhinitis, and asthma.

DIAGNOSIS

Clinical Presentation

History
- **Atopic diseases tend to cluster in individuals and in families,** so careful history taking regarding such diseases is helpful.
  - Major risk factors for AD include either a family or personal history of atopic conditions, including AD, asthma, food allergy, and allergic rhinitis.
  - AD and food allergy typically appear first and reach their highest prevalence within the first 2 years after birth.
- **Identification of environmental exposures** that worsen symptoms is an important part of the history.

Physical Examination
- Affected skin usually appears dry.
- **There are no pathognomonic skin lesions.**
- Acute AD is intensely pruritic and may manifest with **erythematous papules with excoriations, vesicles, and serous exudate.**
- Chronic AD is usually characterized by thickened skin with **lichenification and fibrotic papules.**
- Distribution is age dependent.
  - In infants, the face, scalp, and **extensor surfaces of extremities** are affected with sparing of the diaper area.
  - In older patients, involvement of the **flexural folds of extremities, hands, and feet** is common.

Diagnostic Criteria

- The diagnosis of AD is based on the presence of a constellation of clinical features.
- Major features
  - Pruritus (critical for diagnosis)
  - Facial and extensor surface involvement in infants and children
  - Flexural lichenification in adults
  - Chronic or relapsing dermatitis
  - Personal or family history of atopy

- Minor features
  - Xerosis
  - Cutaneous infections
  - Nonspecific dermatitis of the hands or feet
  - Ichthyosis
  - Palmar hyperlinearity
  - Keratosis pilaris
  - Pityriasis alba
  - Nipple eczema
  - Anterior subcapsular cataracts
  - Elevated serum IgE levels
  - Positive immediate-type allergy skin tests

Differential Diagnosis

- Immunodeficiency should be considered, especially when AD presents in infancy.
  - Immune dysregulation, polyendocrinopathy, enteropathy, X-linked (IPEX) syndrome
  - Wiskott–Aldrich syndrome
  - Hyper-IgE syndrome
  - Severe combined immunodeficiency (SCID)
- Other chronic dermatoses that may be differentiated from AD by history include
  - Seborrheic dermatitis
  - Allergic or irritant contact dermatitis
  - Psoriasis
  - Nummular eczema
  - Lichen simplex chronicus
- Infections
  - Scabies
  - HIV
- Malignancy: Cutaneous T-cell lymphoma should be ruled out in adult-onset eczema without history of childhood eczema.
- Others
  - Zinc deficiency; acrodermatitis enteropathica
  - Netherton syndrome

Diagnostic Testing

Laboratories

- Laboratory tests are of limited value in the diagnosis and management of AD. **There are no definitive diagnostic laboratories for AD.**
  - Total IgE is frequently elevated in AD (but may be normal).
  - Complete blood count (CBC) may show eosinophilia.
- Food-specific IgE concentrations do not identify the type or severity of the reaction and are, therefore, not usually helpful in AD. In vitro measurement of antigen-specific IgE may occasionally be necessary if skin tests are not feasible or contraindicated (e.g., diffuse skin lesions or strong history of food-induced anaphylaxis).

Diagnostic Procedures

- Immediate hypersensitivity skin testing can be important in identifying environmental allergens contributing to comorbid conditions, such as allergic rhinitis.
- In scenarios where a food antigen is suspected of contributing to AD, skin testing can be useful.
  - **Negative testing with proper controls has a high predictive value for ruling out a suspected allergen** (i.e., excellent negative predictive value).

- In contrast, **positive tests have a poor correlation with clinical symptoms** in suspected food allergen–induced AD.
  - Positive skin tests to foods suspected of contributing to AD should be confirmed with a **double-blind, placebo-controlled food challenge,** unless there is a history of anaphylaxis to the suspected food.
- Testing for microbes
  - In patients with suspected *S. aureus* infection, a skin swab and culture should be obtained. Treatment for methicillin-resistant *S. aureus* may be initiated while awaiting results.
  - Recurrent viral skin infections, such as herpes simplex, should be diagnosed and treated promptly.
  - Diagnosis of dermatophytes can be diagnosed clinically or with a KOH preparation.

TREATMENT

Medications

First Line

- If emollients are not completely effective, **topical corticosteroids** are recommended.
  - Topical steroids reduce inflammation and pruritus in both the acute and the chronic forms of AD.
  - **The agent with the lowest effective potency should be used.**
  - Although side effects of appropriately used low- to medium-potency topical corticosteroids are infrequent, skin atrophy and hypopigmentation may occur, especially on the face and intertriginous areas.
  - If a high-potency corticosteroid is indicated for a short time period, the patient must be provided with a lower potency option for maintenance therapy to avoid flares.
  - Once-daily treatment has shown to be effective with fluticasone propionate as well as mometasone furoate.[20]
  - Once control is achieved with a daily corticosteroid regimen, **twice-weekly application of a lower potency corticosteroid to the previously involved areas results in fewer relapses**.
  - Topical steroids are available in various bases, but **ointments have been shown to provide the most optimal medication delivery while preventing evaporative losses.**
  - Topical steroids also decrease *S. aureus* colonization in patients with AD.[21]
  - **Systemic corticosteroids should be avoided** because they are often associated with significant flaring after discontinuation.
- **Topical calcineurin inhibitors**
  - Tacrolimus ointment and pimecrolimus cream are immunomodulatory agents that have anti-inflammatory effects without the side effects of topical corticosteroids.[22]
  - These medications are not associated with skin atrophy and may especially be useful for treatment of the face and intertriginous regions.
  - Patients should be counseled regarding transient localized burning and itching that may occur, because this might limit usefulness in certain patients. Studies have shown that treatment with pimecrolimus cream upon early signs of AD results in a significantly decreased incidence of flares and need for topical corticosteroid rescue.[23]

Second Line

- **PDE-4 inhibitor**, crisaborole[24]
  - Crisaborole reduces levels of proinflammatory cytokines, IL-4, IL-5, and IL-13, and decreased production of IgE.
  - Application twice daily for 28 days in patients aged 2 years and older with mild-to-moderate AD resulted in significant improvement in severity, including decreased erythema, induration, lichenification, and excoriation.

- **Systemic immunomodulating agents** are associated with potential serious adverse effects, but can be beneficial for patients with severe refractory AD; treatments can include
  - **Oral corticosteroids**
  - **Oral cyclosporine A:** Treatment with cyclosporine is associated with reduced skin disease and an improved quality of life.
  - **Mycophenolate mofetil (MMF):** Short-term oral MMF as monotherapy results in clearing of skin lesions in adults with AD resistant to other treatments.
  - **Azathioprine:** Azathioprine is a systemic immunosuppressive agent that has been shown to be effective for severe recalcitrant AD. Its use is limited by a number of side effects and slow onset of action. It is metabolized by thiopurine methyltransferase, so deficiency of this enzyme should be ruled out before initiation of treatment.
- **Vitamin D**
  - Studies have demonstrated the beneficial effects of vitamin D on the innate immune response in patients with AD.[11]
  - Patients with AD who took an oral dose of 4,000 IU of vitamin D daily for 3 weeks had a significant increase in cathelicidin expression, suggesting that supplementation with oral vitamin D could improve the innate antimicrobial protection in patients with AD.[25]
- **Antimicrobial therapy**
  - Secondary infection with *S. aureus* must be treated with 7–10 days of either semisynthetic penicillins or first- or second-generation cephalosporins.
  - Bleach baths with one-half cup bleach per full bathtub have been recommended to reduce skin infections.[26] If the area involved is localized, topical mupirocin applied three times daily for 7–10 days may be effective.
  - Intranasal application of topical mupirocin twice daily for 5 days may reduce nasal carriage.
  - Disseminated eczema herpeticum should be treated with systemic acyclovir.
  - Superficial dermatophytoses can usually be treated with topical antifungal agents.
- **Antipruritic agents**
  - Systemic antihistamines and anxiolytics are especially useful in the evening.
  - Doxepin binds histamine receptors and can be given to adults at night.
  - Second-generation antihistamines have shown only modest clinical benefit in treating pruritus associated with AD.
  - Topical antihistamines and topical anesthetics should be avoided because of the risk of cutaneous sensitization.
- **Biologics**
  - Dupilumab is a humanized monoclonal anti-IL-4Rα that blocks IL-4 and IL-13 signaling. Dupilumab is currently the only FDA-approved biologics for the treatment of moderate-to-severe AD in adults and children aged 12 years and older.[27]
  - Omalizumab, a monoclonal anti-IgE antibody, has shown efficacy in the treatment of severe asthma. To date, it has not been observed to have significant clinical benefit in most patients with AD.[28]
  - Rituximab, a monoclonal anti-CD20 antibody, has shown efficacy in a trial of patients with severe AD who received two doses of 1,000 mg administered 2 weeks apart.[29] In addition, a combined treatment for severe refractory AD with omalizumab and rituximab was found to be effective.[30]
- **Experimental therapies**[31]
  - Tralokinumab, an anti-IL-13 human antibody, met primary end points in a recent phase III clinical trial.
  - Other biologics are in various phases of clinical trials for AD, including
    - Lebrikizumab, an anti-IL-13 humanized monoclonal antibody
    - Tofacitinib, a topical Janus kinase inhibitor
    - Anti-TSLP

- Nemolizumab, a humanized anti-IL-31 receptor monoclonal antibody
- Ustekinumab is a humanized monoclonal antibody to the p40 subunit of the cytokines IL-12 and IL-23. IL-23 is the major inducer of T_H17 T cells, which plays a role in the development of AD.
- Fezakinumab, an IL-22 monoclonal antibody, resulted in consistent improvements in clinical disease scores in adults with moderate-to-severe AD in phase IIa studies.
- Baricitinib, a selective JAK1 and JAK2 inhibitor

- **Allergen immunotherapy (AIT)**
  - AIT may be effective for the treatment of AD associated with allergen sensitivity.
  - Data pooled from eight randomized controlled trials (385 patients) demonstrated that AD patients have benefited from dust mite immunotherapy.[32]
  - However, a 2016 Cochrane systematic review including 12 studies stated that owing to limited evidence, it was insufficient to give conclusive results that AIT may be an effective treatment for AD.[33]
  - AIT may be considered an add-on therapy in patients with associated aeroallergen sensitivity who are not responsive to traditional therapy.[34]

Other Nonpharmacologic Therapies

- **Hydration**
  - Skin hydration is essential because atopic skin shows enhanced water loss and reduced water-binding capacity.
  - **Moisturizers also have an important role in improving skin hydration and should be recommended as a first-line therapy**.
  - Lotions have higher water content than emollient, resulting in more drying of the skin because of an evaporative effect.
  - Because moisturizers should be applied **multiple times daily** on a long-term basis, cost is an obvious concern.
  - **Petroleum jelly** is an inexpensive option that is especially effective as an occlusive to seal in water after bathing.
  - An effective method for improving skin hydration is to soak skin for 10 minutes in warm water, then apply an occlusive agent within a few minutes to retain the absorbed water. For soaking of the face and neck, apply a warm wet washcloth.

- **Tar**
  - Crude coal tar extracts have anti-inflammatory properties that, when used with topical corticosteroids in chronic AD, may reduce the need for more potent corticosteroids.
  - Tar shampoos are often beneficial when the scalp is involved.
  - This should be avoided in acutely inflamed skin because this may result in additional skin irritation.

- **Trigger avoidance**
  - **Irritants** are chemicals or other exposures that can nonspecifically worsen AD (**IgE independent**).
    - Use cleansers with minimal defatting activity and a neutral pH rather than soaps.
    - Launder new clothing before wearing to reduce chemical content.
    - Use a liquid rather than a powder detergent and add an extra rinse cycle.
    - Clothing should be cotton or cotton-blend. Occlusive clothing should be avoided.
    - Shower and wash with a mild soap immediately after swimming in a pool to remove chemicals, immediately followed by application of moisturizer.
    - Nonsensitizing sunscreen should be used before sun exposure.
    - Prolonged sun exposure can result in exacerbation because of evaporative losses and sweating.

- ○ **When a specific antigen is identified that worsens AD, allergen avoidance can be effective.**
  - ■ Food allergy has been implicated in one-third of children with moderate-to-severe AD.[35]
  - ■ If a specific food is implicated in a controlled challenge, avoidance may result in clinical improvement.
  - ■ **Extensive elimination diets are not recommended.** Even patients with multiple positive allergy tests are rarely clinically allergic to more than three foods, based on oral food challenges.
  - ○ Patients with dust mite allergen-specific IgE often demonstrate improvement in their AD after taking measures to reduce dust mite exposure.
- **Wet-wrap dressings**
  - ○ These dressings work by cooling the skin, providing a barrier to scratching, and enhancing penetration of topical corticosteroids.[36]
  - ○ Wet-wrap dressings are most effective when covered with dry dressings or clothing and are often best tolerated at bedtime.
- **Phototherapy**
  - ○ UV light therapy can be useful for chronic recalcitrant AD.
  - ○ Some patients benefit from moderate amounts of natural sunlight.
  - ○ Narrow-band UV-B (peak: 331–313 nm), broadband UV-B (280–320 nm), and UV-A1 (340–400 nm) are commonly used.
  - ○ Photochemotherapy with oral methoxypsoralen followed by UV-A may be helpful in patients with severe AD who do not tolerate topical steroids.
  - ○ Adverse effects include skin erythema, skin pain, and pruritus. Cutaneous malignancy and premature skin aging are potential long-term adverse effects.

COMPLICATIONS

- Eye
  - ○ **Atopic keratoconjunctivitis** (see Chapter 10) is characterized by bilateral eye itching, burning, tearing, and mucoid discharge. It can result in visual impairment from corneal scarring.
  - ○ **Keratoconus** is a conical corneal deformity due to persistent rubbing. Left untreated, keratoconus may lead to the formation of anterior subcapsular cataracts.
- Infections
  - ○ AD confers an increased susceptibility to viruses, including herpes simplex virus (HSV), molluscum contagiosum, and human papillomavirus (HPV).
  - ○ Patients are also at risk for superimposed dermatophytoses.
  - ○ *S. aureus* colonizes the skin of >90% of patients with AD, compared to 5% of normal subjects. This can result in recurrent staphylococcal pustulosis, but invasive *S. aureus* infections are rare.

REFERENCES

1. Boguniewicz M, Leung DY. Atopic dermatitis. In: Adkinson NF, Bochner B, Burks AW, et al., eds. *Middleton's Allergy: Principles and Practice.* 8th ed. Philadelphia, PA: Elsevier Saunders, 2014:540–64.
2. Simpson EL, Irvine AD, Eichenfield LF, et al. Update on epidemiology, diagnosis, and disease course of atopic dermatitis. *Semin Cutan Med Surg.* 2016;35(suppl 5):S84–8.
3. Deckers IA, McLean S, Linssen S, et al. International time trends in the incidence and prevalence of atopic eczema 1990–2010: a systematic review of epidemiological studies. *PloS One.* 2012;7(7):e39803.

4. Bouayad Z, Aichane A, Afif A, et al. Prevalence and trend of self-reported asthma and other allergic disease symptoms in Morocco: ISAAC phase I and III. *Int J Tuberc Lungg Dis.* 2006;10(4):371–7.

5. Ong PY, Ohtake T, Brandt C, et al. Endogenous antimicrobial peptides and skin infections in atopic dermatitis. *N Engl J Med.* 2002;347(15):1151–60.

6. Rodriguez E, Baurecht H, Herberich E, et al. Meta-analysis of filaggrin polymorphisms in eczema and asthma: robust risk factors in atopic disease. *J Allergy Clin Immunol.* 2009;123(6): 1361–70.e67.

7. Gao PS, Rafaels NM, Hand T, et al. Filaggrin mutations that confer risk of atopic dermatitis confer greater risk for eczema herpeticum. *J Allergy Clin Immunol.* 2009;124(3):507–13, 13.e501–7.

8. Ziegler SF. Thymic stromal lymphopoietin and allergic disease. *J Allergy Clin Immunol.* 2012;130(4):845–52.

9. Simon D, Kernland Lang K. Atopic dermatitis: from new pathogenic insights toward a barrier-restoring and anti-inflammatory therapy. *Curr Open Pediatr.* 2011;23(6):647–52.

10. Kantor R, Silverberg JI. Environmental risk factors and their role in the management of atopic dermatitis. *Exp Rev Clin Immunol.* 2017;13(1):15–26.

11. Nizet V, Ohtake T, Lauth X, et al. Innate antimicrobial peptide protects the skin from invasive bacterial infection. *Nature.* 2001;414(6862):454–7.

12. Leung DY, Guttman-Yassky E. Deciphering the complexities of atopic dermatitis: shifting paradigms in treatment approaches. *J Allergy Clin Immunol.* 2014;134(4):769–79.

13. Irvine AD, McLean WH, Leung DY. Filaggrin mutations associated with skin and allergic diseases. *N Engl J Med.* 2011;365(14):1315–27.

14. Eichenfield LF, Tom WL, Chamlin SL, et al. Guidelines of care for the management of atopic dermatitis: section 1. Diagnosis and assessment of atopic dermatitis. *J Am Acad Dermatol.* 2014;70(2): 338–51.

15. Boguniewicz M, Fonacier L, Guttman-Yassky E, et al. Atopic dermatitis yardstick: practical recommendations for an evolving therapeutic landscape. *Ann Allergy Asthma Immunol.* 2018;120(1):10–22.e12.

16. Flohr C, Yeo L. Atopic dermatitis and the hygiene hypothesis revisited. *Curr Probl Dermatol.* 2011;41:1–34.

17. Lowe AJ, Leung DYM, Tang MLK, et al. The skin as a target for prevention of the atopic march. *Ann Allergy Asthma Immunol.* 2018;120(2):145–51.

18. Cabana MD, McKean M, Caughey AB, et al. Early probiotic supplementation for eczema and asthma prevention: a randomized controlled trial. *Pediatrics.* 2017;140(3):e20163000.

19. Panduru M, Panduru NM, Salavastru CM, et al. Probiotics and primary prevention of atopic dermatitis: a meta-analysis of randomized controlled studies. *J Eur Acad Dermatol Venereol.* 2015;29(2):232–42.

20. Pei AY, Chan HH, Ho KM. The effectiveness of wet wrap dressings using 0.1% mometasone furoate and 0.005% fluticasone propionate ointments in the treatment of moderate to severe atopic dermatitis in children. *Pediatr Dermatol.* 2001;18(4):343–4.

21. Peserico A, Stadtler G, Sebastian M, et al. Reduction of relapses of atopic dermatitis with methylprednisolone aceponate cream twice weekly in addition to maintenance treatment with emollient: a multicentre, randomized, double-blind, controlled study. *Br J Dermatol.* 2008;158(4):801–7.

22. Hung SH, Lin YT, Chu CY, et al. *Staphylococcus* colonization in atopic dermatitis treated with fluticasone or tacrolimus with or without antibiotics. *Ann Allergy Asthma Immunol.* 2007;98(1):51–6.

23. Gollnick H, Kaufmann R, Stough D, et al. Pimecrolimus cream 1% in the long-term management of adult atopic dermatitis: prevention of flare progression. A randomized controlled trial. *Br J Dermatol.* 2008;158(5):1083–93.

24. Paller AS, Tom WL, Lebwohl MG, et al. Efficacy and safety of crisaborole ointment, a novel, nonsteroidal phosphodiesterase 4 (PDE4) inhibitor for the topical treatment of atopic dermatitis (AD) in children and adults. *J Am Acad Dermatol.* 2016;75(3):494–503.e496.

25. Mutgi K, Koo J. Update on the role of systemic vitamin D in atopic dermatitis. *Pediatr Dermatol.* 2013;30(3):303–7.

26. Huang JT, Abrams M, Tlougan B, et al. Treatment of *Staphylococcus aureus* colonization in atopic dermatitis decreases disease severity. *Pediatrics.* 2009;123(5):e808–14.

27. Simpson EL, Bieber T, Guttman-Yassky E, et al. Two phase 3 trials of dupilumab versus placebo in atopic dermatitis. *N Engl J Med.* 2016;375(24):2335–48.

28. Wang HH, Li YC, Huang YC. Efficacy of omalizumab in patients with atopic dermatitis: a systematic review and meta-analysis. *J Allergy Clin Immunol.* 2016;138(6):1719–22.e1711.

29. Simon D, Hosli S, Kostylina G, et al. Anti-CD20 (rituximab) treatment improves atopic eczema. *J Allergy Clin Immunol.* 2008;121(1):122–8.

30. Sanchez-Ramon S, Eguiluz-Gracia I, Rodriguez-Mazariego ME, et al. Sequential combined therapy with omalizumab and rituximab: a new approach to severe atopic dermatitis. *J Investig Allergol Clin Immunol.* 2013;23(3):190–6.

31. Boguniewicz M. Biologic therapy for atopic dermatitis: moving beyond the practice parameter and guidelines. *J Allergy Clin Immunol Pract.* 2017;5(6):1477–87.

32. Bae JM, Choi YY, Park CO, et al. Efficacy of allergen-specific immunotherapy for atopic dermatitis: a systematic review and meta-analysis of randomized controlled trials. *J Allergy Clin Immunol.* 2013;132(1):110–7.

33. Tam H, Calderon MA, Manikam L, et al. Specific allergen immunotherapy for the treatment of atopic eczema. *Cochrane Database Syst Rev.* 2016;(2):CD008774.

34. Ridolo E, Martignago I, Riario-Sforza GG, et al. Allergen immunotherapy in atopic dermatitis. *Exp Rev Clin Immunol.* 2018;14(1):61–8.

35. Wang J, Sampson HA. Atopic dermatitis and food hypersensitivity. In: Leung DYM, Szefler SJ, Bonilla FA, et al., eds. *Pediatric Allergy: Principles and Practice.* 3rd ed. New York, NY: Elsevier, 2016:414–9.

36. Devillers AC, Oranje AP. Efficacy and safety of 'wet-wrap' dressings as an intervention treatment in children with severe and/or refractory atopic dermatitis: a critical review of the literature. *Br J Dermatol.* 2006;154(4):579–85.

Allergic Contact Dermatitis

14

Abeer S. Algrafi and Christina G. Kwong

GENERAL PRINCIPLES

- Allergic contact dermatitis (ACD) is an inflammatory skin disease resulting from direct or indirect interaction between the skin and a sensitizing substance.
- ACD comprises approximately 80% of cases of contact dermatitis. Irritant contact dermatitis (ICD) accounts for the other 20%.

Definition

- ACD is an immunologically mediated **delayed-type hypersensitivity reaction** that occurs upon contact with a substance after initial exposure and sensitization.
- Distinguished from ICD, which is a nonimmunological reaction and can occur upon first exposure to triggers such as prolonged wet exposure and detergents

Epidemiology

- Few studies are available on the incidence and prevalence of ACD in the general population. One review of studies from North American and Europe found that ACD prevalence is 20% in the general population.[1]
- Occupational contact dermatitis is estimated to cost over 1 billion dollars per year, of which approximately 20% is from ACD and 80% from ICD.[2]
- Prevalence rate of dermatitis in current workforce from National Institute for Occupational Safety and Health (NIOSH) survey in 2010 was 9.8%, representing approximately 15.2 million workers with dermatitis.[3] Health care professionals attributed to 5.6% of the cases.

Pathophysiology

- ACD is a T-cell-mediated delayed hypersensitivity reaction (type IV). Unlike most allergic diseases, it is a T_H1-type response.
- There are two phases in the development of ACD: sensitization and elicitation.[4]
- The initial response is the **sensitization phase.**
  - Sensitization begins when a topical antigen comes into contact with the skin.
  - Typically molecules that are <500 Da result in ACD because the insulting agent must be small enough to penetrate the stratum corneum (horny layer) of the skin.
  - Once the antigen penetrates the skin, the antigen comes in contact with Langerhans cells (LCs) or other antigen-presenting cells.
  - LCs are then drained by the lymphatic system to local lymph nodes, where they present antigens to helper T lymphocytes.
  - T cells then proliferate via clonal expansion, and eventually memory T cells are created.
  - The production of memory T cells can take 4–7 days, and an individual can stay sensitized for several years.
- The subsequent response is the **elicitation phase**.
  - Reexposure to the same antigen in the skin results in the antigen uptake by LCs and activation of local sensitized CD8+ T lymphocytes resulting in an inflammatory response.

- Several proinflammatory mediators are activated, such as interleukin (IL)-1, IL-2, and interferon (IFN)-γ, leading to chemoattraction of macrophages, mast cells, basophils, eosinophils, and neutrophils to the area of exposure. This leads to the typical eczematous rash associated with contact dermatitis.
- ICD can lead to a barrier defect, which releases proinflammatory mediators by keratinocytes. This increases the risk of subsequent ACD development.

Risk Factors

- Female gender (may be due to increased exposure to chemicals in makeup, fragrances, and jewelry)
- Increasing age
- Concurrent atopic dermatitis or ICD
- Occupation: higher risk in health care workers, construction workers, machinists, chemical industry workers, and beauticians/hairdressers

DIAGNOSIS

Clinical Presentation

History

- A thorough history is often needed to accurately diagnose the cause of the rash. Practitioners may choose to initially obtain a more general history and follow after patch testing with a more focused and comprehensive history.
- ACD typically appears as a chronic eczematous rash with induration that can progress to vesicles and bullae.
  - The most common symptom is pruritus. Sometimes the rash is painful or burns.
  - Symptom onset is typically 4–72 hours after exposure to the allergen.
- The clinician should investigate the course of time the rash developed and/or changed, if the rash has occurred before, and whether it improves when the patient is on vacation or away from work or home.
- A thorough review of the patient's occupation, hobbies, travel, social, and medical history, as well as prescription and over-the-counter medications, is needed to identify any possible exposures to common allergens.
- Common contact allergens
  - **Poison ivy, oak, and sumac**: Reactions to urushiol in the plant sap is the one of the most common allergic reaction in the United States, affecting up to 50 million Americans each year.[5]
  - Review of patch testing results found that the most prevalent contact allergens in the United States are nickel sulfate, methylisothiazolinone (MI), fragrance mix, formaldehyde, methylchloroisothiazolinone (MCI)/MI, balsam of Peru, neomycin sulfate, Bacitracin, paraphenylenediamine (PPD), and cobalt chloride.[6]

Physical Examination

- The appearance and distribution of the rash can provide important diagnostic information.
- ACD can occur on any part of the body.
  - Areas of thin skin such as eyes, neck, and genitalia are the most susceptible to ACD.
  - The areas that are most resistant to sensitization include the palms, soles, and scalp.
  - The most characteristic feature of the rash is that it **occurs at the site of contact** with the allergen.
- Rash appearance depends on the time of the presentation.
  - Initially, an area or erythema develops, followed by eruption of papules or vesicles.
  - Eventually, the vesicle will involute, and crusting and scaling will develop.
  - Patients who are chronically exposed to the allergy develop lichenification, painful fissuring, and skin thickening.

- Distribution of the rash may hold clues as to which allergen is contributing to the rash.
  - Scalp: hair dyes (paraphenylenediamine), hair products
  - Earlobes, neck, wrists: jewelry (nickel, gold, cobalt)
  - Eyelids: cosmetics, nail polish, and other topical hand products
  - Axilla: fragrances and antiperspirants in deodorant
  - Arms/legs with linear streaks: poison ivy/oak/sumac
  - Anogenital: hygiene and contraceptive products
  - Feet: carbamates in footwear rubber
  - Under areas of clothes: allergens in textiles (e.g., formaldehyde, dyes)
  - Sun-exposed skin: photoallergens (e.g., fragrances, topical NSAIDs, and agents in sunscreen like benzophenones)
- **Autosensitization:** secondary distal transfer of skin reaction to a body part from the initial area of the contact allergy (e.g., nail polish or fragrances and preservatives in hair products can cause ACD on the face or ears)
- Systemically administered medications can cross-react with topically applied medications, leading to generalized ACD.

Differential Diagnosis

- Before the diagnosis of ACD is confirmed, other diagnoses need to be excluded.
- The following diseases may have a similar appearance:
  - ICD: usually sharply circumscribed dermatitis; patch test negative
  - Atopic dermatitis: personal/family history of atopy, early age of onset, chronic and recurrent disease, typical distribution
  - Seborrheic dermatitis: distributed in sebaceous gland areas (i.e., scalp, periauricular, glabella, nasolabial folds), dandruff as precursor, greasy-looking scales
  - Dyshidrotic eczema: small vesicles on nonerythematous base; often on the feet and sides of the digits; resolves via desquamation in 2–3 weeks
  - Psoriasis: plaques with dry, thin, silvery-white scales
  - Dermatitis herpetiformis: associated with gluten sensitivity; symmetrically grouped herpetiform papules/vesicles

Diagnostic Testing

- In a few cases, the clinician is able to diagnose ACD and the causative agent from history and physical examination alone. However in the majority of cases, patch testing is necessary to confirm the diagnosis and identify the causative agent.
- Patch testing is the primary diagnostic tool for ACD.
  - The test patch contains a small, nonirritating amount of an allergen in a chamber that is placed on the patient's back.
    - Multiple allergens can be tested at one time with individual chambers used.
    - Commercial preparations are available.
  - After 48 hours, the test patch is removed, and the first reading is obtained to assess the degree of inflammation. A second reading should be done 4–7 days after application.
    - **Crescendo effect**: ACD reactions typically increase in size between 48 and 96 hours.
    - **Decrescendo effect**: Irritant reactions tend to decrease with time.
  - Metals, antibiotics (e.g., neomycin and Bacitracin), and topical corticosteroids are associated with late-peak reactions. If they are suspected, a reading 7–10 days after application is helpful.
  - Photopatch testing consists of duplicate samples of suspected photoallergens placed on the back. After 48 hours, one set is exposed to UV-A light.[2] Test results are then read per usual 4–7 days.
  - Grading of the reactions include[2,6] the following:
    - Negative (−)
    - Doubtful (?+): faint erythema

- Weak positive (1+): nonvesicular erythema, infiltration, possibly papules
- Strong positive (2+): vesicular erythema, infiltration, and papules
- Extreme positive (3+): intense erythema and infiltration, coalescing vesicles, bullous reaction
- Irritant reaction (+/−)
  - Results of a patch test should be interpreted in the setting of the patient's history.
  - Topical products and exposures should be reassessed so that effective elimination of the causative agent can be accomplished.
- Repeat Open Application Test (ROAT) is a test that can be helpful for assessing the clinical relevance of doubtful or weakly positive reactions. A small amount of the suspected substance is applied bid to a localized skin area, such as the antecubital fossa for 1–2 weeks, with monitoring for the development of dermatitis.

TREATMENT

- The **first-line** therapy of ACD is to identify and avoid the triggering allergen.
- Several topical medications are used to treat aggravating symptoms and are not intended to be used for prevention.

Medications

- Topical
  - Topical corticosteroid creams, such as hydrocortisone, triamcinolone, or clobetasol, should be used sparingly because they can cause skin thinning and atrophy.
  - Topical calcineurin inhibitors (i.e., tacrolimus and pimecrolimus) are steroid-sparing agents (indicated in patients aged 2 years and older).
  - Phototherapy with UV-B or psoralen plus UV-A light can be considered for the treatment of chronic ACD that is refractory to corticosteroids and works well in ACD involving hands.[7]
  - In severe cases, wet-wrap therapy might be helpful in conjunction with topical anti-inflammatory medications to minimize the need for systematic medications.
- Systemic therapy
  - Oral antihistamines can be used to treat pruritis or insomnia related to itching.
  - Systemic steroids should be considered in severe cases of ACD that involve large areas of skin and short-term use only.
  - Systemic immunosuppressants, such as cyclosporine, methotrexate, and mycophenolate mofetil, can be considered in cases of severe ACD despite topical treatments.[7] Patient must be monitored for systemic side effects.
  - The role of biologic agents in the treatment of ACD has not yet been established.

Other Nonpharmacologic Therapies

- Topical emollients and moisturization are key to helping restore the skin barrier.
  - Ideally use a preparation that is free from preservatives and fragrances.
  - Cool, moist compresses can provide a soothing effect to areas with weepy lesions.
  - Oatmeal baths can help in symptomatic control of ACD affecting large areas of skin.
  - Drying antipruritic lotions, such as calamine lotion, can be used on localized ACD.
- Topical antihistamines and anesthetics should be avoided because these agents can lead to sensitization.

OUTCOME/PROGNOSIS

- In patients with occupational hand dermatitis, at 7–14 years follow-up, 40% had no issues with dermatitis within the last year and 34% had changed their occupation, 20% were retrained, and 25% were not working.[8]
- If not treated, ACD can progress to chronic eczematous dermatitis.

REFERENCES

1. Thyssen JP, Linneberg A, Menné T, et al. The epidemiology of contact allergy in the general population—prevalence and main findings. *Contact Dermatitis.* 2007;57:287–99.
2. Fonacier L, Bernstein DI, Pacheco K, et al. Contact dermatitis: a practice parameter—update 2015. *J Allergy Clin Immunol Pract.* 2015;3:S1–39.
3. Luckhaupt SE, Dahlhamer JM, Ward BW, et al. Prevalence of dermatitis in the working population, United States, 2010 National Health Interview Survey. *Am J Ind Med.* 2013;56:625–34.
4. Vocanson M, Hennino A, Rozieres A, et al. Effector and regulatory mechanisms in allergic contact dermatitis. *Allergy.* 2009;64:1699–714.
5. Yesul K, Flamm A, ElSohly MA, et al. Poison ivy, oak, and sumac dermatitis: what is known and what is new? *Dermatitis.* 2019;30(3):183–90.
6. DeKoven JG, Warshaw EM, Belsito DV, et al. North American Contact Dermatitis Group patch test results 2015–2016. *Dermatitis.* 2018;29(6):297–309.
7. Welsh E, Golderberg A, Welsh O, et al. Contact dermatitis: therapeutics when avoidance fails. *J Allergy Ther.* 2014;5:1–4.
8. Malkonen T, Alanko K, Jolanki R, et al. Long-term follow-up study of occupational hand eczema. *Br J Dermatol.* 2010;163:999–1006.

Food Allergic Reactions

15

Nora Kabil

GENERAL PRINCIPLES

Definition

Food allergy (FA): Also referred to as **food hypersensitivity**, is an adverse health effect arising from a specific immune response that occurs reproducibly on exposure to a given food. This includes both IgE- and non–IgE-mediated FAs.

- **IgE-mediated FAs** require the presence of food antigen–specific IgE and the development of specific signs and symptoms upon exposure to a specific food.
- **Non–IgE-mediated FAs** are immunologically mediated processes with reproducible signs and symptoms on exposure to a food but without IgE sensitization (see Chapter 16).

Classification

- **Food-induced anaphylaxis** is an IgE-mediated, rapid-onset, potentially fatal systemic reaction that occurs after exposure to food that may result in shock and/or respiratory compromise. Patients may develop a combination of symptoms and signs related to the cutaneous, respiratory, gastrointestinal (GI), and/or cardiovascular systems that constitute anaphylaxis (see Chapter 4).
- **Oral allergy syndrome (OAS) or pollen food allergy syndrome** is a form of contact allergy confined to the lips and oropharynx, affecting pollen-allergic patients. Symptoms of OAS include oral itching, tingling, and/or swelling of the lips, tongue, roof of the mouth, and throat. Offending foods are commonly fresh fruits or vegetables; however, these are typically tolerated in the cooked form.

Epidemiology

- **Food allergies are overreported by patients,** which is one of many obstacles in establishing the true prevalence of FAs.
- **Objective measurements are necessary to make an accurate FA diagnosis.**
- **Milk, eggs, and peanuts account for the vast majority of allergic reactions in young children.**
- **Peanuts, tree nuts, and seafood account for the vast majority of reactions in teenagers and adults.**
- The following data were drawn from a meta-analysis of 51 publications[1]:
  - Self-reported FA to cow's milk, hen's eggs, peanuts, fish, or crustacean shellfish: 13% for adults, 12% for children
  - When objective measures were employed—including skin test, serum IgE, or food challenge—the overall prevalence dropped to 3% for all ages.
- U.S. prevalence rates for specific foods[2]
  - Peanut allergy: 0.4–0.8%
  - Tree nut allergy: 0.4%
  - Seafood allergy: 0.6% in children, 2.8% in adults
- **Most children with FA will eventually tolerate cow's milk, egg, wheat, and soy, but far fewer eventually tolerate peanut and tree nuts.**

132

- Allergy to seafood most commonly develops in adulthood and usually persists.
- A high initial level of allergen-specific IgE to a food is associated with a lower resolution rate over time.
- A decrease in the level of allergen-specific IgE is often associated with the ability to tolerate foods.

Pathophysiology

- In the normal mature gut, about 2% of ingested food antigens penetrate the GI tract barrier and enter the circulation.[3]
- The majority of individuals develop what is known as **oral tolerance** to these antigens, which is a state of **immunologic unresponsiveness**.
- A failure to develop tolerance or a breakdown in this process results in excessive production of food-specific IgE antibodies.
- When food allergens penetrate the mucosal barriers and reach food-specific IgE antibodies bound to mast cells or basophils, mediators are released, which results in symptoms of **immediate hypersensitivity**, including vasodilation, smooth muscle contraction, and mucus secretion (type I hypersensitivity).
- These cells also may release cytokines and other mediators that contribute to a late-phase response.
- The clinical manifestations of IgE-mediated hypersensitivity are widely variable but depend on various host and antigen factors.

Risk Factors

- Family history of a biological parent or sibling with existing, or history of, allergic rhinitis, asthma, atopic dermatitis (AD), or FA increases the risk of FAs.
- Presence of AD, especially when severe and early onset, is associated with increased risk of food sensitization.
- **Asthma is the most commonly identified risk factor associated with severe allergic reactions to foods.**
- Complementary factors that affect the absorption of a food allergen may increase the severity of a reaction and should be taken into account. These include concomitant alcohol consumption, use of NSAIDs, and exercise.

Prevention

- Previous guidelines recommended delayed introduction of highly allergenic solid foods for the purpose of preventing allergic disease in high-risk infants. However, evidence suggests that this practice may increase rather than decrease the incidence of food allergies.
- Currently, the early introduction of highly allergenic solid foods to high-risk infants is recommended. These infants should be at least 4 months of age, be developmentally ready, and have tolerated a few less allergenic complementary foods, such as rice cereal and pureed fruits or vegetables.
- In patients with moderate-to-severe AD despite optimal management and/or symptoms or signs of an immediate allergic reaction while breastfeeding or with the introduction of any food, an allergy evaluation, including a detailed history and possible testing, is recommended before introduction of highly allergenic foods. Evaluation for introducing peanuts may follow the consensus recommendations based on the LEAP and other studies. A suggested approach is as follows[4]:
  ○ In children with recalcitrant or moderate-to-severe AD or egg IgE-mediated FA, evaluation by an allergy specialist is recommended.
  ○ Either peanut skin-prick test (SPT) or peanut IgE testing may be performed.

○ If peanut IgE is <0.35 kUA/L or peanut SPT results in a 0–2 mm wheal, introduction at home or a single supervised in-office feeding is recommended.

○ If peanut IgE is >0.35 kUA/L, refer to an allergy specialist for SPT.

○ If peanut SPT results in a 3–7 mm wheal, supervised in-office feeding or graded oral food challenge is recommended.

○ If a peanut SPT results in a ≥8 mm wheal, the child is probably allergic and should continue evaluation and management by an allergy specialist.

Associated Conditions

• Children with FA are 2.3 times more likely to have asthma, 2.3 times more likely to have AD, and 3.6 times more likely to have respiratory allergies than children without FA.[2]

• Asthmatics with coexisting FAs are more likely to have increased rates of emergency department visits and hospitalization in an intensive care unit for their asthma than non–food allergic asthmatics.

• **Food-dependent, exercise-induced anaphylaxis** is a disorder in which anaphylaxis only occurs if exercise takes place within a few hours of eating and, in most cases, only if a specific food is eaten during the pre-exercise period.

DIAGNOSIS

Clinical Presentation

• Manifestations of an immune-mediated reaction to food can vary widely.

• **Cutaneous reactions to food**

○ **Acute urticaria** is a common manifestation of IgE-mediated FAs, with rapid development, typically within minutes, of polymorphic, round, or irregularly shaped pruritic wheals following the ingestion of the offending food.

○ **Angioedema** is also a common manifestation of IgE-mediated FA that usually occurs in combination with urticaria. This is a nonpitting, nonpruritic, well-defined swelling of the subcutaneous tissue, abdominal organs, or upper airway.

○ **Acute contact urticaria:** Direct skin contact with the offending food results in urticaria. In addition to the common allergens, fresh fruits and vegetables are among the food that have been implicated in this form of reaction.

• **Food-induced anaphylaxis** is the most common serious consequence of FA.

○ Typically IgE mediated and believed to involve systemic mediator release from sensitized mast cells and basophils

○ Significantly underrecognized and undertreated

○ Prompt recognition and management are essential to ensure a favorable outcome.

○ Fatalities can occur within 30 minutes of exposure and usually result from respiratory compromise.

Differential Diagnosis

• Acute allergic reactions triggered by other allergens, such as medications or insect stings

• AD flares triggered by other irritants

• Food poisoning due to bacterial toxins or scombroid poisoning

• Chronic GI symptoms due to lactose intolerance, gastroesophageal reflux, infection, anatomical abnormalities, or metabolic disorders

• Gustatory flushing syndrome is an erythematous band on the cheek in the distribution of the auriculotemporal nerve, triggered by tart foods.

- Chemical and irritant effects of foods, such as gustatory rhinitis due to neurologic responses to temperature or capsaicin
- Pharmacologic effects such as tryptamine in tomatoes and food additives may mimic allergic symptoms of the skin and GI tract.
- Mental/behavioral disorders resulting in food aversion

Diagnostic Testing

- Diagnostic testing is based on a comprehensive history, which should suggest whether or not the reaction was IgE or non–IgE mediated. This determines the kind of testing to pursue and the possible food involved.
- **Testing should not be comprised of general broad panels of food allergens.**

Laboratories

- **Total serum IgE:** Although it is often elevated in atopic individuals, it is not a sensitive or specific test for FAs.
- **Food allergen–specific serum IgE**
  - Formerly measured using the radioallergosorbent test (RAST), **specific IgE levels are now measured by more sensitive fluorescence enzyme-labeled assays.**
  - Similar to SPT, these tests are useful in identifying foods that may provoke IgE-mediated food allergic reactions but are **not diagnostic of FA alone.**
  - These tests determine allergic sensitization and the presence of allergen-specific antibodies, which directly correlate with the likelihood of clinical reactivity,[5] but not always with clinical allergy.
  - Especially useful when SPT cannot be done, either due to clinical contraindications or because of failure to discontinue antihistamines prior to the test.
- **Component testing**
  - These tests measure specific IgE responses to individual proteins as opposed to a mixture of proteins.
  - This can help determine which patients are at higher risk for allergic reactions vs. those who are sensitized but clinically tolerant.
  - It may also distinguish those who are at risk for severe reactions vs. milder symptoms.
  - Depending on the specific component target(s) of IgE reactivity (see Table 15-1), a patient may be at low, variable, or high risk of a true allergy.[6–10]
- **Mast cell and basophil mediators**
  - Histamine and tryptase are rarely used to support the diagnosis of food-induced anaphylaxis.
  - **Tryptase lacks specificity and may not be elevated in food-induced anaphylaxis.**

Diagnostic Procedures

- The SPT assists in the identification of foods that potentially induce IgE-mediated reactions but is **not diagnostic of FA when used alone.**
- SPT reflects the presence of IgE bound to cutaneous mast cells.
- SPT has a **low positive predictive value (PPV),** as many patients have IgE to specific foods without clinical FA.
- When the patient provides a history suspicious for FA, an SPT is valuable in identifying the food responsible and, therefore, has a **high sensitivity and a high negative predictive value (NPV)** in this clinical setting.
- Results are immediately available, making SPT the most commonly performed procedure in the evaluation of IgE-mediated FA.
- The patient **must be off all antihistamine medications for 1 week** prior to the procedure to insure the reliability of the test.

TABLE 15-1 WHOLE FOOD AND COMPONENTS[6-10]

Whole food	Component proteins	Meaning of positive IgE reaction (Component IgE profiles)
Milk	Casein (protein stable when heated)	High risk of reaction to all forms of cow's milk
	α-Lactalbumin and β-lactoglobulin (protein unstable when heated)	High risk of reaction to fresh cow's milk Low risk of reaction to baked food containing cow's milk
Egg	Ovomucoid (protein stable when heated)	High risk of reaction to all forms of egg
	Ovalbumin (protein unstable when heated)	High risk of reaction to fresh eggs Low risk of reaction to baked eggs
Peanut	Ara h 1,2,3	High risk of systemic reaction including anaphylaxis Ara h 2 is nearly always associated with clinical allergy
	Ara h 8	Low risk of systemic reactions (associated with local or no reactions)
	Ara h 9	Variable risk of strong allergic reaction (often accompanied by sensitization to other peanut proteins)
Tree nuts Cashew Hazelnut Brazil nut Walnut	Cashew Ana o 3 Hazelnut Cor a 9,14 Brazil nut Ber e 1 Walnut Jug r 1	High risk of systemic reactions including anaphylaxis
	Hazelnut Cor a 8 Walnut Jug r 3	Associated with mild local reactions, as well as systemic reactions
	Hazelnut Cor a 1	Low risk of systemic reactions Associated with local reactions or no reaction at all

Other
- **A double-blind, placebo-controlled oral food challenge is the gold standard for diagnosing FA,** but its use is limited by time and cost.
- Single-blind and open food challenges are frequently used to screen patients for FA (see Table 15-2).
- These challenges should be designed and performed under medical supervision and avoided in patients with a recent life-threatening reaction to a particular food.[11-20]

TABLE 15-2 RECOMMENDED ORAL GRADED FOOD CHALLENGE CUTOFFS[11-20]

Food	Wheal (mm) PPV	Wheal (mm) NPV	Specific IgE PPV	Specific IgE NPV	Component resolved diagnosis (CRD) (kU/L)
Wheat					
Cow's milk	≥8 mm 95% PPV		≥26 kU/L 74% PPV	<26 kU/L 87% NPV	
Heated cow's milk		<7 mm 100% NPV <12 mm 90% NPV	≥15 kU/L or ≥5 kU/L if <1 year old 95% PPV >35 kU/L 85% PPV	≤2 kU/L 50% NPV <5 kU/L 90% NPV	Casein 0.94 kU/L 96% NPV Casein 4.95 kU/L 89% NPV
Egg white	≥4 mm 95% PPV	≤3 mm 50% NPV	≥7 kU/L 95% PPV	≤2 kU/L 50% NPV	
Heated egg	>11 mm 95% PPV	<10 mm 100% NPV	≥50 kU/L 88% PPV	<0.85 kU/L 96% NPV <50 kU/L 86% NPV	Ovalbumin 6.33 kU/L 84% NPV Ovomucoid 4.40 kU/L 86% NPV
Peanut	≥8 mm 95% PPV	<8 mm 80% NPV	≥14 kU/L 95% PPV	<2 kU/L and history of prior reaction 50% NPV <5 kU/L and no history of prior reaction 50% NPV	Ara h 2 1.28 kU/L Specificity 0.97 Sensitivity 0.78
Tree nuts	≥8 mm 95% PPV		≥15 kU/L 95% PPV		
Sesame seed	≥8 mm 95% PPV	<7 mm 83% NPV	≥7 kU/L 50% PPV	<7 kU/L 81% NPV	

NPV, negative predictive value; PPV, positive predictive value.

TREATMENT

- **Management of acute reactions**
  - Isolated symptoms such as flushing, urticaria, mild angioedema, or OAS not associated with additional signs or symptoms of an allergic reaction can be treated with antihistamines.
  - If progression is noted, epinephrine should be given immediately.
  - If the patient has a history of prior severe allergic reaction, epinephrine should be given earlier in the course.
  - **Acute systemic allergic reactions (anaphylaxis) to food should be managed as outlined in Chapter 4.**
- **Epinephrine**
  - Prompt and rapid IM epinephrine after onset of symptoms of food-induced anaphylaxis is **first-line therapy.**
  - **Benefits of epinephrine far outweigh the risks,** and delays in epinephrine administration are associated with increased morbidity and death.
  - Dosing
    - Autoinjector (IM): 0.1 mg for infants and toddlers 7.5–15 kg, 0.15 mg for children 10–30 kg, and 0.3 mg for those >30 kg
    - Epinephrine IM 1:1,000 solution: 0.1 mg/kg, maximum dose of 0.3 mg
  - Epinephrine is the only first-line treatment for anaphylaxis, and there is no substitute.
  - Adjunctive medications are frequently used to alleviate symptoms in anaphylaxis, but there are little or no data demonstrating their effectiveness.
- **Discharge therapy**: Epinephrine autoinjector prescription/instructions, allergen avoidance education, and follow-up with primary care physician or referral to an allergist should be provided to all patients with confirmed or suspected food-induced anaphylaxis.
- **Oral immunotherapy**
  - Oral immunotherapy (OIT) describes protocols that are used to prevent severe reactions to food allergens.
  - OIT protocols rely on administering escalating amounts of a food allergen daily until a maintenance dose is achieved. This maintenance dose is generally continued indefinitely.
  - Patients successfully undergoing OIT are probably protected from accidental ingestion of small amounts of an allergen.
  - OIT protocols probably **do not induce long-term tolerance,** and the food must be continuously ingested to maintain protection from accidental exposures.
  - Adverse side effects from OIT are common.
  - The Food and Drug Administration (FDA) has recently approved a powdered peanut allergen (Palforzia) for OIT.

Lifestyle/Risk Modification

- **Strict allergen avoidance is currently the safest strategy for managing IgE- and non–IgE-mediated FA.**
- Food allergen avoidance in patients with documented FA may reduce the severity of associated comorbid conditions, such as AD.

SPECIAL CONSIDERATIONS

Vaccinations in Patients with Egg Allergy

- Many vaccines are grown in chick embryos and may contain small, variable amounts of egg protein.
- The MMR (measles, mumps, and rubella) and MMRV (measles, mumps, rubella, and varicella) vaccines are safe in egg-allergic children, even in those with a history of severe reaction to eggs.

- Influenza vaccine: Egg-allergic patients of any severity should receive their annual influenza vaccine, and **no** special precautions are required.
- Rabies and yellow fever vaccines should **not** be given to patients with an egg allergy, unless an allergy evaluation and testing to the vaccine have been done.

PATIENT EDUCATION

- **Food labeling**
  - Patients with FAs and their caregivers must be educated on the interpretation of ingredient lists on food labels to optimize trigger avoidance.
  - In 2004, a law was passed by the U.S. Congress requiring that **products containing any of the eight major food allergens clearly list them on the labels in simple English.** This includes peanut, tree nuts, egg, milk, soy, wheat, fish, and shellfish.
- **Emergency management**
  - Patients with FAs and their caregivers should be informed on the risk of anaphylaxis and be able to recognize signs and symptoms early.
  - Families should be equipped with the knowledge and skills to handle such medical emergencies, including understanding of and ready access to an anaphylaxis emergency action plan.
  - Epinephrine autoinjector teaching should be done in the office, and the clinician should ensure that patients/caregivers are familiar with the sequence of events according to the action plan.
  - Patients should wear medical identification jewelry or carry an anaphylaxis wallet card.

MONITORING/FOLLOW-UP

- Annual testing of pediatric patients is reasonable to evaluate whether they have outgrown allergies to foods that are likely to resolve over time (e.g., milk, egg, wheat, soy), provided that the patient has not had a recent reaction to the food.
- Testing for ongoing allergies to peanut, tree nuts, fish, and shellfish should be performed less frequently, because allergies to these foods are not typically outgrown.

REFERENCES

1. Rona RJ, Keil T, Summers C, et al. The prevalence of food allergy: a meta-analysis. *J Allergy Clin Immunol.* 2007;120:638–46.
2. Boyce JA, Assa'ad A, Burks AW, et al. Guidelines for the diagnosis and management of food allergy in the United States: report of the NIAID-sponsored expert panel. *J Allergy Clin Immunol.* 2010;126:S1–58.
3. Sampson HA, Burks AW. Adverse reactions to foods. In: Adkinson N, Busse W, Bochner B, et al., eds. *Middleton's Allergy: Principles and Practice.* 7th ed. Philadelphia, PA: Elsevier, 2009:1139–63.
4. Tobias A, Cooper SF, Acetal ML, et al. Addendum guidelines for the prevention of peanut allergy in the United States: report of the NIAID-sponsored expert panel. *J Allergy Clin Immunol.* 2017;139:22–44.
5. Sampson HA. Utility of food-specific IgE concentrations in predicting symptomatic food allergy. *J Allergy Clin Immunol.* 2001;107:891–6.
6. Canonica GW, Ansotegui IJ, Pawankar R, et al. A WAO—ARIA—GA2LEN consensus document on molecular-based allergy diagnostics. *World Allergy Organ J.* 2013;6:1–17.
7. Kleine-Tebbe J, Jakob T. *Molecular Allergy Diagnostics: Innovation for a Better Patient Management.* Switzerland: Springer International Publishing, 2017.
8. Matricardi PM, Kleine-Tebbe J, Hoffmann HJ, et al. EAACI molecular allergology user's guide. *Pediatr Allergy Immunol.* 2016;27(suppl 23):1–250.
9. Sastre J. Molecular diagnosis in allergy. *Clin Exp Allergy.* 2010;40(10):1442–60.
10. Treudler R, Simon JC. Overview of component resolved diagnostics. *Curr Allergy Asthma Rep.* 2013;13(1):110–7.

11. Eller E, Bindslev-Jensen C. Clinical value of component-resolved diagnostics in peanut-allergic patients. *Allergy.* 2013;68(2):190–4.
12. Permaul P, Stutius LM, Sheehan WJ, et al. Sesame allergy: role of specific IgE and skin-prick testing in predicting food challenge results. *Allergy Asthma Proc.* 2009;30(6):643–8.
13. Cortot CF, Sheehan WJ, Permaul P, et al. Role of specific IgE and skin-prick testing in predicting food challenge results to baked egg. *Allergy Asthma Proc.* 2012;33(3):275–81.
14. Bartnikas LM, Sheehan WJ, Hoffman EB, et al. Predicting food challenge outcomes for baked milk: role of specific IgE and skin prick testing. *Ann Allergy Asthma Immunol.* 2012;109(5):309–13.e1.
15. Sampson HA, Aceves S, Bock SA, et al. Food allergy: a practice parameter update-2014. *J Allergy Clin Immunol.* 2014;134(5):1016–25.e43.
16. Nowak-Wegrzyn A, Bloom KA, Sicherer SH, et al. Tolerance to extensively heated milk in children with cow's milk allergy. *J Allergy Clin Immunol.* 2008;122(2):342–7.e1–2.
17. Caubet JC, Nowak-Węgrzyn A, Moshier E, et al. Utility of casein-specific IgE levels in predicting reactivity to baked milk. *J Allergy Clin Immunol.* 2013;131(1):222–4.e4.
18. Ando H, Movérare R, Kondo Y, et al. Utility of ovomucoid-specific IgE concentrations in predicting symptomatic egg allergy. *J Allergy Clin Immunol.* 2008;122(3):583–8.
19. Peters RL, Allen KJ, Dharmage SC, et al. Skin prick test responses and allergen-specific IgE levels as predictors of peanut, egg, and sesame allergy in infants. *J Allergy Clin Immunol.* 2013;132(4):874–80.
20. Clark AT, Ewan PW. Interpretation of tests for nut allergy in one thousand patients, in relation to allergy or tolerance. *Clin Exp Allergy.* 2003;33(8):1041–5.

Non–IgE-Mediated Food Allergy

16

Christopher J. Rigell and Anthony Kulczycki, Jr.

GENERAL PRINCIPLES

Definition

Non–IgE-mediated food allergies are immunologically mediated processes with reproducible signs and symptoms on exposure to a food but without evidence of IgE sensitization. They differ from IgE-mediated food allergies as symptoms are predominantly gastrointestinal (GI) related and are delayed in onset.

Classification

- **Eosinophilic esophagitis (EoE):** chronic localized eosinophilic inflammation of the esophagus involving both IgE- and non–IgE-mediated mechanisms, resulting in esophageal dysfunction. Proton-pump inhibitor responsive esophageal eosinophilia (PPI-REE) clinically, endoscopically, and histologically resembles EoE that resolves with PPI use, but not secondary to gastroesophageal reflux disease (GERD). It is now thought to be part of an EoE continuum rather than a distinct disease.[1]
- **Eosinophilic gastrointestinal diseases (EGIDs):** group of rare diseases involving portions of the GI tract distal to the esophagus that includes **gastritis, gastroenteritis, and colitis**
- **Food protein–induced enterocolitis syndrome (FPIES):** non–IgE-mediated food hypersensitivity often resulting in delayed-onset emesis and diarrhea
- **Food protein–induced allergic proctocolitis (FPIAP):** non–IgE-mediated eosinophilic inflammation of the lower GI tract (distal sigmoid and rectum) resulting in blood and mucus in the stool of otherwise healthy children
- **Food protein–induced enteropathy (FPE):** non–IgE-mediated reaction involving the small bowel resulting in chronic diarrhea and malabsorption

Epidemiology

- **EoE**[2]
  - Increasing in prevalence and now estimated to be 1 in 1,000–1 in 2,000
  - Male predominance (approximately 3:1) exists.
  - In children, milk, egg, and wheat are the most common food triggers.
  - In adults, milk and wheat are the most common food triggers.
- **Eosinophilic gastritis, gastroenteritis, and colitis**[3]
  - Prevalence ranges from 3.5 to 8.3 per 100,000.
  - No gender predilection
  - Peak age of diagnosis is in the third decade of life.
- **FPIES**[4,5]
  - Likely underreported, but an Australian population study reported an incidence of 15.4/100,000 per year.
  - Most common food triggers include cow's milk and soy proteins.
  - Most common solid foods include rice and oats.
  - Extremely rare in exclusively breast-fed infants.

○ Triggers to a single food occur in 65-80% of cases, whereas 5–10% have more than three food triggers.
○ Acute presentation occurs within the first 3 months of life, often 1–4 weeks after introduction of formula.
○ Can be delayed if secondary to solid foods.

- **FPIAP**[4]
  ○ Thought to be a transient, benign condition.
  ○ One cohort study in Israel showed prevalence of 0.16%.
  ○ Often presents within the first 2–8 weeks of life.
  ○ Milk, soy, and egg are the most common causes.
  ○ May occur in breast-fed infants.
- **FPE**[4]
  ○ Rare and thought to be decreasing in prevalence owing to increased rates of breastfeeding, as it is mostly associated with formula.
  ○ Often presents within the first 2 months of life.
  ○ Cow's milk is the most common cause.

Pathophysiology

- **EoE**[2,6]
  ○ A chronic, immune-mediated esophageal disease mediated predominantly, but not exclusively, by food antigens. Complete histologic reversal of refractory esophageal eosinophilia was seen in eight children after exclusive feeding of an amino acid–based formula for at least 6 weeks. The use of H2 antihistamines did not result in this reversal.[7]
  ○ The ultimate cause(s) remain(s) unknown despite increased understanding of pathogenesis.
  ○ Eosinophils are found throughout the GI tract in normal individuals, except in the esophagus.
  ○ Rate of increased incidence suggests environmental factors are prominent.
  ○ Esophageal epithelial damage is caused by acid and allergens (food and environmental).
  ○ This damage results in production of thymic stromal lymphopoietin (TSLP) and eotaxin-3.
  ○ The production of these cytokines leads to an influx of eosinophils, mucosal tryptase–positive mast cells and basophils, innate lymphoid cells, and adaptive B and T lymphocytes.
  ○ Long term, this increased T_H2 response results in remodeling and ultimately leads to fibrosis, angiogenesis, and smooth muscle hypertrophy if not treated.
  ○ Although not directly IgE mediated, EoE is a T_H2-driven disease with shared pathways.
  ○ Interleukin (IL)-5, as the major eosinophil growth factor, and IL-13, through its induction of eotaxin-3, play important roles.
- **EGIDs**
  ○ Similar to EoE, thought to involve T_H2 cytokines.
  ○ There is an association with peripheral eosinophilia.[8]
  ○ Similar association with atopy suggests exposure to food or environmental allergens may drive eosinophil accumulation.
  ○ Some studies have shown differences in pathophysiology compared to EoE, meaning they may not share a common pathogenesis.[3]
- **FPIES/FPIAP/FPE**[5,9,10]
  ○ Thought to be immunologic and cell mediated but incompletely understood.
  ○ FPIES: Reaction to a food antigen results in GI tract inflammation that causes increased intestinal permeability and a fluid shift.
  ○ Lack of humoral immune response has been demonstrated, but increased IL-8 and tryptase suggest possible neutrophil and mast cell involvement.

Risk Factors

- *TSLP*, *calpain 14*, *eotaxin-3*, and *STAT6* are possible candidate genes related to the development of EoE.[2,11]
- Aeroallergen sensitization to pollens and indoor allergens can trigger EoE and/or lessen the effectiveness of therapy.
- Oral immunotherapy for food and aeroallergens appears to initiate or unmask EoE.
- Perinatal risk factors include maternal or newborn fever, antibiotic use, PPI use, cesarean delivery, and admission into the neonatal intensive care unit.
- An inverse relationship with *Helicobacter pylori* has been seen, but no causation has been proven. One thought is *H. pylori* infection tends to polarize toward a T_H1 response and absence results in skewing toward a T_H2 response.[12]

Prevention

There is insufficient evidence to support routine food allergy testing prior to the introduction of allergenic foods or alternations in maternal diet during pregnancy or lactation.

Associated Conditions

- EGIDs
  - Approximately 75% of patients with EoE or EGIDs are atopic.[2]
  - Patients with IgE-mediated food allergy are significantly more likely to have EoE compared to the general population.
  - Presence of asthma and allergic rhinitis in children is associated with subsequent development of EoE.[13]
  - There is a higher prevalence of oral allergy syndrome in patients with EoE.
  - Some EoE patients have increased co-occurrence of autoimmune conditions.
- FPIES/FPIAP/FPE patients may have IgE-mediated food allergy and other atopic conditions.

DIAGNOSIS

Clinical Presentation

History

- **EoE**
  - Children tend to have food refusal, severe reflux symptoms, failure to thrive, vomiting, chest, and abdominal pain.
  - Adults tend to have more dysphagia and food impaction, but may present with chest pain.
  - Typically there is no temporal relationship with offending foods unlike IgE-mediated food allergy. Rather, foods that are dry or incompletely chewed (breads, meats) may cause symptoms because of mechanical obstruction.
- **EGIDs**
  - Eosinophilic gastritis presents with abdominal pain, early satiety, nausea, and vomiting.
  - Eosinophilic gastroenteritis presents with diarrhea, anemia, and/or hypoalbuminemia.
  - Eosinophilic colitis presents with diarrhea or hematochezia.
  - One classification system groups symptoms based on the layer of inflammation with mucosal involvement resulting in diarrhea, malabsorption, GI bleeding, vomiting, and abdominal pain; muscular layer involvement resulting in vomiting, abdominal distention, and pain; serosal layer involvement resulting in abdominal distention, ascites, and peritonitis.[3]
- **FPIES**
  - Acute presentation consists of profuse, repetitive emesis within 1–3 hours after food ingestion. Diarrhea may occur within 2–10 hours.
    - Patients may become lethargic and dehydrated.
    - Severe cases may result in cyanosis and hypotension.
    - Symptoms resolve within 24 hours, and patients are well in between episodes.

- Chronic presentation may consist of intermittent emesis, bloody diarrhea, lethargy, dehydration, failure to thrive, and abdominal distension.
- No reported FPIES-related deaths.
- **FPIAP**: Presents with blood and mucus in the stool of an otherwise healthy infant.
- **FPE**: Presents with failure to thrive.

Diagnostic Criteria

- **EoE**
  - Symptoms related to esophageal dysfunction.
  - ≥15 eosinophils per high-power field in an eosinophil-rich area on biopsy isolated to the esophagus.[1,6]
  - Previously, persistence after high-dose PPI therapy was considered part of the diagnostic criteria, but now PPI-REE and EoE are thought to be nearly indistinguishable.[1]
  - GERD is no longer viewed as being mutually exclusive with EoE.[1]
  - Secondary causes of esophageal eosinophilia have been ruled out.
  - Is a response to treatment.
- **EGIDs**
  - Owing to the low prevalence, there are not well-established diagnostic criteria.
  - Patients should have recurrent GI symptoms and eosinophilic infiltration in the GI tract that are not attributable to a secondary cause.
  - There is a gradient of expected eosinophils with none in the esophagus, a maximum of 26 eosinophils per high-power field in the duodenum, a maximum of 50 eosinophils per high-power field in the ascending colon, and approximately 30 eosinophils per high-power field in the distal aspects of the colon.[3]
- **FPIES**
  - Acute FPIES should have major and three or more minor criteria.
  - Major criteria: vomiting 1–4 hours after ingestion of culprit food and absence of IgE-mediated respiratory and cutaneous symptoms
  - Minor criteria[5] include
    - two or more episodes of repetitive vomiting to same suspected food,
    - repetitive vomiting after eating a different food,
    - extreme lethargy,
    - marked pallor,
    - need for emergency department (ED) visit,
    - need for IV hydration,
    - diarrhea within 24 hours,
    - hypotension,
    - hypothermia.
  - Major criterion for chronic FPIES includes resolution of symptoms within days following elimination of offending food(s) and acute recurrence of symptoms upon reintroduction. Onset of vomiting in 1–4 hours and diarrhea within 24 hours.[5]

Differential Diagnosis

- **EoE**: There are many other causes of esophageal eosinophilia including GERD, PPI-REE, infectious esophagitis, hypereosinophilic syndrome, parasitic infection, inflammatory bowel disease (IBD), drug-associated esophagitis, achalasia, connective tissue disorders, and graft-vs.-host disease.
- **FPIES**: GI obstruction, infectious gastroenteritis, sepsis, necrotizing enterocolitis, anaphylaxis, inborn errors of metabolism, lactose intolerance, cyclic vomiting, severe GERD, Hirschsprung, IBD, celiac, EGIDs, food aversion, primary immunodeficiencies
- **FPIAP**: anal fissure, necrotizing enterocolitis (mainly in premature infants), Meckel diverticulum

Diagnostic Testing

Testing should not be comprised of general broad panels of food allergens.[14,15]

Laboratories

- **EoE**
  - No studies have identified the predictive values for specific IgE to foods.
  - Peripheral eosinophilia and elevated total IgE may be demonstrated but are often normal.
  - IgG4 levels have been found to be increased in active EoE, but it is not established whether this elevation is pathogenic or an epiphenomenon.
  - There is a 96-gene panel based on the EoE transcriptome that helps to differentiate from GERD and can also differentiate active vs. quiescent disease.
- **EGIDs**
  - Should rule out parasitic infection with stool ova and parasites.
  - Peripheral eosinophilia and elevated total IgE may be demonstrated.
- **FPIES**
  - White blood cell differential may show neutrophilia and thrombocytosis.
  - Severe cases may result in methemoglobinemia and metabolic acidosis.
  - Chronic presentations may result in anemia, hypoalbuminemia, and eosinophilia.

Diagnostic Procedures

- **EoE**
  - Allergy testing–based diets and empiric elimination–based diets have been used in treatment of EoE, although both have limitations. Allergy testing has high negative predictive value, except for milk, but poor positive predictive value.
  - Skin testing for aeroallergens is necessary to assess whether aeroallergen sensitivity contributes to symptoms.
  - Atopy patch testing has been demonstrated to detect culprit foods 50% of the time and has a >90% negative predictive value, except for milk. However, it is time-consuming and has generally fallen out of favor.
- **EGIDs:** Ascitic fluid Gram stains can demonstrate eosinophilia, as can tissue samples from endoscopic biopsies.
- **FPIES**
  - Allergy skin tests to food and serum IgE antibodies to foods are most often negative, but can be done if clinical history is concerning for IgE-mediated process or other atopic history. Atopy patch testing is not recommended.
  - Oral food challenge is the gold standard if diagnosis cannot be made on clinical history alone.
    - Considered positive if meets major criteria and two minor criteria (lethargy, pallor, diarrhea 5–10 hours after ingestion, hypotension, hypothermia, increased neutrophil count of at least 1,500 above baseline).
    - Most protocols give 0.06–0.6 g/kg (average 0.3 g/kg) of food protein in two to three doses every 15 minutes, with maximum total dose of 3 g protein or 10 g food. The patient is then monitored for 4 hours.
    - Peripheral IV access should be obtained in the event IV fluids are needed.
- **FPIAP**
  - Hemoccult testing of stool should be performed if no evidence of gross blood.
  - Stool samples can demonstrate neutrophils and eosinophils.
  - Although not required, colonic biopsies typically show higher than expected numbers of eosinophils.

Endoscopy

- **EoE**
  - Endoscopic findings may show longitudinal furrowing, friability, whitish exudates, longitudinal shearing, transient or fixed rings, edema, and raised white specks, although 17% of patients may have normal gross endoscopic findings.[16]

- Six biopsies should be taken from different locations in the esophagus (proximal as well as distal).
- Histologically should see at least 15 eosinophils per high-power field in an eosinophil-rich area. May also see eosinophilic microabscesses, basal zone hyperplasia, lamina propria fibrosis, and increased mast cells

TREATMENT

Medications

Systemic steroids, although effective, should be avoided if at all possible because of their adverse side effects.

First Line
- **EoE**
  - No medications have been Food and Drug Administration (FDA) approved specifically for EoE.
  - PPIs
    - Start with standard dose.
    - Some patients may require high-dose PPIs for 8 weeks (in adults, omeprazole 20–40 mg twice daily or equivalent and in children 1–2 mg/kg twice daily or equivalent).
  - Orally administered topical corticosteroids reduce esophageal eosinophil count in most patients, and budesonide and fluticasone are the most well studied.[1,6]
    - Adult dose: viscous budesonide slurry 1 mg twice daily or swallowed fluticasone propionate 220 μg two puffs twice daily for a 3-month period
    - There is a risk of esophageal candidiasis.
- **EGIDs**: no randomized controlled trials, but some reports of benefit with swallowed topical corticosteroids (budesonide slurry or capsule and swallowed fluticasone)
- **FPIES**: oral rehydration if mild with one or two episodes of emesis and no lethargy. IV rehydration if moderate-to-severe reaction. May need supportive care in the ED

Second Line
- **EoE**
  - Ongoing trials to evaluate role of monoclonal antibodies against IL-4 receptor and IL-13 have shown preliminary promise. Monoclonal antibodies against IgE and IL-5 have largely been ineffective.[17]
  - Future targets include TSLP, eotaxins, and transforming growth factor (TGF)-β1.
- **FPIES**: IM or IV ondansetron or a single dose of IV methylprednisolone (1 mg/kg)

Surgical Management

In EoE, endoscopic dilation can provide symptomatic relief due to strictures.

Lifestyle/Risk Modification
- **EoE**
  - Elemental diet for 6 weeks leads to a resolution rate of >90%.
  - Six-food empiric elimination diets usually consist of most common allergenic food groups (milk, egg, soy, wheat, fish/shellfish, peanut/tree nuts) and are effective in 72% of cases.[18]
  - Fish/shellfish and nuts rarely cause EoE.
  - Owing to the severe restriction, attempts at empiric four-food (cow's milk, gluten-containing cereals, eggs, and legumes) and two-food elimination diets (milk and gluten) have also been attempted with improvement rates of 54–64% and 43%, respectively.[18]

- ○ The use of allergy testing to guide elimination inconsistently leads to improvement. More useful in children than adults.
- ○ Step-up therapy from two-food elimination to four-food elimination to six-food elimination based on response has led to a reduced number of endoscopies and a shortening in the time to diagnosis.[19]
- ○ Patients who require more foods to be eliminated have been found to be more likely to have multiple food triggers.
- ○ Goal is to identify culprit foods to avoid for life and to reintroduce other foods.
- **EGIDs**: no randomized controlled trials, but some evidence that elemental diets led to improvement in symptoms[3]
- **FPIES**
  - ○ The offending food should be removed from the diet and avoided.
  - ○ Unlike with IgE-mediated food allergy, the ability to tolerate baked forms of cow's milk and egg is unclear and should not be assumed.
  - ○ Maternal avoidance of culprit food should not be recommended if the infant is thriving and asymptomatic.[5]
- **FPIAP**: Use an amino acid or extensively hydrolyzed formula. Can also eliminate cow's milk from maternal diet.

COMPLICATIONS

- **EoE:** esophageal remodeling and fibrosis causing strictures
- **FPIES:** may develop IgE-mediated allergy

REFERRAL

- Counseling by a nutritionist may be helpful in developing dietary plans.
- Occupational therapy and speech language pathologists may be necessary to help with eating technique.
- Gastroenterology for diagnostic endoscopies and if dilation of strictures is needed.

PATIENT EDUCATION

- Providing an action plan for FPIES can be helpful because of unfamiliarity with the diagnosis.
- Patients and their caregivers must be educated on the interpretation of ingredient lists on food labels to optimize trigger avoidance.
- In 2004, a law was passed by the U.S. Congress requiring that **products containing any of the eight major food allergens must clearly list them on the label in simple English.** This includes peanut, tree nuts, egg, milk, soy, wheat, fish, and shellfish.[20]

MONITORING/FOLLOW-UP

- **EoE**
  - ○ Efficacy of treatment should be assessed after 6–12 weeks with a repeat endoscopy.
  - ○ Duration of PPI or topical steroids is not well established. Maintenance therapy may be considered for patients with severe dysphagia, relapse after therapy cessation, or history of stricture.
  - ○ Dietary avoidance of culprit foods may preclude the need for long-term pharmacologic treatment.
- **FPIES**: Oral food challenges should be conducted 12–18 months after the initial reaction to determine if resolved.

OUTCOME/PROGNOSIS

- EoE is a chronic condition and, if untreated, can lead to esophageal remodeling and strictures.
- FPIES typically resolved by 3–5 years of age. If evidence of IgE sensitization, less likely to resolve.
- FPIAP typically resolves by 1–2 years of age.
- FPE typically resolves by 1–3 years of age.

ADDITIONAL RESOURCES

- Patient advocacy groups for EoE
  - American Partnership for Eosinophilic Disorders
  - Campaign Urging Research for Eosinophilic Diseases (CURED)
- Patient advocacy group for FPIES: FPIES Foundation

REFERENCES

1. Lucendo AJ, Molina-Infante J, Arias A, et al. Guidelines on eosinophilic esophagitis: evidence-based statements and recommendations for diagnosis and management in children and adults. *United European Gastroenterol J.* 2017;5:335–58.
2. Spergel J, Aceves SS. Allergic components of eosinophilic esophagitis. *J Allergy Clin Immunol.* 2018;142:1–8.
3. Egan M, Furuta GT. Eosinophilic gastrointestinal diseases beyond eosinophilic esophagitis. *Ann Allergy Asthma Immunol.* 2018;121(2):162–7.
4. Leonard SA. Non–IgE-mediated adverse food reactions. *Curr Allergy Asthma Rep.* 2017;17:84.
5. Nowak-Wegrzyn A, Chehade M, Groetch ME, et al. International consensus guidelines for the diagnosis and management of food protein-induced enterocolitis syndrome: Executive summary—Workgroup Report of the Adverse Reactions to Foods Committee, American Academy of Allergy, Asthma & Immunology. *J Allergy Clin Immunol.* 2017;139:1111–26.
6. Dellon ES, Gonsalves N, Hirano I, et al. ACG clinical guideline: evidence based approach to the diagnosis and management of esophageal eosinophilia and eosinophilic esophagitis (EoE). *Am J Gastroenterol.* 2013;108:679–92.
7. Kelly KJ, Lazenby AJ, Rowe PC, et al. Eosinophilic esophagitis attributed to gastroesophageal reflux: improvement with an amino acid-based formula. *Gastroenterology.* 1995;109:1503–12.
8. Caldwell JM, Collins MH, Stucke EM, et al. Histologic eosinophilic gastritis is a systemic disorder associated with blood and extragastric eosinophilia, T_H2 immunity, and a unique gastric transcriptome. *J Allergy Clin Immunol.* 2014;134:1114–24.
9. Leonard SA, Pecora V, Fiocchi AG, et al. Food protein-induced enterocolitis syndrome: a review of the new guidelines. *World Allergy Organ J.* 2018;11:4.
10. Cherian S, Varshney P. Food protein-induced enterocolitis syndrome (FPIES): review of recent guidelines. *Curr Allergy Asthma Rep.* 2018;18:28.
11. Rochman M, Azouz NP, Rothenberg ME. Epithelial origin of eosinophilic esophagitis. *J Allergy Clin Immunol.* 2018;142:10–23.
12. Jensen ET, Dellon ES. Environmental factors and eosinophilic esophagitis. *J Allergy Clin Immunol.* 2018;142:32–40.
13. Hill DA, Grundmeier RW, Spergel JM. Eosinophilic esophagitis is a late manifestation of the allergic march. *J Allergy Clin Immunol Practice.* 2018;6(5):1528–33.
14. Sampson HA, Burks AW. Adverse reactions to foods. In: Adkinson N, Busse W, Bochner B, et al., eds. *Middleton's Allergy: Principles and Practice.* 7th ed. Philadelphia, PA: Elsevier, 2009:1139–63.
15. Sampson HA, Aceves S, Bock SA, et al. Food allergy: a practice parameter update-2014. *J Allergy Clin Immunol.* 2014;134:1016–25.
16. Kim HP, Vance RB, Shaheen NJ, et al. The prevalence and diagnostic utility of endoscopic features of eosinophilic esophagitis: a meta-analysis. *Clin Gastroenterol Hepatol.* 2012;10:988–96.
17. Wechsler JB, Hirano I. Biological therapies for eosinophilic gastrointestinal diseases. *J Allergy Clin Immunol.* 2018;142:24–31.

18. Molina-Infante J, Lucendo AJ. Dietary therapy for eosinophilic esophagitis. *J Allergy Clin Immunol.* 2018;142:41–7.
19. Molina-Infante J, Arias A, Alcedo J, et al. Step-up empiric elimination diet for pediatric and adult eosinophilic esophagitis: the 2-4-6 study. *J Allergy Clin Immunol.* 2018;141(4):1365–72.
20. U.S. Food and Drug Administration. Food Allergen Labeling and Consumer Protection Act of 2004. (Public Law 108-282, Title II) Section 201(qq). Published October 2006. Last Accessed 5/5/20. https://www.fda.gov/food/food-allergensgluten-free-guidance-documents-regulatory-information/food-allergen-labeling-and-consumer-protection-act-2004-falcpa

Drug Allergy and Desensitization

Abeer S. Algrafi and Jennifer Marie Monroy

GENERAL PRINCIPLES

Definition

- A drug allergy or hypersensitivity is a type of adverse drug reaction (ADR).
- An **ADR** is an undesired or unintended response that occurs when a drug is given for the appropriate purpose.
- Hypersensitivity should be used to describe **objectively reproducible symptoms or signs initiated by exposure to a defined stimulus at a dose tolerated by normal persons.**[1]
- **Allergy is a hypersensitivity reaction initiated by specific immunologic mechanisms.**[1] This can refer to **IgE-mediated or T-cell-mediated reactions**. Usually will occur upon reexposure to the offending drug.

Classification

- ADRs can be divided into two major types: type A and type B.
  - **Type A reactions** are **predictable** adverse reactions secondary to the pharmacologic proprieties of the drug and are often dose dependent.
    - It is the most common type of ADR and accounts for >80% of ADRs.
    - Examples include overdosage (e.g., arrhythmia due to theophylline overdose), known side effects (e.g., nausea with codeine), indirect effects (e.g., *Clostridium difficile* infection resulting from clindamycin administration for a skin infection), and drug–drug interactions (e.g., sildenafil increasing the hypotensive effects of isosorbide mononitrate).
  - **Type B reactions** are **unpredictable** adverse reactions that are usually dose independent and unrelated to the drug's pharmacokinetics.
    - Accounts for about 10–15% of ADRs
    - Divided into drug intolerance, drug allergy, and nonallergic reactions with immunologic manifestations (previously known as **pseudoallergic or anaphylactoid reactions**), which involve IgE-independent degranulation of mast cells
- The different immunologic mechanisms for drug allergy are characterized in the Gell and Coombs classification of hypersensitivity, as shown in Table 2-1.
  - **Type I** reaction: IgE-mediated and immediate onset, usually within an hour of drug administration. Presents as anaphylaxis, urticaria, angioedema, asthma, and rhinitis
  - **Type II** reaction: IgG antibody-mediated resulting in cytotoxic destruction of cells; onset can occur within hours of drug administration. Includes immune cytopenias
  - **Type III** reaction: IgG antibody–antigen complexes with complement activation. Onset delayed >1 week after drug exposure. Presents as serum sickness, vasculitis, or drug fever
  - **Type IV** reaction: T-cell mediated and onset occurs days to weeks after first exposure to the drug. Divided into four subtypes. Presents as various exanthems, fixed drug eruptions, contact dermatitis, and severe cutaneous adverse reactions (SCARs), which include Stevens–Johnson syndrome (SJS), toxic epidermal necrolysis (TEN), acute generalized exanthematous pustulosis (AGEP), and drug rash with eosinophilia and systemic symptoms (DRESS)

Epidemiology

- A meta-analysis from studies conducted in the United States from 1966 to 1996 showed 15.1% of hospitalized patients experienced an ADR with an incidence of 3.1–6.2% of hospital admissions because of ADRs.[2]
- Within ADRs, allergic drug reactions occur approximately 6–10% of the time.[3]
- Death from ADRs occur in about 0.2–0.4% of hospitalized patients.[2]
- Anaphylaxis-related deaths in the United States were due to medications in 58.8% of the approximately 2,500 patients reported in a ten-year period.[4]
- Cutaneous reactions are the most common adverse drug event with an annual incidence of 2.26/1,000 persons.[5]

Pathophysiology

- High-molecular-weight (HMW) drugs, usually >4,000 Da, are large enough to elicit an immune response independently, whereas low-molecular-weight (LMW) drugs, typically <1,000 Da, create an immune response by interacting with other molecules.
- There are three models of immune activation by a small molecule
  - Hapten/prohapten model: A small molecule such as a drug or its metabolite can form a covalent bond with a larger protein creating a hapten–carrier complex.
  - Pharmacologic interaction (p-i) model: The drug cannot bind covalently to a carrier protein and instead binds noncovalently to the T-cell receptor (TCR) on T cells and/or the major histocompatibility complex (MHC) on antigen-presenting cells.[6]
  - Altered peptide repertoire model: The drug will bind in the class I HLA peptide-binding cleft and change the specificity of the HLA peptide presentation. The altered peptides are seen as foreign by T cells and trigger an immune response.[7]

Risk Factors

- **Drug factors**
  - **Size and structure:** HMW drugs and the ability of a drug or its metabolites to bind to carrier proteins are more immunogenic.
  - **Route of exposure:** Cutaneous administration is the most immunogenic.[8] Penicillin (PCN) and sulfonamides are no longer available topically because of this reason. Once sensitized, parental administration is associated with anaphylaxis more than oral administration.
  - **Dose, duration, and frequency:** Higher dose, longer duration of therapy, and increased frequency of therapy all contribute to immunogenicity.
  - MRGPRX2 is a G-protein-coupled receptor on human mast cells that is involved in a dose-dependent interaction with a drug that can elicit a nonallergic reaction with immunologic manifestations.[9] Drugs associated include vancomycin, fluoroquinolones, neuromuscular blocking agents, and opioids.
- **Patient-related factors**
  - **Gender:** Women are affected more frequently than men. However, there are no significant differences in the clinical presentation or severity between genders.
  - **Age:** Children are less likely to be exposed to a drug repeatedly, which reduces the risk of sensitization and overall incidence rate.
  - **Genetic factors:** Both genetics and environmental factors play a role in determining an individual's sensitivity to a drug.
    - **Atopy:** Presence of atopic diseases is not a risk factor for drug allergy. However, atopic individuals may be at an increased risk to develop nonallergic reactions with immunologic manifestations, in particular with radiocontrast media (RCM).[10]

- **Acetylators and hydroxylators:** There is a higher risk for ADRs in patients who are slow acetylators or hydroxylators. Increased risk of drug-induced lupus (DIL) to isoniazid, hydralazine, and procainamide in slow acetylators.
- **HLA type:** There are some HLA genotype variants that play a key role in the development of drug hypersensitivity.
  - For example, abacavir was found to bind to the antigen-presenting groove of MHC class I molecules in patients carrying the HLA-B*57:01 allele. Testing for this HLA genotype is standard of care prior to prescribing abacavir.
  - Other HLA associations include HLA-B*15:02 allele and carbamazepine-induced SJS/TEN in Asian populations and HLA-B*58:01 allele and allopurinol-induced SJS/TEN in Asian populations.
- **Family history of multiple drug allergies**
- **Prior history of drug reactions** may confer a predilection to more than one non–cross-reacting medication.
- **Concurrent medical illness:** Some medical conditions, especially infections, predispose to an increased risk for ADRs.
  - Trimethoprim–sulfamethoxazole (TMP–SMX) hypersensitivity occurs in 5% of HIV-negative patients and in 60% of patients with HIV.[11]
  - In an Epstein–Barr viral (EBV)-infected individual, administration of ampicillin produces a nearly universal maculopapular rash.[12]
- **Concurrent medical therapy:** Patients treated with β-blocking agents may be diagnosed with an allergic reaction later into the reaction. β-Blockers can also impede treatment with epinephrine.

Prevention

- Prevention is vital to reduce the incidence of allergic drug reactions.
- It is important to only prescribe medications that are clinically essential.
- Minimizing polypharmacy also decreases the incidence of allergic drug reactions.
- If an allergy to a drug is in question, use skin testing when possible or a graded dose challenge can help delineate if the drug can be safely used at a therapeutic dose.
- Patients who have had an allergic drug reaction should be informed of the reaction and how to avoid further exposure, including the drug and any agents that may cross-react. The patient may carry a card or wear a medical alert bracelet.
- HLA testing can be used if the patient is high risk for development of SCARs to a drug (e.g., abacavir and carbamazepine).

DIAGNOSIS

Clinical Presentation

History
- A thorough history is essential for making the diagnosis of an allergic drug reaction.
- Questions should be directed at establishing the following information:
  - Sign and symptoms: Where and in what order did the symptoms begin, progress, and resolve?
  - Timing of the reaction: from the first dose of the suspected drug, to the peak of the reaction, and then the resolution after discontinuing the suspected drug
  - How was the drug reaction treated?
  - Purpose of drug: Was it prescribed for the appropriate treatment and can the signs and symptoms be explained by a concurrent illness?
  - Other medications the patient is receiving: This includes all over-the-counter drugs and dietary supplements.

○ Prior exposure to the drug or another drug in the same or related class: If so, when was it given and what was the outcome?

○ History of other allergic drug reactions: Did the patient ever see an allergist and receive skin testing? What was the reaction and how long ago did it occur?

• The history obtained will then help decide the appropriate diagnostic test to evaluate the allergic drug response.

Clinical Features of Drug Allergy

• **Type I reactions (IgE-mediated reaction)**

  ○ Symptoms usually begin within 30 minutes to 8 hours after reexposure to the drug.

    ▪ **Anaphylaxis** is discussed in detail in Chapter 4. It is important to remember that nonallergic reactions with immunologic manifestations can be indistinguishable from anaphylaxis but are not mediated by IgE.

    ▪ **Urticaria and angioedema** are discussed in detail in Chapter 12 and are examples of a type I hypersensitivity and the second most frequent drug-induced skin eruption.

  ○ Commonly implicated drugs include β-lactam drugs, platinum-based chemotherapy (e.g., carboplatin and oxaliplatin), neuromuscular blocking agents, and foreign proteins (e.g., chimeric monoclonal antibody, cetuximab, contains α-gal and will trigger anaphylaxis when administered to a person sensitized to α-gal after a tick bite from a lone-star tick).

• **Type II reactions (complement-dependent cytotoxic reaction involving IgG/IgM)**

  ○ Mostly present with hematologic manifestations without any other symptoms

  ○ The onset can occur a week after exposure and resolves in 1–2 weeks after discontinuing the drug. Reexposure to drug can cause symptoms within hours.

    ▪ **Drug-induced eosinophilia:** can be caused by gold salts, allopurinol, aminosalicylic acid, ampicillin, tricyclic antidepressants, capreomycin sulfate, carbamazepine, digitalis, phenytoin, sulfonamides, vancomycin, and streptomycin.

    ▪ **Drug-induced thrombocytopenia:** can present with petechial bleeding in skin and oral mucosa. Sequestration of platelets in the liver and spleen can result in splenomegaly and hepatomegaly. The most implicated drugs are gold salts, quinidine, sulfonamides, vancomycin, carbamazepine, NSAIDs, abciximab, and heparin.

    ▪ **Drug-induced hemolytic anemia**: can present with dyspnea, fatigue, pallor, dark urine, and splenomegaly. The list of common causative drugs includes PCN, cephalosporins, NSAIDs, cisplatin, tetracycline, methyldopa, levodopa, mefenamic acid, procainamide, tolmetin, quinidine, chlorpropamide, nitrofurantoin, probenecid, rifampin, streptomycin, isoniazid, erythromycin, triamterene, and phenacetin.

    ▪ **Drug-induced neutropenia or agranulocytosis**: presents days to weeks after starting offending drug and patient presents clinically with symptoms related to an infection. The list of common causative drugs includes clozapine, sulfonamides, sulfasalazine, propylthiouracil, methimazole, semisynthetic PCNs, quinidine, procainamide, flecainide, dapsone, phenytoin, phenothiazines, and rituximab.

• **Type III reactions (IgG antigen–antibody complex deposition)**

  ○ A reaction that develops after the drug binds to a specific IgG molecule and forms immune complexes that can activate complement and precipitate out into several tissues and organs

  ○ The reaction can be rapid and more severe upon reexposure to a similar drug.

  ○ **Serum sickness**

    ▪ Symptoms begin 6–21 days after administration of the drug and include fever, malaise, skin eruptions (palpable purpura or urticaria), arthralgias/myalgias, arthritis, lymphadenopathy, glomerulonephritis, and leukopenia.

- Laboratory findings include low serum complement and elevated erythrocyte sedimentation rate (ESR).
- Once the offending drug is discontinued, symptoms resolve completely in a few days to weeks depending on the severity.
- It is commonly seen in serum immunotherapy, including rabies, botulism, and venom antitoxins.
- β-Lactams are the most commonly associated nonserum drug to cause serum sickness.
○ **Vasculitis**
  - Cutaneous vasculitis commonly presents with palpable purpuric lesions on the legs and varies in size.
  - The most common affected areas are the buttocks, upper extremities, or the trunk.
  - To a lesser extent, other organs are involved, such as the gastrointestinal tract or kidneys.
  - Systemic symptoms, such as malaise, arthralgia, and fever, are less common.
  - Vasculitic lesions typically develop within several weeks of the initiation of the causative drug.
  - The most common culprits are PCNs, cephalosporins, sulfonamides phenytoin, diltiazem, furosemide, and allopurinol.
  - An Arthus reaction is a localized reaction involving immune complexes deposited on small blood vessels and results in infiltration of neutrophils and localized skin necrosis. Symptoms start in a few hours and peak 24 hours at sites where a vaccine booster was injected. Has been documented to occur with tetanus and diphtheria vaccines.[13]
○ **Drug fever**
  - Fever may be the only manifestation of a drug allergy, diagnosis is one of exclusion.
  - In nonsensitized individuals, the onset of fever is highly variable and differs among drug classes, but most commonly appears 7–10 days after starting a drug, and defervescence occurs 2–3 days after discontinuation of the drug.
  - Rechallenge with the offending agent will usually cause recurrence of fever within a few hours, confirming the diagnosis.
  - Etiology is unknown but suspected to include immune complex and T-cell-mediated reactions.
  - Medications associated with drug fever include azathioprine, sulfasalazine, minocycline, TMP–SMX, sirolimus, and tacrolimus.
- **Type IV reactions (cell mediated)**
  ○ The onset of these reactions is delayed for at least 2 days to a few weeks after exposure to the culprit drug.
  ○ **Maculopapular or morbilliform skin eruptions**
    - The most common drug-induced skin eruption
    - Rash typically is symmetric beginning in areas of pressure and spares the palms and soles. It is confluent with erythematous macules and papules.
    - Begins 4–7 days after initiating a drug
  ○ **Fixed drug eruption**
    - **Skin lesions that occur in the same area upon reexposure to a drug**
    - It is characterized by sharply demarcated solitary or multiple, round to oval erythematous patches with dusky red to brown centers, some of which may progress to bulla formation after readministration of the incriminating drug.
    - Typically, symptoms begin 30 minutes to 8 hours after reexposure to the drug.
    - After stopping the offending drug, the lesion will resolve in 2–3 weeks leaving an area of desquamation and then hyperpigmentation.
    - Drugs commonly implicated in fixed drug reactions include barbiturates, acetaminophen, NSAIDs, quinine, sulfonamides, PCNs, tetracycline, and carbamazepine.

- ○ **Contact dermatitis**: discussed in further detail in Chapter 14, is a type IV hypersensitivity reaction from exposure of a topically applied drug
- ○ **Erythema multiforme (EM)**
  - A skin eruption that is generally self-limited. Presents with a combination of macules, papules, vesicles, bullae, and target shaped lesions.
  - Lesions are predominantly on the extremities and involve the palms and soles, but rarely the scalp or face.
  - Mucosal involvement is usually limited to the oral cavity. Rash resolves in 2–4 weeks and may have residual hyperpigmentation.
  - EM is due to infections most of the time, but drugs associated with EM include NSAIDs, sulfonamides, antiepileptics, PCNs, and allopurinol.
- ○ **Stevens–Johnson syndrome**
  - Characterized by fever, mucosal involvement, and sloughing of <10% of the epidermis. Ocular involvement is common.
  - It may manifest as erythematous or violaceous patches, atypical target shaped lesions, bullae, erosions, and ulcers. The bullae usually show a positive Nikolsky sign.
  - Symptoms begin 1–3 weeks after starting the drug. Recovery can last 6 weeks. Mortality is around 10% in severe cases.
  - Discontinuing the offending drug and starting high-dose corticosteroids reduce morbidity and mortality.[14]
  - **If the putative drug is readministered, symptoms will recur and thus any drug challenge (including graded challenge) is contraindicated.**
  - Drugs that commonly cause SJS include sulfonamides, anticonvulsants including lamotrigine, barbiturates, nevirapine, piroxicam, and allopurinol.
- ○ **Toxic epidermal necrolysis**
  - TEN is life-threatening and characterized by fever, diffuse necrosis, and sloughing of >30% of epithelial surface.
  - SJS/TEN overlap involves 10–30% of epithelial surface.
  - TEN has a mortality rate of up to 40%.[15] Treating TEN with cyclosporine has been shown to be decrease mortality.[16]
  - As with SJS, **any drug challenge (including graded challenge) with the offending agent is contraindicated.**
  - Drugs associated with TEN include sulfonamides, allopurinol, barbiturates, carbamazepine, phenytoin, and NSAIDs.
- ○ **Drug reaction with eosinophilia and systemic symptoms (DRESS)**
  - Reaction typically starts 2–6 weeks after starting the offending drug.
  - Features associated with DRESS include widespread rash (can vary in appearance), eosinophilia, involvement of viscera (e.g., kidney and liver), high fever, facial edema, atypical lymphocytes, mucosal involvement that is mild, and lymphadenopathy.
  - Associated with reactivation of human herpes virus (HHV)-6 more commonly than HHV-7, cytomegalovirus (CMV), and EBV.
  - Mortality is approximately 10%.
  - Young patients can develop autoimmune diseases (e.g., thyroiditis, type 1 diabetes, hemolytic anemia) as a long-term complication, whereas elderly patients are more vulnerable to end-organ failure (e.g., kidney failure).[17]
  - Drugs associated with DRESS include allopurinol, aromatic antiepileptics, sulfonamides, olanzapine, nevirapine, vancomycin, minocycline, and dapsone.
- ○ **Acute generalized exanthematous pustulosis (AGEP)**
  - Reaction occurs hours to days after starting the offending drug.
  - Eruption of diffuse nonfollicular sterile pustules on an erythematous base
  - Begins on the face or skin folds and quickly spreads to the trunk and limbs

- Can be associated with fever and leukocytosis
- Drugs associated with AGEP include diltiazem, PCNs, quinolones, sulfonamides, hydroxychloroquine, pristinamycin, and terbinafine.

○ **Drug-induced lupus erythematosus (DILE or DIL)**
- Symptoms may not appear for months after initiating a drug.
- It is characterized by typical general lupus-like symptoms with fever, malaise, arthralgias, and pleurisy. Unlike idiopathic systemic lupus erythematosus (SLE), it is rare to have a butterfly malar rash, discoid lesions, oral ulcers, Raynaud phenomenon, alopecia, and renal or neurologic involvement.
- DIL is seen in older individuals, with males and females equally affected. It is a milder disease than SLE.
- Patients have a positive ANA or IgG anti-[(H2A-H2B)-DNA] antibodies, which include antichromatin, antinucleosome antibodies, or antihistone antibodies that can help confirm a diagnosis of DIL.
- Symptoms improve generally within days or weeks after discontinuation of therapy.
- Drugs with the highest risk of DIL are hydralazine, procainamide, quinidine, minocycline, penicillamine, isoniazid, and anti–tumor necrosis factor α (TNF-α) therapy.

○ **Drug-induced liver injury (DILI)**
- Begins 1–5 weeks after initiating drug. Liver damage may result from cholestasis or hepatocellular injury or a mixture of both.
- Patient may develop icterus, fever, rash, and eosinophilia in addition to abnormalities in the liver function tests.
- Recovery can be expected after removal of the offending drug, if irreversible cell damage has not occurred.
- Commonly offending agents for immune-mediated liver injury include amoxicillin-clavulanate, phenytoin, diclofenac, allopurinol, phenothiazines, halothane, and sulfonamides.

○ **Drug-induced acute interstitial nephritis (AIN)**
- Symptoms start days to weeks after initiating the drug. Associated with fever, rash, and eosinophilia.
- Renal involvement includes mild proteinuria, microhematuria, and eosinophiluria.
- Renal insufficiency resolves once the offending drug is removed.
- Drugs seen in AIN are β-lactams (especially methicillin), rifampin, NSAIDs, sulfonamides, captopril, allopurinol, methyldopa, anticonvulsants, cimetidine, ciprofloxacin, and proton-pump inhibitors.

○ **Drug-induced interstitial lung disease (DILD)**
- Reactions are variable and can occur days to years after treatment.
- Proposed mechanisms include an immune-mediated response by T cells.
- There are many clinical patterns, ranging from benign infiltrates to life-threatening acute respiratory distress syndrome.
- The clinical manifestations of DILD are nonspecific and include cough, fever, dyspnea, and hypoxemia.
- Discontinuation of the drug can help aid in the diagnosis, and challenging with the offending drug is not practical because the pulmonary damage caused by DILD can be irreversible.
- Drugs that can cause DILD include TNF-α inhibitors, rituximab, bleomycin, cyclophosphamide, methotrexate, minocycline, and hydroxyurea.

Diagnostic Criteria

Table 17-1 presents the clinical criteria for an allergic drug reaction.[18]

TABLE 17-1 CLINICAL CRITERIA OF ALLERGIC DRUG REACTIONS

1. Allergic reactions occur in only a small percentage of patients receiving the drug and cannot be predicted from animal studies.
2. The observed clinical manifestations do not resemble known pharmacologic actions of the drug.
3. In the absence of prior exposure to the drug, allergic symptoms rarely appear before 1 week of continuous treatment. After sensitization, even years previously, the reaction may develop rapidly on reexposure to the drug. As a rule, drugs used with impunity for several months or longer are rarely the culprits. This temporal relationship is often the most vital information in determining which of many drugs being taken needs to be considered most seriously as the cause of a suspected drug hypersensitivity reaction.
4. The reaction may resemble other established allergic reactions, such as anaphylaxis, urticaria, asthma, and serum sickness–like reactions. However, various skin rashes (particularly exanthems), fever, pulmonary infiltrates with eosinophilia, hepatitis, AIN, and lupus syndrome have been attributed to drug hypersensitivity.
5. The reaction may be reproduced by small doses of the suspected drug or other agents possessing similar or cross-reacting chemical structures.
6. Eosinophilia may be suggestive if present.
7. Rarely, drug-specific antibodies or T lymphocytes have been identified that react with the suspected drug or relevant drug metabolite.
8. As with adverse drug reactions in general, the reaction usually subsides within several days after discontinuation of the drug.

AIN, acute interstitial nephritis.

Reprinted from Ditto AM. Drug allergy: introduction, epidemiology, classification of adverse reactions, immunochemical basis, risk factors, evaluation of patients with suspected drug allergy, patient management considerations. In: Grammer LC, Greenberger PA, eds. *Patterson's Allergic Diseases.* 8th ed. Philadelphia, PA: Wolters Kluwer, 2018, with permission.

Diagnostic Testing

- Diagnostic tests for allergies are discussed in further detail in Chapter 3.
- In vitro testing consists of various laboratory tests to aid in the assessment of drug allergy.
  - **Tryptase levels** are usually elevated up to 4 hours after an anaphylactic event and are more sensitive than serum or urine histamine levels.
  - Decreases in total hemolytic complement (CH50) or C3 and C4 levels can be seen in drug reactions involving complement activation.
  - Total IgE levels are not useful for drug allergy.
  - If DRESS is suspected, evaluate for eosinophilia with complete blood count (CBC), atypical lymphocytes on peripheral smear, and liver or kidney injury with comprehensive metabolic panel (CMP). Reactivation of HHV-6/7, EBV, and CMV can be present in DRESS as well.
  - Skin biopsy can be useful to evaluate for SCARs.
  - In vitro measurement of **antigen-specific IgE** can be helpful in diagnosing drug allergy.
    - In general, measuring in vitro antigen-specific IgE is less sensitive than skin testing.
    - It requires the knowledge of which drug metabolite is immunogenic, and this is not known for many drugs.

- In vitro antigen-specific IgE has been validated for the major (penicilloyl) determinant of PCN, but not for the minor determinants.
- **The lack of an in vitro antigen-specific IgE to a drug does not rule out drug allergy.**
  - Other in vitro tests that are used in research for diagnosing drug allergy are
    - Basophil activation test (BAT) measures activation of the markers CD63 and CD203c that are on the surface of basophils after incubation with the drug.
    - Lymphocyte transformation test (LTT) can help diagnose delayed T-cell hypersensitivity as it measures T-cell proliferation when cultured with a drug.
- In vivo testing involves skin testing and test dosing the patient with the suspected drug.
  - **Prick and intradermal cutaneous tests** help to measure an IgE response by measuring a wheal-and-flare response on the skin to the drug tested.
    - HMW drugs such as antisera, egg-containing vaccines, monoclonal antibodies, latex, and toxoids can be used directly as skin testing reagents.
    - There are published nonirritating concentrations for many common drugs implicated in type I drug reactions.[19]
    - It is important for patients to abstain from using antihistamines and tricyclic antidepressants, which can interfere with the wheal-and-flare response.
    - There is a refractory period of 4–6 weeks after an episode of acute anaphylaxis where skin tests are invalid.
    - A negative test does not rule out a drug allergy.
  - **Patch testing** (discussed in Chapter 14) and **delayed intradermal testing** (read at 24 hours) can be used to assess for a type IV hypersensitivity.
  - **Graded dose challenge** (provocative test dosing)
    - Provides a direct challenge to determine whether a suspected drug caused the clinical manifestations
    - Graded challenges are generally performed when there is low probability of a true drug allergy.
    - However, this approach has the risk of a potentially serious adverse reaction and must be performed by a person with experience in managing hypersensitivity reactions.
    - In graded challenges, the dose of medication is incrementally raised until therapeutic dose is achieved. The most common approach used in clinical practice gives 10% of the dose, followed by 90% of the dose. For a history of a delayed skin reaction (not SCARs), a dose challenge can be expanded to last for days.
    - If a patient tolerates a graded challenge without any adverse reaction, the patient does not have a drug allergy to the medication. Future doses of the same medication can be administered without further testing.
    - If the risk of an adverse reaction is felt to be too high to risk a graded challenge, a drug desensitization can be performed.
    - Graded dose challenges are faster than desensitization but carry a higher risk of adverse reaction.

TREATMENT

- **Withdrawing the suspected culprit drug is the most important step in managing an ADR.**
- Most ADRs due to allergy will resolve with discontinuation of the offending agent.
- Follow practice guidelines for treatment of anaphylaxis (Chapter 4), urticaria, angioedema (Chapter 12), bronchospasm (Chapter 5), and contact dermatitis (Chapter 14).
- Serum sickness reactions can be treated with antihistamines and NSAIDs. A prednisone taper can be given for severe reactions.

TABLE 17-2	PRETREATMENT PROTOCOL FOR RADIOCONTRAST MEDIA	
	Drug and dose	
Time before the procedure (hour)	Prednisone[a]	Diphenhydramine[b]
13	50 mg PO or IV	
7	50 mg PO or IV	
1	50 mg PO or IV	50 mg PO or IV

[a]Or methylprednisolone, 40 mg IV.
[b]Or chlorpheniramine, 10–12 mg.

- SJS, drug fever, DRESS (with kidney or lung involvement), and DIL can be treated with corticosteroids.
- In TEN, corticosteroids are not effective, but cyclosporine may help decrease mortality.
- In patients with a suspected or known drug allergy, you can administer an alternative drug that does not cross-react, administer a potentially cross-reactive drug under close supervision, perform a graded dose challenge to the suspected drug, or perform a drug desensitization.
- For nonallergic reactions with immunologic manifestations, the risk of a reaction can be minimized by premedications before the drug is given. Table 17-2 provides a commonly used premedication protocol for RCM.

Drug Desensitization
- Drug desensitization allows for a temporary state of tolerance to a drug.
- Mechanisms underlying drug desensitization are not fully understood.
- This procedure has to be done under close medical observation by a trained professional. Table 17-3 provides a sample desensitization protocol.[20]
- The drug is given in 10- to 15-minute intervals for IV preparations and 20–30 minutes for oral preparations. The starting dose is $1/10,000^{th}$ or $1/1,000^{th}$ the target dose, and typically the dose is doubled until the target dose is achieved.
- Patients will be tolerant to the medication only as long as the drug continues to be given. In general, if the patient goes longer than 48 hours without a dose, then the desensitization will need to be performed again.
- β-Blockers should be withheld or tapered before procedure.
- Antihistamines are withheld prior to the procedure because they can mask early symptoms of anaphylaxis.
- The choice to perform a graded dose challenge or desensitization should be based on the assessment of an experienced clinician.
- Desensitization is contraindicated for drugs triggering SCARs and serum sickness.
- For a non–IgE-mediated reaction, pretreatment with H1 and H2 blockers, montelukast, and/or glucocorticoids can be used.

SPECIAL CONSIDERATIONS

Penicillin Allergy
- Anaphylaxis has been reported to occur in 1:100,000 with serious allergic reactions in 4.6/10,000 administrations.[21]
- About 8% of patients report having a PCN allergy.[22]

TABLE 17-3	PROTOCOL FOR ORAL PENICILLIN DESENSITIZATION	
Time (minute)	Units	Route
0	100	PO
15	200	PO
30	400	PO
45	800	PO
60	1,600	PO
75	3,200	PO
90	6,400	PO
105	12,500	PO
120	25,000	PO
135	50,000	PO
150	100,000	PO
165	200,000	PO
180	400,000	PO
195	50,000	SC
210	100,000	SC
225	200,000	SC
240	400,000	SC
255	800,000	SC
270	1,000,000	IM
285	100,000	IV
300	200,000	IV
315	400,000	IV

Adapted from Sullivan TJ, Wedner HJ. Drug allergy. In: Wedner HJ, Korenblat PE, eds. *Allergy Theory and Practice.* 2nd ed. Philadelphia, PA: WB Saunders, 1992:548.

- Hospitalized patients with a history of PCN allergy have been shown to have a longer hospital stay with increased incidence of vancomycin-resistant *Enterococcus*, methicillin-resistant *Staphylococcus aureus*, and *C. difficile* infections compared to patients without a reported PCN allergy.[23]
- About 90% patients with history of PCN allergy will be able to tolerate PCN because most patients outgrow their allergy overtime (typically after 5 years).[24] Antibiotic stewardship programs have been developed to help decrease the use of β-lactam alternatives, given the lower likelihood of having a true PCN allergy.
- PCN reactions can be stratified by time course (Table 17-4). Immediate (<1 hour) and accelerated reactions (1–72 hours) are IgE mediated.
- The most frequently reported PCN allergy is a maculopapular rash, which occurs in 2–3% of treatments. The next most common reactions include urticaria, fever, and bronchospasm.
- PCN requires conjugation with proteins to elicit an immune response, given it is a LMW drug.

TABLE 17-4 PENICILLIN REACTIONS BY TIME COURSE

Immediate (<1 hour)	Accelerated (1–72 hours)	Delayed (>72 hours)
Anaphylaxis	Urticaria	Maculopapular rash
Urticaria	Bronchospasm	Fever
Angioedema	Erythema multiforme	Serum sickness
Bronchospasm	Maculopapular rash	Recurrent myalgias or urticaria
	Serum sickness	

- **The major antigenic determinant is a penicilloyl moiety** formed by PCN covalently binding to lysine residues in serum or cell surface proteins. This occurs in approximately 93% of PCN molecules.
- The minor antigenic determinants are all remaining PCN conjugates (7%), which include PCN, penicilloate, and penilloate.
- **Skin testing**
  - The major antigenic determinant can be tested with Pre-Pen. It was withdrawn from the market in 2004 because of the lack of a manufacturer but has been Food and Drug Administration (FDA) approved again in 2009. **Pre-Pen is the only FDA-approved skin test for drug allergy.**
  - A standardized test for minor antigenic determinants is not commercially available. A fresh solution of benzylpenicillin can be used for skin testing.
  - Skin testing will not help predict the occurrence of a non–IgE-mediated reaction.
  - The predictive value of a history of PCN allergy combined with skin testing in determining PCN hypersensitivity shows that 19% of patients with a positive history will have a positive skin test. In patients with a negative history of PCN allergy, 4–7% had a positive skin test. The incidence of reaction among skin test–negative subjects is <1% when evaluating for minor antigenic determinants.[25,26]
- **Cross-reactivity**
  - The cross-reactivity between β-lactam antibiotics is variable and largely determined by their side-chain structure attached to the β-lactam nucleus.
  - **Cephalosporins** had higher cross-reactivity to PCN before 1980s because they were contaminated with small amounts of PCN.[27]
  - Risk of a cross-reaction between a PCN and cephalosporin that do not share the same side chain is <2%. Cross-reactivity between PCN and monobactams is 0%, between PCN and carbapenems is <1%, and between cephalosporins and carbapenems is <1%.[28]
  - Patients with **amoxicillin allergy** should avoid cefadroxil, cefprozil, and cefatrizine because all these drugs share same R-group side chain.
  - The monobactam **aztreonam** does share an identical R1-group side chain with ceftazidime and is cross-reactive.[29]
- **Desensitization** is performed if there is no alternative drug available and the patient has a positive skin test. Table 17-3 presents a sample PCN protocol.

Sulfonamide Allergy

- Allergies to sulfonamides are increased in patients with HIV compared to the general population. TMP–SMX hypersensitivity occurs in 5% of HIV-negative patients and in 60% of patients with HIV.[11]

- The most common reaction is a **maculopapular rash** that develops 7–12 days after initiating the drug. This may be associated with a fever. Urticaria can be seen, but anaphylaxis is rare. SJS and TEN are known to be caused by sulfonamides.
- Aromatic sulfonamides (usually antimicrobial) such as SMX, sulfadiazine, sulfisoxazole, and sulfacetamide have an aromatic amine at N4 position and a substituted ring at N1 position. This differs from other sulfonamide-containing drugs, such as thiazide diuretics and sulfonylurea antiglycemic drugs, and these two different groups of sulfonamides do not cross-react.[30]
- Sulfonamides are metabolized primarily by *N*-acetylation and secondarily by cytochrome P450 *N*-oxidation.
- **Slow acetylators are at increased risk of drug reaction** because they preferentially metabolize sulfonamide antibiotics by *N*-oxidation, resulting in reactive nitroso metabolites that cause cellular damage and react with protein to become immunogenic. This switch in metabolism is because of decreased glutathione reductase, which is also known to be diminished in HIV patients.[31]
- There are no standardized skin tests to evaluate sulfonamide drug allergy, but protocols have been reported for skin testing as well as for desensitization.

Local Anesthetics

- True allergy to local anesthetics (LAs) drugs is rare. The patient may have experienced a side effect of the epinephrine given with the LA or a vasovagal reaction.
- LAs are divided into two classes based on the structure. Table 17-5 lists LAs.
  - Group I: *p*-aminobenzoic acid (PABA)-containing LAs (esters) cross-react with one another, including benzocaine, procaine, and tetracaine.
  - Group II: Non–PABA-containing LAs (amides) do not cross-react with one another.
- If the LA causing the previous reaction is known, then choose another LA that does not cross-react.
- If the LA is unknown and the patient is to undergo a procedure, then refer to an allergist to test the LA of choice. Multiple LAs can be tested at once using dilutions of the drug with epicutaneous and intradermal testing. This is then followed by SC challenge of the drug.
- It is important not to use a preparation containing epinephrine or preservatives for skin testing. Epinephrine may cause false-negative skin tests, and parabens may cause false-positive skin tests. Patients with a previous reaction should use preservative-free preparations in the future.
- If the reported allergic reaction was delayed in onset, then patch testing can be used.

Monoclonal Antibodies

- Anaphylaxis is not common among monoclonal antibodies, but has been reported (e.g., rituximab, cetuximab, trastuzumab).

TABLE 17-5 CLASSES OF LOCAL ANESTHETICS

PABA containing	Non-PABA containing
Chloroprocaine (Nesacaine)	Bupivacaine (Marcaine)
Procaine (Novocain)	Etidocaine (Duranest)
Tetracaine (Pontocaine)	Lidocaine (Xylocaine)
	Mepivacaine (Carbocaine)
	Prilocaine (Citanest)

PABA, *p*-aminobenzoic acid.

- Hypersensitivity reactions to monoclonal antibodies can be divided into five types[32]
  - **Infusion reaction** with cytokine release from lymphocytes causing fever, chills/rigors, nausea, pain, headache, dyspnea, hypertension/hypotension. Symptoms can occur with the first infusion and will improve with subsequent infusions along with premedications.
  - **Type I IgE/non-IgE mediated** involving mast cell and basophil release with flushing, pruritus, rash, urticaria, shortness of breath, gastrointestinal symptoms, back pain, cardiovascular collapse
  - **Cytokine release** (TNF-α, interleukin [IL]-6, IL-1β) from T cells that remain persistent through subsequent infusions
  - **Mixed reactions** of type 1 IgE mediated and cytokine release with symptoms listed earlier.
  - **Type IV reactions** with delayed maculopapular rash
- Skin testing protocols are available to evaluate for a type I drug reaction, although they are not standardized.
- Drug desensitization has shown to be helpful in treating patients with type I IgE-mediated/non–IgE-mediated reactions, mixed reactions, and type IV reactions.

NSAIDs/Aspirin

- NSAIDs can induce various types of hypersensitivity reactions, including IgE-mediated and non–IgE-mediated urticaria and angioedema, fixed drug eruptions, maculopapular eruptions, contact dermatitis, and SCARs.
- Aspirin-exacerbated respiratory disease (AERD) or Samter triad consists of chronic rhinosinusitis with nasal polyps (CRSwNP), asthma, and hypersensitivity reaction to aspirin and other NSAIDs.
  - Reaction is not IgE mediated but results from the decrease in prostaglandin E_2 owing to the blockade of its production from cyclooxygenase type 1 inhibition. Aspirin can also release mediators from mast cells and eosinophils.
  - Diagnosis is made typically based on history. If there is not a clear history, then a challenge to aspirin can be performed.[33]
    - Challenges should occur only if the patient's asthma is stable and forced expiratory volume at 1 second (FEV_1) is >70% of the predicted value or <1.5 L.
    - Oral challenge consists of doubling the dose of aspirin and monitoring for 1–2 hours after each dose for a decrease of FEV_1 >20% of baseline (positive reaction) or decrease of FEV_1 <15% with no nasal or ocular symptoms (negative reaction).
    - Bronchial challenge test starts with increasing doses of lysine aspirin using a dosimeter-controlled nebulizer every 30 minutes and measuring FEV_1 10 minutes after administration with same criteria for a positive and negative reaction as earlier.
    - Nasal aspirin challenge is safer to perform because it rarely will produce systemic symptoms and can be used in patients with severe asthma. It is not as sensitive as the oral or bronchial challenge. A ketorolac or lysine-aspirin solution is delivered into the nose at increasing doses every 30 minutes. Reaction is based on symptom score, rhinomanometry, and/or acoustic rhinometry or peak nasal inspiratory flow.
  - Aspirin desensitization can help improve asthma symptoms and sense of smell as well as decrease the need for polyp surgery, use of corticosteroids, and the incidence of sinus infections.[34]
    - The protocols vary and can last 1–5 days. Most protocols aim for 650–1,300 mg of aspirin daily. If nasal symptoms are controlled after 1 month, then the aspirin is decreased to 325 mg bid. Monitor for side effects of higher doses of aspirin include gastritis.
    - Daily aspirin doses at 325 mg and greater allow for use of other NSAIDs that can be used to treat rheumatologic disorders and chronic pain.

REFERENCES

1. Johansson SG, Bieber T, Dahl R, et al. Revised nomenclature for allergy for global use: report of the nomenclature review committee of the World Allergy Organization, October 2003. *J Allergy Clin Immunol.* 2004;113:832–6.
2. Lazarou J, Pomeranz BH, Corey PN. Incidence of adverse drug reactions in hospitalized patients: a meta-analysis of prospective studies. *JAMA.* 1998;279:1200–5.
3. Solensky R, Phillips EJ. Drug allergy. In: Burks AW, Holgate ST, O'Hehir RE, et al., eds. *Middleton's Allergy Principles and Practice.* 9th ed. Philadelphia, PA: Elsevier; 2020:1261–82.
4. Jerschow E, Lin RY, Scaperotti MM, et al. Fatal anaphylaxis in the United States, 1999–2010: temporal patterns and demographic associations. *J Allergy Clin Immunol.* 2014;134(6):1318–28.
5. Koelblinger P, Dabade TS, Gustafson CJ, et al. Skin manifestations of outpatient adverse drug events in the United States: a national analysis. *J Cutan Med Surg.* 2013;17(4):269–75.
6. Pichler WJ, Adam J, Daubner B, et al. Drug hypersensitivity reactions: pathomechanism and clinical symptoms. *Med Clin North Am.* 2010;94:645–64.
7. Illing P, Vivian J, Dudek N, et al. Immune self-reactivity triggered by drug-modified HLA-peptide repertoire. *Nature.* 2012;486:554–8.
8. Adkinson NF. Risk factors for drug allergy. *J Allergy Clin Immunol.* 1984;74(4):567–72.
9. McNeil BD, Pundir P, Meeker S, et al. Identification of a mast-cell-specific receptor crucial for pseudo-allergic drug reactions. *Nature.* 2015;519:237–41.
10. Enright T, Chua-Lim A, Duda E, et al. The role of a documented allergic profile as a risk factor for radiographic contrast media reaction. *Ann Allergy.* 1989;62(4):302–5.
11. Phillips E, Mallal S. Drug hypersensitivity in HIV. *Curr Opin Allergy Clin Immunol.* 2007;7(4):324–30.
12. Bierman CW, Pierson WE, Zeitz SJ, et al. Reactions associated with ampicillin therapy. *JAMA.* 1972;220(8):1098–100.
13. Siegrist CA. Mechanisms underlying adverse reactions to vaccines. *J Comp Path.* 2007;137:S46–50.
14. Tripathi A, Ditto AM, Grammer LC, et al. Corticosteroid therapy in an additional 13 cases of Stevens-Johnson syndrome: a total series of 67 cases. *Allergy Asthma Proc.* 2000;21(2):101–5.
15. Roujeau JC, Kelly JP, Naldi L, et al. Medication use and the risk of Stevens-Johnson syndrome or toxic epidermal necrolysis. *N Engl J Med.* 1995;333:1600–7.
16. Ng QX, De Deyn MLZQ, Venkatanarayanan N, et al. A meta-analysis of cyclosporine treatment for Stevens-Johnson syndrome/toxic epidermal necrolysis. *J Inflamm Res.* 2018;11:135–42.
17. Chen YC, Chang CY, Cho YT, et al. Long-term sequelae of drug reaction with eosinophilia and systemic symptoms: a retrospective cohort study from Taiwan. *J Am Acad Dermatol.* 2013;68:459–65.
18. Ditto AM. Drug allergy: introduction, epidemiology, classification of adverse reactions, immunochemical basis, risk factors, evaluation of patients with suspected drug allergy, patient management considerations. In: Grammer LC, Greenberger PA, eds. *Patterson's Allergic Diseases.* 7th ed. Philadelphia, PA: Lippincott Williams & Wilkins, 2009:238–275.
19. Brockow K, Garvey LH, Aberer W, et al. Skin test concentrations for systemically administered drugs—an ENDA/EAACI Drug Allergy Interest Group position paper. *Allergy.* 2013;68:702–12.
20. Sullivan TJ, Wedner HJ. Drug allergy. In: *Allergy Theory and Practice.* 2nd ed. Philadelphia, PA: WB Saunders, 1992:548.
21. Johannes CB, Ziyadeh N, Seeger JD, et al. Incidence of allergic reactions associated with antibacterial use in a large, managed care organisation. *Drug Saf.* 2007;30:705–13.
22. Macy E. Penicillin and beta-lactam allergy: epidemiology and diagnosis. *Curr Allergy Asthma Rep.* 2014;14:476.
23. Macy E, Contreras R. Health care use and serious infection prevalence associated with penicillin "allergy" in hospitalized patients: a cohort study. *J Allergy Clin Immunol.* 2014;133:790–6.
24. del Real GA, Rose ME, Ramirez-Atamoros MT, et al. Penicillin skin testing in patients with a history of beta-lactam allergy. *Ann Allergy Asthma Immunol.* 2007;98:355–9.
25. Green GR, Rosenblum AH, Sweet LC. Evaluation of penicillin hypersensitivity: value of clinical history and skin testing with penicilloyl-polylysine and penicillin G. *J Allergy Clin Immunol.* 1977;60:339–45.
26. Sogn DD, Evans R, Shepherd GM, et al. Results of the National Institute of Allergy and Infectious Diseases Collaborative Clinical Trial to test the predictive value of skin testing with major and minor penicillin derivatives in hospitalized adults. *Arch Intern Med.* 1992;152:1025–32.
27. Khan DA, Solensky R. Drug allergy. *J Allergy Clin Immunol.* 2010;125(2 suppl 2):S126–37.
28. Chiriac AM, Banerji A, Gruchalla RS, et al. Controversies in drug allergy: drug allergy pathways. *J Allergy Clin Immunol Pract.* 2019;7:46–60.

29. Frumin J, Gallagher JC. Allergic cross-sensitivity between penicillin, carbapenem, and monobactam antibiotics: what are the chances? *Ann Pharmacother.* 2009;43:304–15.

30. Strom BL, Schinnar R, Apter A, et al. Absence of cross-reactivity between sulfonamide antibiotics and sulfonamide nonantibiotics. *N Engl J Med.* 2003;349:1628–35.

31. Davis CM, Shearer WT. Diagnosis and management of HIV drug hypersensitivity. *J Allergy Clin Immunol.* 2008;121:826–32.

32. Isabwe GAC, Neuer MG, de las Vecillas Sanchez L, et al. Hypersensitivity reactions to therapeutic monoclonal antibodies: phenotypes and endotypes. *J Allergy Clin Immunol.* 2018;142:159–70.

33. Nizankowska-Mogilnicka E, Bochenek G, Mastalerz L, et al. EAACI/GA2LEN guideline: aspirin provocation tests for diagnosis of aspirin hypersensitivity. *Allergy.* 2007;62:11118.

34. Berges-Gimeno MP, Simon RA, Stevenson DD. Long-term treatment with aspirin desensitization in asthmatic patients with aspirin-exacerbated respiratory disease. *J Allergy Clin Immunol.* 2003;111:180–6.

Insect Allergy

Mark Alan Pinkerton, II and Tiffany Dy

18

GENERAL PRINCIPLES

- Insects cause several types of reactions in individuals in the United States. Most stings produce a transient local reaction. A smaller subset can develop serious or life-threatening reactions.[1]
- Most stings are caused by insects in the order Hymenoptera, which includes bees, yellow jackets (YJs), wasps, hornets, and ants.
- Sting evaluations require careful history taking, a physical examination, and classification of reactions.
- Treatment depends on reaction type and can range from symptomatic treatment for local reactions to injectable epinephrine for anaphylaxis.
- In addition to lifestyle modifications and prescription of auto-injectable epinephrine, referral to an allergist-immunologist is recommended for venom immunotherapy (VIT) consideration following a severe reaction.
- This chapter focuses on allergy to stinging insects and venom-mediated reactions. Reactions to biting insects, such as mosquitoes, ticks, flies, and fleas, as well as those caused by environmental aeroallergens (e.g., cockroaches), can be found in other chapters of this book.

Definition

- Hymenoptera (Latin for membranous wings) includes insects with two pairs of wings, antennae, and an ovipositor that is used to deliver the venom. Families of interest include Apidae, Vespidae, and Formicidae.
- Apidae includes **honeybees** (HBs) and **bumblebees.**
  - Domestic HBs are usually found in commercial hives, and stings are usually occupational.
  - Wild HBs build their nests in buildings, tree hollows, or old logs. They are typically not aggressive if not around their nests.
  - When they sting, a barbed stinger with venom sac is often left behind. Because most other insects do not leave a stinger, the presence of one suggests, but is not pathognomonic of, the HB.
  - **Africanized HBs** can be found in the Southwestern states including California, Arizona, New Mexico, Texas, and Nevada. They attack in swarms and are much more aggressive than the domestic HB. Given their swarming nature, multiple stings may occur simultaneously, causing a toxic reaction.[1]
- Vespidae includes YJs, wasps, and hornets.
  - **YJs** live in the ground, wall tunnels, logs, or crevices. **They are aggressive and responsible for most reported reactions.** They do not require much provocation for stinging, particularly around food.
  - **Hornets** build large paper-mâché nests that are often found in shrubs or trees. They are also aggressive and may chase if provoked.
  - **Wasps** have smaller hives in a honeycomb shape. These can be found under eaves, patio furniture, and in shrubs.
  - All three of these insects are attracted to human food and can be found at outdoor events or around garbage.[1]

- Formicidae include fire ants and harvester ants.
  ○ **Fire ants,** particularly those in the genus *Solenopsis,* are most commonly found in the Southeastern and south-central states, but they are native to South America.
  ○ *Solenopsis invicta* venom causes a sterile pustule, which is pathognomonic for a fire ant bite.[2]
  ○ Formicidae differ from other Hymenoptera in that they are wingless and sting in a circular pattern.

Classification

- **Local reactions** are either small or large and immediate or delayed.
  ○ Typically, the area is swollen, red, and painful.
  ○ By definition, a local reaction must be contiguous with the site of the sting.
  ○ Immediate reactions occur within <4 hours.
- **Large local reactions** are defined by a diameter >10 cm with symptoms peaking in 24–48 hours.[3]
  ○ These reactions can last for 5–10 days and can be so large as to include an entire extremity.
  ○ Involved areas are contiguous.
  ○ Reactions can have associated lymphangitic streaks toward inguinal or axillary lymph nodes and can be mistaken for cellulitis.[4]
  ○ These reactions may be accompanied by fever, fatigue, and malaise.
- **Cutaneous systemic reactions** are similar to large local reactions, except they are non-contiguous (e.g., a sting to the foot with a separate reaction appearing on the hand in a noncontiguous manner). Signs are confined to the dermis and may include urticaria and angioedema.
- **Systemic reactions** include both cutaneous systemic reactions and anaphylaxis.
  ○ Multiple systems can be involved, including cardiovascular (hypotension and tachycardia), respiratory (bronchospasm, laryngeal edema, tongue swelling, or throat swelling), neurologic (seizures), and gastrointestinal (nausea, emesis, diarrhea, abdominal pain).
  ○ Anaphylaxis generally requires two or more body systems to be involved (see Chapter 4).
  ○ If bradycardia is present, a vasovagal reaction should be considered, though anaphylaxis can occasionally present with bradycardia.[5]

Epidemiology

- Systemic reactions in U.S. adults have a prevalence of approximately 3%. About 40 deaths occur in the United States each year secondary to insect stings.[1]
- Those who experience a cutaneous systemic reaction have about a 10% chance of developing a systemic reaction if restung. Subsequent reactions are most likely to be cutaneous, and fewer than 3% will have severe anaphylaxis.[1]
- Large local reactions occur more frequently and worldwide have a prevalence of 2.4–10%.
  ○ Beekeepers have a higher prevalence, up to 38%.
  ○ Those who sustain a large local reaction have a 5–15% chance of a systemic reaction if stung by the same type of insect again.[3]
- Positive serum or skin test results for venom-specific IgE are present in >20% of healthy adults; however, only 5–15% of those with asymptomatic sensitization will have a systemic reaction upon a subsequent sting.[6]
- **YJ or HB** will be positive on either skin or serum testing in 10–20% of all adults.[6] Of those evaluated for YJ or HB reaction, 30–50% will have a positive skin test to both.[7]
- **Fire ants** sting up to half of those they come in contact with each year.[8]

Pathophysiology

- Reactions to insect bites are caused by different mechanisms.
  - Most hypersensitivity reactions are mediated by venom-specific IgE antibodies.
  - Other immune reactions have also been reported, including serum sickness–like responses, neuritis, encephalitis, glomerulonephritis, and vasculitis.
  - When stung by multiple insects simultaneously, the venom may cause a **toxic reaction.**
    - These reactions may appear clinically similar to anaphylaxis and can cause death.
    - Multiple stings, particularly with Africanized HB or fire ants, can be incited by disturbing a hive or nest.[1]
  - Components of venom that produce a damaging effect, but do not necessarily induce IgE-mediated hypersensitivity, include hyaluronidase, melittin, mast cell–degranulating peptide, mastoparan-C, histamine, dopamine, norepinephrine, acetylcholine, and kinins.[3,6]
- **Venom allergens causing IgE-mediated hypersensitivity reactions consist of proteins.**
  - The major protein in **HB,** *Api mellifera,* is Api-m-1.
  - The major protein in **YJ,** *Vespula vulgaris,* is Ves-v-5.
  - The fire ant (*S. invicta*) protein Sol-i-3 is similar to Ves-v-5.[7]
- **Solenopsin is the toxic component from fire ant venom.**[9]
  - The alkaloid portion of this venom is responsible for burning, edema, and pustule formation. Laboratory tests in rodents demonstrated central nervous system (CNS) and cardiac effects when injected IV, including dizziness, seizures, and death.
  - It has been postulated that heart failure after a large number of fire ant stings could be secondary to this property of solenopsin.[8]
- Reactions to biting insects, such as mosquitoes, flies, gnats, scabies, and ticks, commonly cause papular urticaria.
  - Mosquito bites can cause large local reactions and systemic symptoms.
  - Anaphylaxis has been reported with mosquito, tick, and horse fly bites.[10]
- Cross-reactivity patterns vary depending on familial classification.
- **Vespids have significant cross-reactivity** (YJ, hornet, wasp).
  - Different species in the same genera of ants will cross-react; however, they do not have much cross-reactivity across genera (e.g., different species of fire ant [*Solenopsis*] cross-react with each other, but not with harvester ants [*Pogonomyrmex*]).
  - HBs have very limited cross-reactivity with bumblebees.[6]

Risk Factors

- Risk for systemic reaction is based on the severity of a previous reaction, type of insect allergy, and time since previous reaction.
  - The more severe the reaction, the greater the chance a subsequent reaction will also be severe.
  - For an anaphylactic reaction, if the patient is restung in the next 9 years, the risk of experiencing another anaphylactic response is 60%. Without intervention, this risk decreases to 40% if it has been 10–20 years since the previous sting.
  - HB allergy confers a higher risk of systemic reaction compared to other Hymenoptera.[6]
- Occupation and hobbies can put you at risk for stings.
  - Beekeepers have the highest risk.
  - Gardeners, campers, farmers, and horseback riders are also at increased risk.
  - Risk for a sting also increases in outdoor areas where food is present.
- Risk of systemic reaction is increased by[5]
  - Angiotensin-converting enzyme (ACE) inhibitors
  - Baseline tryptase levels >5 ng/L
  - Male sex
- Elevation of baseline tryptase is an independent risk factor for severe anaphylaxis to a sting.[11]

- An increase in baseline serum tryptase levels has been correlated with increasing age, potentially increasing the risk for severe systemic reactions in the elderly.[12]
- Patients with mastocytosis have been reported to have a higher risk for more severe reactions after stings, and up to 39% of these patients have an allergy to Hymenoptera venom.[13]
- There is higher risk of anaphylaxis if a patient had a serum sickness reaction and toxic reaction, had multiple stings at once, or had a previous sting within a few weeks.

DIAGNOSIS

- History is very important in helping to distinguish the type of insect.
- Physical characteristics of the reaction help determine future risk and what, if any, diagnostic workup needs to be pursued.
- Hymenoptera allergy is confirmed through allergen-specific IgE testing.

Clinical Presentation

History
- A key element of the history is attempting to find out **what insect** stung the patient.
  - Both the nature and location of the activity occurring at the time of sting are important.
  - Any characteristics the patient can use to describe the insect are helpful, such as size, color, or whether a stinger was left in the skin.
  - If the patient can bring in the insect, then an accurate diagnosis can be made.
- It is also important to note whether the patient actually saw an insect, or if there is an insect bite on examination. This assists in differential diagnosis, as 25% of the general population are sensitized to venom.[6]
- Other important elements of history include assessment of
  - Time from sting to reaction (**latency**)
  - **Duration** of the reaction
  - History of **previous stings** (and by what insects)
- A thorough history of the patient's activities, hobbies, and other medical problems will help tailor treatment.
- Medical comorbidities and current medications can be prognostic. For example, patients on β-blockers can have protracted anaphylaxis.

Physical Examination
- Physical examination should focus on the type of reaction (local or systemic) and severity (large local, cutaneous systemic, anaphylaxis).
- **Cardiovascular** collapse is responsible for 25% of fatalities. Important signs include flushing, tachycardia, hypotension, and vascular collapse/shock.
- **Respiratory** obstruction is responsible for 60% of fatalities. Important signs include lip, tongue, and/or throat angioedema; wheezing; stridor; and respiratory distress or failure.
- **Cutaneous** symptoms include pain and pruritus.
  - Distribution and contiguity of swelling, flushing, urticaria, and whether there is angioedema of lip, throat, or tongue should be assessed.
  - Pustules present at the bite area are pathognomonic of fire ants.
  - Size of the area of swelling and contiguity are very important in determining whether the reaction is local, large local, or systemic.
- **Gastrointestinal** symptoms include nausea and abdominal cramping. Signs include emesis and diarrhea.
- **Other general signs and symptoms** are dizziness, fainting, seizures, malaise, fever, fatigue, rashes indicative of vasculitis, joint pain, renal, mental, or sensory complaints.
- Evaluate for signs of secondary **infection** at bite site(s). Septicemia causes 2% of associated deaths.

Differential Diagnosis

- Other illnesses can be confused with an insect sting, particularly if the insect was not seen.
- Alternate diagnoses to consider include
  - Local reactions
    - Cellulitis
    - Vasculitis
    - Boils
    - Abscesses
  - Systemic reactions
    - Vasovagal reaction
    - Myocardial infarction
    - Pulmonary embolism
    - Sepsis
    - Drug reaction
    - Food allergy
    - Other cause of anaphylaxis

Diagnostic Testing

- The goal of diagnostic testing is to identify the culprit insect so that VIT may be instituted. Diagnosis involves skin testing or in vitro venom-specific serum IgE testing in special cases.
- Presence of venom-specific IgE in the absence of a history of a systemic reaction is not sufficient to make a diagnosis of venom allergy, nor is it predictive of severity of a future reaction. Approximately 27–40% of individuals in the general population will have detectable venom-specific IgE.[14]
- Further diagnostic testing to identify the type of insect is indicated in anaphylaxis, systemic cutaneous reactions, and some large local reactions.
- **Testing should be performed to all members of Hymenoptera, unless the patient can absolutely identify fire ant as the stinging insect.** If fire ant is identified, testing with venom to other stinging insects is not indicated.[1]
- Diagnostic testing typically begins with immediate hypersensitivity skin testing with positive and negative controls. **It is preferable to wait 3–6 weeks after having a reaction before skin testing is performed to prevent false-negative results.**
- **Skin-prick testing** can be performed to several insects and is preferred over in vitro venom-specific IgE testing because of its greater sensitivity.
  - In the United States, testable venom proteins include yellow hornet, white-faced hornet, YJ, wasp, and HB.
  - Whole-body extracts are used for fire ant testing rather than purified venom protein alone.[15]
  - Epicutaneous testing is performed initially, and if negative, followed by intradermal skin testing, starting at 0.001–0.01 µg/mL of venom with incremental 10-fold increases in concentrations every 20–30 minutes.
  - Testing is considered positive if a response occurs at or before 1 µg/mL of venom or 1:500 (wt/vol) for fire ant extract.
  - The size of a positive skin test does not necessarily correlate with the severity of the reaction.
- Indications for in vitro venom-specific IgE testing with ImmunoCAP include
  - Presence of strong clinical history with negative skin testing
  - Presence of severe skin conditions or dermatographism
  - Inability to discontinue use of medications that may render the skin inactive, such as antihistamines or tricyclic antidepressants
  - Inconsistent results of skin testing and clinical history

TREATMENT
Medications
Immediate Therapy for a Sting

- HB stings leave embedded stingers behind. There is variation in total amount of venom injected per sting, but most of the venom is injected in under 30 seconds. If a stinger is removed very quickly, a reaction could theoretically be minimized. However, a long search and removal of the stinger is not recommended because this may delay additional treatment.[16,17]
- Local reactions are treated symptomatically.
  - Pain relief can be obtained with cold compresses and oral analgesics.
  - Oral antihistamines may alleviate itching.
- Patients with large local reactions can also be treated with **oral antihistamines and analgesics.**
- **Oral steroids** (40–60 mg prednisone as a single dose or rapidly tapered over 2–5 days) can be prescribed if edema is spreading, limbs are not functioning properly, or edema involves the lip or face.[3,6]
- **For anaphylaxis, epinephrine is the treatment of choice.** In a life-threatening situation, there is no contraindication for epinephrine.[1]
- If the diagnosis of anaphylaxis is in question, a **serum tryptase** can be drawn within 1–3 hours after the event and followed up after the patient is stabilized. However, a normal level *does not* exclude diagnosis.
  - If anaphylaxis occurs, the patient should be monitored for at least 3–6 hours for a late-phase reaction or protracted anaphylaxis, particularly if they are taking β-blockers.
  - Glucagon may be helpful for patients taking β-blockers.[6]
- **Auto-injectable epinephrine** is available by prescription at doses of 0.3 mg administered IM or 0.15 mg administered IM. Individuals weighing >30 kg should receive 0.3 mg dosing.
- Individuals who are prescribed auto-injectable epinephrine should be educated on how to use these devices properly.

Venom Immunotherapy

- VIT is a potentially life-saving treatment for patients with systemic reactions to Hymenoptera and can decrease the risk of future systemic reactions to <5%.[1]
- VIT is composed of the venoms (or whole-body extract in the case of fire ant) to which a patient is allergic.
  - Components of VIT are determined by antigen-specific IgE testing.
  - All venoms to which a patient tests positive are generally used.
- Table 18-1 summarizes who should receive VIT.
- **VIT is indicated in patients who have had anaphylaxis and in some patients who have experienced non–life threatening, cutaneous systemic reactions, and large local reactions. Patients must demonstrate the presence of venom-specific IgE, either by skin or in vitro testing.**
- Previous recommendations advised VIT for patients >16 years of age with nonlife-threatening systemic cutaneous reactions. In 2016, practice guidelines were modified to recommend VIT only for patients with severe anaphylaxis.[18]
- Exceptions do exist if a patient desires VIT or if the patient is at high risk for frequent or multiple stings.[1]
- Patients who have cutaneous systemic reactions and large local reactions who work in an occupation or participate in hobbies with high risk for multiple or frequent stings should be considered for VIT.[7]
- **VIT is contraindicated in patients with uncontrolled asthma.**[12]
- Special consideration should be given for certain patient populations.
  - Pregnant patients
    - VIT may be continued if initiated prior to pregnancy.

TABLE 18-1	GENERAL GUIDELINES FOR VENOM IMMUNOTHERAPY	
Reaction	Result of skin test or venom-specific IgE test	Is venom immunotherapy indicated?
Local reaction (<4 inches or 10 cm in diameter, <24-hour duration)	Positive or negative	No
Large local reaction (>4 inches or 10 cm in diameter, >24-hour duration)	Positive or negative	Usually no, but exceptions made for those with frequent exposures
Nonlife-threatening, widespread cutaneous systemic reactions (generalized urticarial, angioedema, erythema, pruritus)	Positive	Usually no, but exceptions made for those with medical conditions or medications that would affect outcome of anaphylaxis, frequent exposures, or impaired quality of life
Systemic, life-threatening reaction	Positive	Yes
No history of reaction	Positive	No

- VIT should not be initiated during pregnancy secondary to risk of effect of systemic reactions on the fetus.
- Dose should be maintained and not escalated in those pregnant women who are already on VIT.
  ○ Patients requiring β-blockers or ACE inhibitors
    - The patient and physician should weigh the small risk of a systemic reaction to VIT against risk of anaphylaxis to an insect sting.
    - Alternatives to treatment with ACE inhibitors and β-blockers should be considered.
    - If there is no acceptable alternative, and both ACE inhibitors or β-blockers and VIT are indicated, consider risk vs. benefit on a case-by-case basis.
    - Patients receiving these medications during the buildup phase of VIT should be closely monitored. Consider holding these medications for 24 hours before each injection.
  ○ Patients with known mast cell disorders
    - Patients with mastocytosis are at increased risk of systemic reactions to VIT.
    - Pretreatment with omalizumab can be considered.[19]
- VIT requires multiple treatments over a prolonged period.
  ○ Injections are generally administered once weekly until a few weeks after the maintenance dose is reached (100-μg venom or 0.5 mL of 1:100 [wt/vol] fire ant extract) after which dosing is spaced to 4-week intervals.
  ○ It can take up to 28 weeks to reach maintenance, assuming there are no reactions during the buildup phase.
  ○ VIT should be continued for at least 5 years.
  ○ VIT should be continued indefinitely for patients with the following:
    - History of life-threatening reactions to venom

- HB venom allergy
- Systemic reactions to VIT
- Elevated baseline serum tryptase or systemic mastocytosis
- The decision of when to discontinue VIT is still being debated and should be a decision between the patient and the physician based on numerous factors, such as the type of insect, future risk of stings, and the type of reaction to insect sting.[1,20]
- Reactions to VIT can be local or systemic.
  - The majority are local, though 5–15% can have systemic reactions.
  - Pretreatment with oral antihistamines may help reduce all reactions.[6]
- Given the risk of severe reactions, VIT should be administered in a medical office capable of treating anaphylaxis.

Lifestyle/Risk Modification

- Day-to-day preventive measures include the following:
  - Have a professional exterminate nests in the area.
  - Watch for new nests.
  - Avoid bright or floral clothing when outside.
  - Do not walk barefoot outside.
  - If working outside, wear clothing that covers skin, including gloves, long pants/sleeves, head covering, and socks with shoes.
  - Exercise caution in high-risk areas such as attics, bushes, or picnics.
  - Keep insecticides for use if a stinging insect is identified.
- Those with a history of systemic reaction or anaphylaxis should:
  - Wear a medical alert necklace or bracelet.
  - Carry auto-injectable epinephrine.
    - It should be reinforced that this medication should be **easily available,** and if a sting occurs, its use should **not be delayed.**
    - Antihistamines are not a suitable substitute for epinephrine.
- It is prudent to discuss an emergency plan and remind patients to go to an emergency facility for monitoring if a sting occurs.
- For those who might be candidates for VIT, it is important to refer them to an allergist-immunologist for venom-specific IgE testing.[1]

REFERRAL

See Table 18-2 for indications for referral.

TABLE 18-2	INDICATIONS FOR REFERRAL TO ALLERGIST-IMMUNOLOGIST
Patients who have	
Systemic reaction to a sting (cutaneous or anaphylactic)	
Anaphylaxis with insect sting in the differential of causative factors	
A reaction that may require venom immunotherapy	
A comorbidity making anaphylaxis difficult to treat (e.g., on β-blocker)	
A need for further education on avoidance and treatment	
A specific request to see an allergist-immunologist	

MONITORING/FOLLOW-UP

- Duration of initial monitoring after a systemic reaction should be at least 3–6 hours.
- Patients with systemic reactions should be referred to an allergist-immunologist for venom-specific IgE testing.
- Patients undergoing VIT receive monitoring during injections. They receive weekly injections for several months, then monthly injections for several years.

OUTCOME/PROGNOSIS

- For patients who have reactions to insect stings, the severity of future reactions is predicted by the severity of past reactions.
- Approximately 5–10% of those with large local reactions will have a systemic reaction in the future.[7]
- Most deaths due to insect stings occur **within 4 hours** of the sting, though 10% are delayed.
- Epinephrine use is critical in a life-threatening systemic reaction.
- VIT greatly improves prognosis and decreases the risk of a systemic reaction to <5%.
- For those who have had a systemic reaction and do not receive VIT, the risk for further systemic reaction can approach 60%.[1]

REFERENCES

1. Moffitt JE, Golden DB, Reisman RE, et al. Stinging insect hypersensitivity: a practice parameter update. *J Allergy Clin Immunol.* 2004;114:869–86.
2. Hoffman DR. Ant venoms. *Curr Opin Allergy Clin Immunol.* 2010;10:342–6.
3. Severino M, Bonadonna P, Passalacqua G. Large local reactions from stinging insects: from epidemiology to management. *Curr Opin Allergy Clin Immunol.* 2009;9:334–7.
4. Golden DB. Large local reactions to insect stings. *J Allergy Clin Immunol Pract.* 2015;3:331–4
5. Demain JG, Minaei AA, Tracy JM. Anaphylaxis and insect allergy. *Curr Opin Allergy Clin Immunol.* 2010;10:318–22.
6. Golden DB. Insect allergy. In: Adkinson NF, Busse WW, Holgate ST, et al., eds. *Middleton's Allergy: Principles and Practice.* 7th ed. Philadelphia, PA: Mosby/Elsevier, 2009:1005–18.
7. Hamilton RG. Diagnosis and treatment of allergy to hymenoptera venoms. *Curr Opin Allergy Clin Immunol.* 2010;10:323–9.
8. deShazo RD. My journey to the ants. *Trans Am Clin Climatol Assoc.* 2009;120:85–95.
9. Touchard A, Aili SR, Fox EG, et al. The biochemical toxin arsenal from ant venoms. *Toxins.* 2016;8:30.
10. Lee H, Halverson S, Mackey R. Insect allergy. *Prim Care Clin Office Pract.* 2016;43:417–31.
11. Rueff F, Przybilla B, Bilo MB, et al. Predictors of severe systemic anaphylactic reactions in patients with Hymenoptera venom allergy: importance of baseline serum tryptase-a study of the European Academy of Allergology and Clinical Immunology Interest Group on Insect Venom Hypersensitivity. *J Allergy Clin Immunol.* 2009;124:1047–54.
12. Nittner-Marszalska M, Cichocka-Jarosz E. Insect sting allergy in adults: key messages for clinicians. *Pol Arch Med Wewn.* 2015;125:929–37.
13. Ollert M, Blank S. Anaphylaxis to insect venom allergens: role of molecular diagnostics. *Curr Allergy Asthma Rep.* 2015;15:26.
14. Sturm GJ, Schuster C, Kranzelbinder B, et al. Asymptomatic sensitization to Hymenoptera venom is related to total immunoglobulin E levels. *Int Arch Allergy Immunol.* 2009;148;261–4.
15. Khurana T, Bridgewater, J, Rabin R. Allergenic extracts to diagnose and treat sensitivity to insect venoms and inhaled allergens. *Ann Allergy Asthma Immunol.* 2017;118:531–6.
16. Brown TC, Tankersley MS. The sting of the honeybee: an allergic perspective. *Ann Allergy Asthma Immunol.* 2011;107:463–71.

17. Fitzgerald KT, Flood AA. Hymenoptera stings. *Clin Tech Small Anim Pract.* 2006;21:194–204.
18. Golden DB, Demain J, Freeman T, et al. Stinging insect hypersensitivity: a practice parameter update 2016. *Ann Allergy Asthma Immunol.* 2017;118(1)28–54.
19. Rueff F, Przybilla B, Bilo M, et. al. Predictors of side effects during the buildup phase of venom immunotherapy for Hymenoptera venom allergy: the importance of baseline serum tryptase. *J Allergy Clin Immunol.* 2010;126(1):105–11.e5.
20. Golden DB. Discontinuing venom immunotherapy. *Curr Opin Allergy Clin Immunol.* 2001;1:353–56.

Eosinophilia

19

Benjamin D. Solomon and Maleewan Kitcharoensakkul

GENERAL PRINCIPLES

Definition

- **Eosinophilia** is defined as an absolute peripheral blood eosinophil count >500 cells/µL (0.5×10^9 cells/L).
- Eosinophilia is often further categorized by degree:
  - Mild: 500–1,500 cells/µL
  - Moderate: 1,500–5,000 cells/µL
  - Severe: >5,000 cells/µL
- **Hypereosinophilia** is generally used to refer to eosinophilia >1,500 cells/µL.
- **Hypereosinophilic syndrome (HES)** refers specifically to a spectrum of eosinophilic disorders in which hypereosinophilia is associated with organ damage and other causes have been ruled out.

Classification

- There are several ways to classify eosinophilia, with no clear consensus. Table 19-1 lists disorders associated with eosinophilia.
- **Reactive eosinophilia** vs. **primary eosinophilic disorders**: Distinguishes eosinophilia secondary to a primary disease process from eosinophilia due to a hematologic disorder of eosinophils.
- HES has been divided into several variants, as seen in Table 19-2.[1]

Epidemiology

- Allergic diseases, especially drug reactions, are the most common etiology of eosinophilia in North America, but parasitic infection is the most common etiology globally.
- Most features of eosinophilic disorders are similar between children and adults. However, the pediatric population has a higher frequency of immunodeficiency-associated cases and more gastrointestinal (GI) and pulmonary presentations.[2]

Pathophysiology

- Eosinophils are bone marrow–derived granulocytes involved in allergic and nonallergic inflammation.
- >90% of eosinophils are located in tissues, particularly the GI tract and lymphoid tissue. Compared to the average survival in peripheral circulation of 6–12 hours, tissue survival time can reach several weeks.
- Eosinophils contain and can release large amounts of preformed cytotoxic proteins from intracellular granules, including major basic protein, eosinophil cationic protein, eosinophil peroxidase, and eosinophil-derived neurotoxin. Eosinophils can also produce superoxide, leukotrienes, and various inflammatory cytokines.
- Eosinophil growth factor cytokines include interleukin (IL)-5, IL-3, and granulocyte macrophage colony-stimulating factor (GM-CSF). Maturation is mediated by the transcription factors GATA-1 and PU.1.

TABLE 19-1 GENERAL DIFFERENTIAL OF EOSINOPHILIA

Allergic	Atopy (asthma, allergic rhinitis, atopic dermatitis) Aspirin-exacerbated respiratory disease Allergic bronchopulmonary aspergillosis
Drug reactions	Drug reaction with eosinophilia and systemic symptoms (DRESS) Acute interstitial nephritis
Neoplastic	Hypereosinophilic syndromes Reactive eosinophilia secondary to mastocytosis, malignancy
Infectious	*Schistosoma* *Strongyloides* HIV Hookworms
Immunodeficiency	Omenn syndrome Hyper-IgE syndrome Autoimmune lymphoproliferative syndrome (ALPS) Immune dysregulation, polyendocrinopathy, enteropathy, X-linked (IPEX)
Rheumatologic	Eosinophilic granulomatosis with polyangiitis (EGPA) IgG4-related disease Sarcoidosis Diffuse fasciitis with eosinophilia
Tissue specific	Gastrointestinal: eosinophilic gastrointestinal diseases Pulmonary: eosinophilic pneumonia, hypersensitivity, pneumonitis Dermatologic: Kimura syndrome

TABLE 19-2 HYPEREOSINOPHILIC SYNDROME (HES) CLASSIFICATION

Subtype	Molecular characteristics
Myeloproliferative HES	May be due to mutations in *PDGFRB, JAK2,* and *FGFR1* or a 4q12 deletion resulting in a *FIP1L1-PDGFRA* fusion protein
Lymphocytic HES	Aberrant T cells producing IL-5
Familial HES	Autosomal dominant due to 5q31–33 mutation
Organ-restricted HES	Eosinophilic gastrointestinal diseases, eosinophilic pneumonia
Specific syndromes associated with hypereosinophilia	EGPA
Idiopathic HES	Unknown

EGPA, eosinophilic granulomatosis with polyangiitis; FGFR1, fibroblast growth factor receptor 1; FIP1L1, Fip1-like1; JAK2, Janus kinase 2; PDGFRA, platelet-derived growth factor receptor α; PDGFRB, platelet-derived growth factor receptor β.

- Mechanisms of eosinophilic disease
  - Inflammation and tissue damage: Eosinophil activation results in releases of inflammatory cytokines and tissue-toxic proteins.
  - Fibrosis: Eosinophils can promote fibroblast proliferation and activation, leading to fibrosis. Seen in endocardial pathology of eosinophilic granulomatosis with polyangiitis (EGPA) and epithelial fibrosis in eosinophilic esophagitis (EoE).
  - Infiltration: An elevated tissue burden of eosinophils can directly lead to organ dysfunction. Can lead to obstructive and hypoxic disorders of the affected organs.

DIAGNOSIS

Clinical presentation

Eosinophilic disorders may affect many organ systems, as described in Table 19-3.

History
- Symptoms
  - Constitutional: Fever, chills, weight loss can be associated with malignant, infectious, or immune etiologies. Weight loss can also result from nutritional deficiencies associated with GI eosinophilia.
  - Pulmonary: Wheezing and shortness of breath are associated with asthma, infection, and immune-mediated lung diseases.
  - Cardiovascular: Shortness of breath can also be associated with heart failure in EGPA or HES.
  - Neurological: Peripheral neuropathy can be seen in EGPA or HES. Focal symptoms can occur with certain infections.
  - Dermatological: Rashes including urticaria are nonspecific and can be seen in many eosinophilic disorders.
  - GI: Dysphagia, dyspepsia, abdominal pain, and diarrhea are seen with GI tissue eosinophilia and infections.
  - Hematological: Disruption of hematopoiesis leading to cytopenic symptoms can be seen in HES.
- Travel history: crucial in the diagnosis of parasitic infections. Specific patterns of travel can help discriminate causative organisms.
- Past medical history: Eosinophilia most commonly occurs as a component of a larger disease process, and isolated eosinophilia is rarely the initial presentation of such disorders.
- Family history: Though purely hereditary eosinophilia is rare, family history is a risk factor in disease states, such as allergic diseases, immunodeficiency, and rheumatologic disorders.
- Medication history: crucial for identifying drug reactions. It is important to pay attention to supplements, over-the-counter medications, and brief medication courses (e.g., NSAIDs and antibiotics). Previous uneventful use of a medication does not exclude the possibility of a new-onset drug reaction.
- Social history: can identify occupational or home allergen exposures

Physical Examination
- HEENT (head, eye, ears, nose, throat): Otitis media, rhinitis/sinusitis, nasal polyps, and ulcers may be seen in allergic and immunologic diseases.
- Cardiac: gallops, murmurs, and signs of heart failure in HES and rheumatologic etiologies
- Pulmonary: prolonged expiratory phase or wheeze in asthma and infection
- Abdomen: splenomegaly in myeloproliferative and immune disorders
- Dermatologic: eczema, urticaria, vasculitis
- Lymphatic: lymphadenopathy in many etiologies
- Neurologic: neuropathies in HES and rheumatologic causes

TABLE 19-3	EOSINOPHILIA DIFFERENTIAL DIAGNOSIS BASED ON PRESENTING SYMPTOMS
Dermatologic	• DRESS • HES • Atopic dermatitis • Parasites • Omenn syndrome • Hyper-IgE syndrome
Pulmonary	• Asthma • AERD • Löffler syndrome • ABPA • EGPA
GI	• Schistosomiasis • *Strongyloides* • IPEX • EGIDs
Hematologic/lymphatic	• HES • Filariasis • Hyper-IgE syndrome • ALPS
Renal/GU	• AIN • EGPA • *Schistosoma*
Cardiac	• HES • EGPA
Recurrent infections	• Omenn syndrome • Hyper-IgE syndrome • WAS • HIV
Endocrine	• IPEX
CNS	• Eosinophilic meningitis • DOCK8 deficiency
MSK	• *Trichinella*

ABPA, allergic bronchopulmonary aspergillosis; AERD, aspirin-exacerbated respiratory disease; AIN, acute interstitial nephritis; ALPS, autoimmune lymphoproliferative syndrome; CNS, central nervous system; DRESS, drug reaction with eosinophilia and systemic symptoms; EGID, eosinophilic gastrointestinal disorders; EGPA, eosinophilic granulomatosis with polyangiitis; GI, gastrointestinal; GU, genitourinary; HES, hypereosinophilic syndrome; IPEX, immune dysregulation, polyendocrinopathy, enteropathy, X-linked; MSK, musculoskeletal; WAS, Wiskott–Aldrich syndrome.

Differential Diagnosis

• **Medication-induced causes**
  ○ Peripheral eosinophilia is not an uncommon laboratory finding in patients receiving antibiotics, especially penicillin, cephalosporins, and fluoroquinolones. However, most patients are asymptomatic, and the eosinophilia does not necessarily require discontinuation of the medication.[3]

- Drug reaction with eosinophilia and systemic symptoms (DRESS)
  - DRESS, also known as **drug-induced hypersensitivity syndrome**, is a multiorgan inflammatory response that may be life-threatening.
  - Common culprit drugs are anticonvulsants, antibiotics, sulfonamides, minocycline, and allopurinol.
  - Pathogenesis is likely multifactorial, including drug metabolites, specific HLA alleles, reactivation of human herpesvirus 6 (HHV-6), and immune system activation.[4]
  - Incidence is 1/5,000–10,000 exposures.[4]
  - The onset of symptoms usually occurs 2–6 weeks after initiation of culprit drugs. Common manifestations included cutaneous eruptions, fever, and visceral involvement.
  - The diagnosis of DRESS is purely clinical and based on consistent clinical symptoms, history of exposure to culprit drugs, and exclusion of other diseases. Lab results that support the diagnosis include leukocytosis, presence of atypical lymphocytes in peripheral blood, and hepatic abnormalities.[5] RegiSCAR and J-SCAR scoring systems have been developed and used in establishing the diagnosis.
  - The main treatment is removal of culprit drugs. Systemic corticosteroids may be used and frequently require a gradual dose reduction to prevent symptoms recurrences.
- **Acute interstitial nephritis**
  - Immune-mediated, tubulointerstitial injury caused by medications (antibiotics, NSAIDs, diuretics, and others), infection, and others
  - Patients typically present with nonspecific symptoms of acute renal failure.
  - The classic triad of fever, skin rash, and arthralgias has been described in acute interstitial nephritis (AIN) associated with β-lactams and cephalosporins.
  - Urinalysis may reveal proteinuria, hematuria, and eosinophiluria.[6]
- Others drug reactions associated with eosinophilia are acute generalized exanthematous pustulosis (AGEP), hypersensitivity myocarditis, drug-induced hepatitis, and drug-induced gastroenterocolitis.
- **Allergic Diseases**
  - **Asthma** (see Chapter 5 for further details)
    - Clinical and molecular subtyping of asthma is an area of ongoing investigation. However, eosinophilic asthma with airway eosinophilia is often recognized as a unique category of asthma.[7]
    - Airway eosinophilia is associated with increased airway remodeling, basement membrane thickening, and smooth muscle hypertrophy.
    - A small proportion (<20%) of all asthma patients exhibit peripheral eosinophilia.[8]
    - Eosinophilic asthma can be associated with severe features despite maximal inhaled corticosteroid (ICS) therapy, with increased hospitalization frequency, likelihood of intubation, and mortality.[9]
    - Eosinophilic asthma is usually defined by a sputum eosinophil frequency of >1%, but sputum analysis is not routinely recommended owing to difficulty with reliability.[10]
    - Peripheral eosinophilia and FeNO may moderately predict airway eosinophilic airway inflammation, but less reliably predict asthma severity.[7]
  - **Aspirin-exacerbated respiratory disease (AERD)**
    - AERD is a non–IgE-dependent sensitivity to cyclooxygenase 1 (COX-1) inhibitors, including aspirin.
    - The mechanism is unclear but may result from overproduction of cysteinyl leukotrienes and underproduction of prostaglandin E2 as a result of COX-1 antagonism.
    - The overall prevalence is <2.5%, but this increases to nearly 15% in those with severe asthma.

- Clinical history includes the combination of asthma and rhinosinusitis with nasal polyposis in the setting of aspirin and COX-1 inhibitor use. Acute symptoms can occur minutes to hours after ingestion and are often dose dependent.[11]
- Asthma can be severe and treatment refractory.
- Nasal polyps can grow aggressively and frequently recur.
- Up to 7% of patients experience life-threatening eosinophilia-associated coronary artery vasospasm, presenting as chest pain.[12]
- Provocation challenge with COX-1 inhibitors is the gold standard of diagnosis.
- Peripheral eosinophilia is seen in approximately one-third of patients.[13]
- Presentation can resemble eosinophilic asthma, and polyposis can be confused for chronic sinusitis.
- Treatment includes avoidance of COX-1 inhibitors, use of leukotriene inhibitors (montelukast), 5-lypoxygenase (5LO) inhibitors (zileuton), and oral corticosteroids, and desensitization protocols to COX-1 inhibitors. Dupilumab may also be used to treat asthma and nasal polyposis. Anti-IL5 therapies can also be used to treat asthma in these patients.
  ○ **Atopic dermatitis** (see Chapter 13 for further details)
    - Nearly all patients show tissue eosinophilia and peripheral eosinophilia that correlate with disease severity.
    - Evaluation of eosinophilia does not routinely factor into diagnosis or treatment, and therapies targeting eosinophils have not been effective.[14]
  ○ **Allergic rhinitis** (see Chapter 9 for further details)
    - Eosinophilia is seen in allergic rhinitis (AR), nonallergic rhinitis with eosinophilia syndrome (NARES), and chronic rhinosinusitis.
    - Many patients have peripheral and mucosal eosinophilia, which increases with concomitant asthma.[15]
  ○ **Allergic bronchopulmonary aspergillosis (ABPA)**
    - This hypersensitivity to *Aspergillus*, seen primarily in asthma and cystic fibrosis patients, presents as recurrent exacerbations of respiratory symptoms refractory to standard therapy.
    - **APA is a result of colonization with *Aspergillus*, not active infection.**
    - In severe cases, patients can develop mucous plugs, hemoptysis, and pulmonary fibrosis.
    - Diagnosis is based on a combination of history, radiologic features, and *Aspergillus* sensitivity.
    - Systemic steroids are first-line therapy, with antifungal azoles generally reserved for those who are unable to taper corticosteroids.[16]
- **Infectious Diseases**
  ○ **Outside North America and Europe, helminth infections are the most common cause of peripheral eosinophilia.**
  ○ Only 5% of recent travelers seeking medical care present with eosinophilia, whereas up to 27% of immigrants present with eosinophilia.[17,18]
    - In travelers, the most identified causes of eosinophilia are *Schistosoma* (6%), hookworm (3%), and *Strongyloides* (2%).[17]
    - In recent immigrants, the most identified causes of eosinophilia are filariasis (53%), *Strongyloides* (47%), and *Schistosoma* (29%).[18]
  ○ Most cases of eosinophilia secondary to infection are asymptomatic.
  ○ Dermatologic, GI, and pulmonary symptoms are the most common manifestation of eosinophilic infections (Table 19-4).
  ○ Travel history can be particularly useful in differential diagnosis (Table 19-5).
  ○ ***Schistosoma* spp.**

TABLE 19-4	DIFFERENTIAL DIAGNOSIS OF PARASITIC INFECTION BY SYSTEM
GI	• *Schistosoma* • Hookworms • *Strongyloides* • *Echinococcus* • *Ascaris*

Pulmonary	• ABPA
	• Löffler syndrome
	  • Hookworm
	  • *Strongyloides*
	  • *Ascaris*
	• *Coccidioides*

Skin	• Hookworms • Cutaneous larva migrans • *Strongyloides* • *Coccidioides*
MSK	• *Trichinella* • *Coccidioides*
GU	• *Schistosoma haematobium*
CNS	• *Angiostrongyliasis* • *Gnathostomiasis* • *Baylisascaris* • *Schistosoma* • *Coccidioides*

CNS, central nervous system; GI, gastrointestinal; GU, genitourinary; MSK, musculoskeletal.

TABLE 19-5	OMENN SYNDROME CRITERIA

- Generalized skin rash
- Absence of maternal engraftment
- CD3 T cells >300/µL
- T-cell proliferation to antigen <30% of normal *or* 4 of the following, including at least one marked (*):
  - (*) Oligoclonal T cells
  - (*) >80% of T cells are CD45RO+
  - (*) T-cell proliferation to mitogen <30% of normal
  - (*) T-cell proliferation to mixed leukocyte reaction <30% of normal
  - (*) Mutation in SCID-causing gene
  - Hepatomegaly
  - Splenomegaly
  - Lymphadenopathy
  - Elevated IgE
  - Increase in absolute eosinophil count

- Presentation may include swimmer's itch, acute febrile illness, urinary symptoms, or chronic intestinal or hepatosplenic infection.
- Half of individuals infected with a *Schistosoma* spp. will develop mild eosinophilia.[19] Nearly all patients with acute schistosomiasis will develop moderate-to-severe eosinophilia.[20]
- Serology is the most sensitive screening test. Stool microscopy and serum molecular testing can be used to support the diagnosis and quantify parasite burden.

○ *Strongyloides*
- An occasional cause of eosinophilia in recent travelers, but more common in immigrants with eosinophilia (48 vs. 10%)[21]
- In North America, the infection is associated with socioeconomically disadvantaged, institutionalized, and rural populations.
- Symptoms
  □ Most infections are asymptomatic. Peripheral eosinophilia may be the only abnormality.
  □ Common GI symptoms include abdominal pain, vomiting, diarrhea, and malabsorption.
  □ Intradermal migration of larvae can result in serpiginous, pruritic tracts on the skin.
  □ **Löffler syndrome**: pulmonary migration of larvae with dry cough, wheeze, and hemoptysis. Can also be caused by hookworms and *Ascaris*.
  □ Hyperinfection syndrome: life-threatening sepsis from larval dissemination in immunosuppressed patients, most commonly because of corticosteroids
- Nearly all patients develop peripheral eosinophilia.[17]
- Serologic and stool polymerase chain reaction (PCR) assays have the highest sensitivity, but other helminth infections can cause false-positive results.[22]
- Two doses of ivermectin spaced 3–4 weeks apart can result in pathogen clearance in nearly all individuals.[22]

○ **Hookworm and cutaneous larva migrans**
- "Hookworm" most commonly refers to the human hookworms, *Ancylostoma duodenale* or *Necator americanus*.
- Symptoms
  □ Dermatologic symptoms: focal, pruritic, maculopapular rash at the site of larval penetration. **Cutaneous larva migrans** specifically refers to serpiginous, highly pruritic lesions associated with animal hookworm species.
  □ GI symptoms include abdominal pain, vomiting, and diarrhea. Local tissue damage can lead to GI bleeding, anemia, and malabsorption.
- Most human hookworm infections present with a high degree of eosinophilia (>3,000/μL).[17]
- Diagnosed by stool microscopy
- Unlike other hookworm infections, cutaneous larva migrans can be treated with a one-time dose of ivermectin.[23]

○ **Filariasis: *Wuchereria bancrofti* and *Brugia* spp.**
- Asymptomatic infection is found in 2% of return travelers with eosinophilia.[17]
- Filaria are transmitted between human hosts by *Aedes* and *Mansonia* mosquitoes.
- May present with lymphatic filariasis ("elephantiasis"): dramatic proximal extremity edema or scrotal swelling with painful lymphadenopathy. Less commonly presents with tropical pulmonary eosinophilia, which is asthma-like with nocturnal cough and wheezing, occurring in <1% of infected individuals.
- Most patients present with eosinophilia, but those with pulmonary infection nearly all present with eosinophil count >3,000 cells/μL.[24]

- Antigen testing is the most sensitive test.
- Both lymphatic and pulmonary symptoms respond to diethylcarbamazine (DEC).[25]
- Onchocerciasis and Loa loa infection must be excluded because DEC can precipitate infection, leading to blindness and encephalopathy, respectively.
- Addition of steroids can be helpful for pulmonary symptoms, but *Strongyloides* must be excluded.
  ○ **Others**
    - *Ascaris*: related to hookworms with a similar distribution. Less common infection, but most common cause of Löffler syndrome. Approximately half of infected individuals develop eosinophilia.[26] Typical treatment involves 3 days of albendazole.
    - *Trichinella*: acquired from ingestion of encysted larvae in undercooked meat. Contaminated pork is most common, but also seen in meat from wild game. Notably presents with myalgia, fever, and periorbital/fascial edema. Eosinophilia is nearly always present. Frequent creatine phosphokinase (CPK) and lactate dehydrogenase (LDH) elevation. Confirmed by serology, while muscle biopsy is reserved for diagnostic uncertainty. Mild cases are self-limiting. Severe infections may require albendazole.[27]
    - *Echinococcus*: transmitted by ingestion of material contaminated with feces of infected dogs. Infection can remain dormant as cysts for years. Liver involvement most common with biliary obstruction, pancreatitis, and portal hypertension. Pulmonary symptoms also frequent with cough, chest pain, and hemoptysis. Rupture of cysts can result in anaphylaxis. Eosinophilia is due to intermittent cyst leakage and thus infrequently detected. Treatment involves albendazole, cyst aspiration, and resection.[28]
    - *Coccidioides*: fungal infection seen primarily in Southwestern United States and is often subclinical. Primarily presents as pneumonia, but it can develop constitutional symptoms, arthralgias, erythema nodosum, and erythema multiforme. Eosinophilia is seen in up to 30% of patients and should heighten suspicion in otherwise typical appearing pneumonia.[33] Serological screening is most sensitive but may be negative early on, requiring fungal culture for diagnosis. Most cases self-resolve. For patients with systemic symptoms, azoles and amphotericin may be warranted.
    - HIV: 10–30% of HIV patients can develop eosinophilia, particularly in those with low CD4 counts. Parasitic coinfection is identified only in a minority. Eosinophilia correlates with increased frequency of cutaneous symptoms.[29]
    - Eosinophilic meningitis: defined as ≥10 eosinophils/μL of cerebrospinal fluid (CSF) or eosinophils ≥10% of central nervous system (CNS) leukocytes. Rare and almost all cases due to infection. The most common organisms are *Angiostrongyliasis*, *Gnathostomiasis*, *Baylisascaris*, but many others have been documented. Often acquired through undercooked meat. Angiostrongyliasis causes vague CNS symptoms including headache, neck pain, and vomiting, but without fever. Gnathostomiasis and *Baylisascaris* are more likely to produce focal symptoms including seizures, paresthesias, and paralysis, with positive CNS imaging. Infectious causes of eosinophilic meningitis almost always have peripheral eosinophilia as well. Diagnosis and treatment vary based on etiology.[30,31]
- **Eosinophilia in Immunodeficiency**
  ○ Immunodeficiencies, particularly those with eosinophilia, are more likely to present during childhood.[32]
  ○ The degree of eosinophilia does not help distinguish different primary immunodeficiencies (PIDs). Absolute eosinophilia count (AEC) can vary substantially within a single PID. However, Omenn syndrome and hyper-IgE syndrome (HIES) have the most documented cases with severe eosinophilia.
  ○ **Hyper-IgE syndromes**
    - Typically present with eczema and recurrent infections with elevated serum IgE levels (general >1,000 IU/mL)

- Dermatitis and infections can present during infancy, whereas structural abnormalities continue to develop through adulthood.
- Autosomal dominant (AD-HIES, formerly Job syndrome): *STAT3* deficiency. Most common form.[33] Unique presentation features include
  - Cutaneous manifestations: eczema, newborn rash
  - Recurrent infections: skin abscesses, pneumonia/pneumatoceles, thrush. Predominantly *Staphylococcus aureus*, though frequent fungal infections.
  - Connective tissue abnormalities: facial features including broad nasal bridge, "coarse/doughy" facies, retained primary teeth, scoliosis, and pathologic fractures.
- Autosomal recessive (AR-HIES): includes *DOCK8* deficiency and more rarely, *TYK2*, *PGM3*, or *SPINK5* deficiency.[34] Unique presentation features include
  - Susceptibility to viral skin infection: molluscum contagiosum warts, herpes zoster, and recurrent herpes simplex infections
  - Neurologic complications: viral meningitis and progressive multifocal leukoencephalopathy
  - Autoimmunity: hemolytic anemia and vasculitis
  - Atopy: environmental and food allergies, in addition to eczema
  - Lack of skeletal or dental abnormalities, absence of pneumatoceles
- Diagnosis
  - National Institutes of Health (NIH) HIES scoring system can aid in the diagnosis of AD-HIES. Initially created for patients with a family history and AD-HIES–type presentation. Weighted scores specific for DOCK8 or STAT3 deficiency are available.[35,36]
  - Laboratory abnormalities may include elevated IgE, eosinophilia, and decreased $CD45RO^+$ memory T cells, $CD27^+$ memory B cells, and T_H17 cells.
  - Eosinophilia is present in almost all patients.[33]
  - Definitive diagnosis requires genetic testing.
- Treatment
  - Primary treatment involves screening and management of disease manifestations, including skin infections, atopy, and malignancy.
  - Prophylaxis for staphylococcal skin infections can decrease risk of severe infections.
  - Screening for AR-HIES can include testing for herpes simplex virus (HSV), cytomegalovirus (CMV), and Epstein–Barr virus (EBV).
  - Definitive treatment for AR-HIES is bone marrow transplantation, which has generally been ineffective for AD-HIES.[33]

○ **Omenn syndrome**
- Subset of "leaky" severe combined immunodeficiency disease (SCID), resulting in expansion of autoreactive, oligoclonal lymphocyte populations (see Chapter 21 for further details)
- Almost all mutations affect VDJ recombination. Most commonly involve RAG1 and RAG2. Natural killer (NK) cell involvement is uncommon.
- Features that distinguish Omenn syndrome from classic SCID include generalized erythroderma, lymphadenopathy, and hepatosplenomegaly.
- Diagnostic criteria are seen in Table 19-5.[37,38]

○ **Autoimmune lymphoproliferative syndrome (ALPS)**
- Mutations in Fas (TNFRSF6), Fas ligand, or CASP10 lead to uncontrolled immune activation because of impaired lymphocyte apoptosis.[39] This presents with chronic lymphadenopathy and splenomegaly, multilineage cytopenias due to sequestration and autoimmune destruction, and a 50-fold risk of lymphoma.[40]
- As of 2011, over 500 cases have been reported.[41]
- Diagnostic criteria are seen in Table 19-6.[42] Eosinophilia is present in 16% of patients and correlates with an increased need for splenectomy, severe infections, and mortality.

TABLE 19-6 2009 ALPS WORKSHOP CRITERIA

Definitive diagnosis: Both required criteria plus one primary accessory criterion
Probable diagnosis: Both required criteria plus one secondary accessory criterion

Required criteria
- Chronic lymphadenopathy/splenomegaly for >6 months, noninfectious, nonmalignant
- Blood CD3$^+$ TCRαβ$^+$ CD4$^-$CD8$^-$ T cells >1.5% of all lymphocytes or >2.5% of all CD3$^+$ cells

Primary accessory criteria
- Defective lymphocyte apoptosis in ×2 assays
- Somatic or germline mutations in *FAS, FASLG,* or *CASP10*

Secondary accessory criteria
- Serum FASL >200 pg/mL
- IL-10 >20 pg/mL
- Vitamin B12 >1,500 ng/L
- IL-18 >500 pg/mL
- Autoimmune cytopenia with hypogammaglobulinemia
- Consistent histopathology
- Family history of noninfectious, nonmalignant lymphadenopathy

ALPS, autoimmune lymphoproliferative syndrome; IL, interleukin; TCR, T-cell receptor.

Adapted from Oliveira JB, Bleesing JJ, Dianzani U, et al. Revised diagnostic criteria and classification for the autoimmune lymphoproliferative syndrome (ALPS): report from the 2009 NIH International Workshop. *Blood.* 2010;116:e35–40.

- Control of cytopenia and lymphoma surveillance are the core components of management.[41] Cytopenias refractory to steroids may respond to mycophenolate mofetil, sirolimus, or rituximab.
- The utility of serial imaging for lymphoma surveillance is currently unsettled.
- Splenectomy is avoided because of disease recurrence and high rates of sepsis compared to even the general postsplenectomy patient.

○ **Immune Dysregulation, Polyendocrinopathy, Enteropathy, X-linked (IPEX)**
- This extremely rare, potentially fatal X-linked recessive disorder is caused by mutations in *FOXP3*, the master transcription factor of immunosuppressive regulatory T cells (Tregs).
- IPEX presents in male infants with a classic triad of intractable diarrhea, type 1 diabetes, and eczema. Severe diarrhea is the most common presenting feature and develops in almost all individuals, often resulting in failure to thrive.[43] Additional autoimmune manifestations include thyroiditis, hemolytic anemia, nephropathy, and hepatitis.
- Eosinophilia is present in nearly all patients. Definitive diagnosis requires gene sequencing.
- Treatment involves immunosuppressive agents, including glucocorticoids, calcineurin inhibitors, and sirolimus, with consideration for hematopoietic stem cell transplant.[44]

○ **Wiskott–Aldrich Syndrome (WAS)**
- Classic triad of severe eczema, thrombocytopenia, and recurrent pyrogenic infections
- Caused by mutations in WAS, leading to defect in cytoskeletal polymerization

- ○ **Loeys–Dietz Syndrome**
  - Presentation is similar to AD-HIES with atopy, elevated IgE, and musculoskeletal abnormalities. Unique vascular abnormalities including aneurysms and tortuosity.
  - Caused by mutations in transforming growth factor (TGF)-β signaling pathway, leading to connective tissue abnormalities and lymphocyte dysfunction
  - Eosinophilia can be associated with eosinophilic gastrointestinal disorders (EGIDs).
- **Rheumatologic causes of eosinophilia**
  - ○ **Eosinophilic granulomatosis with polyangiitis (EGPA, formerly Churg–Strauss)**
    - Vasculitis of small- and medium-sized vessels diagnosed at mean age of 40 years, with proposed diagnostic criteria in Table 19-7.[45]
    - Atopy and sinopulmonary disease: asthma seen in 90% of patients and can precede EGPA diagnosis by 4–9 years. Can also present with AR and nasal polyps.
    - Parenchymal lung disease: fleeting peripheral pulmonary infiltrates and alveolar hemorrhage
    - Vasculitis: can result in purpura, nodules, ulcerating lesions, and livedo reticularis from skin involvement and motor and sensory neuropathies due to involvement of peripheral nerves
    - Renal: segmental, necrotizing, crescentic glomerulonephropathy without immune complex deposition. Indistinguishable from that seen in granulomatosis with polyangiitis (GPA) and microscopic polyangiitis (MPA).
    - Cardiac: cardiomyopathy, myocarditis, pericarditis, endocarditis, and valvulitis. Represents the main cause of patient mortality. Patients with cardiac manifestations have higher peripheral eosinophilia (9,000 vs. 3,000 cells/μL).[46]
    - **Antineutrophil cytoplasmic antibody (ANCA) is only found in a minority of patients.**
    - Differential
      - □ AERD: Lung infiltrates and systemic manifestations are uncommon.
      - □ GPA and MPA vasculitis: Asthma and eosinophilia are uncommon.
    - Glucocorticoids are often sufficient to achieve remission. Steroid-sparing agents, including cyclophosphamide, azathioprine, and methotrexate, are warranted to maintain remission in patients with organ-threatening disease.[47] Mepolizumab may result in decreased relapse frequency.[48]

TABLE 19-7	**1990 AMERICAN COLLEGE OF RHEUMATOLOGY EGPA DIAGNOSTIC CRITERIA**

Criteria
- Asthma
- Peripheral eosinophilia >10%
- Neuropathy
- Transient pulmonary infiltrates
- Paranasal sinus disease
- Extravascular eosinophilia

Diagnostic probability
- Presence of ≥4 criteria has sensitivity of 85% and specificity of 99.7%

EGPA, eosinophilic granulomatosis with polyangiitis.
Modified from Masi AT, Hunder GG, Lie JT, et al. The American College of Rheumatology 1990 criteria for the classification of Churg-Strauss syndrome (allergic granulomatosis and angiitis). *Arthritis Rheum.* 1990;33:1094–100.

○ **IgG4-related disease (IgG4RD)**

- IgG4RD involves systemic, multisystem, fibrotic inflammation with infiltrating IgG4+ plasma cells. Relevance of IgG4 to pathogenesis is unclear.
- Prevalence is 2.2/100,000, predominantly affecting adult males.
- Initial presentation is often a subacute mass or enlargement of one or more organs. Systemic symptoms are typically absent. IgG4RD can affect any organ system, most commonly the pancreas, salivary/lacrimal glands, lymph nodes, biliary tree, and kidney.[49]
- Evaluation includes serum immunoglobulin levels, imaging for evidence of organ involvement, and biopsy confirmation.
  □ IgG4 is frequently elevated, but not diagnostic; >135 mg/dL has 90% sensitivity and 60% specificity, >270 mg/dL has 35% sensitivity and 91% specificity.[50]
  □ Eosinophilia (>500 cells/μL) is seen in 38% of patients.[51]
- Glucocorticoids are first-line treatment and result in partial to full remission in 89% of patients.[50] Rituximab may be useful for patients who fail steroids.

○ **Diffuse fasciitis with eosinophilia (formerly Shulman disease)**

- This extremely rare disease involves abrupt-onset skin erythema and swelling. Can progress to *peau d'orange* with pitting edema and depressed veins ("groove" sign). Skin manifestations are typically symmetric and localized to the extremities.[52]
- Additional symptoms include inflammatory polyarthritis, myalgia, weakness, weight loss, and carpal tunnel.
- Long-term complications can include joint contractures (e.g., "prayer" sign) and restrictive lung disease.
- Peripheral eosinophilia is seen in 60–90% of patients.[53] Inflammatory markers are often elevated. Aldolase is often elevated, while creatine kinase (CK) remains normal.
- Differential
  □ Systemic sclerosis: Sclerodactyly, telangiectasia, and Raynaud phenomenon are unique to systemic sclerosis.
  □ Toxic oil syndrome and eosinophilia-myalgia syndrome: very rare and suggested by epidemiology
  □ Nephrogenic systemic fibrosis: rare adverse reaction to gadolinium-based MRI contrast in patients with renal failure
- Glucocorticoids result in partial or complete remission in the majority of patients.[53]
- Combination of methotrexate and glucocorticoids results in higher portion of complete remission.

○ **Sarcoidosis**

- Sarcoidosis is a multisystem, noncaseating granulomatous disorder.
- Prevalence is 10–20/100,000 individuals, highest in black Americans.
- Almost half of patients present asymptomatically with incidental radiologic findings.[54] Common presenting symptoms include cough, dyspnea, and chest pain.
- Extrapulmonary symptoms, seen in one-third of patients, include uveitis, arthralgia and myalgia, splenomegaly, lymphadenopathy, and nonspecific skin lesions. **Löfgren syndrome** is the specific combination of hilar lymphadenopathy, arthritis, and erythema nodosum and carries a good prognosis.
- Sarcoidosis is diagnosed by unique radiologic findings and other laboratory abnormalities, including
  □ Bilateral hilar lymphadenopathy or reticular opacities
  □ Involvement of at least one additional organ system
  □ Exclusion of alternative etiologies
- In equivocal cases, evidence of noncaseating granulomas on tissue biopsy is required.

- Elevated angiotensin-converting enzyme (ACE) levels and hypercalcemia/hypercalciuria are nonspecific findings, but frequently seen in patients.
- Up to 41% of patients display peripheral eosinophilia.[55]
- Differential diagnosis
  - Infectious lung disease: similarly present as a granulomatous lung disease. Histology must include acid-fast staining to rule out.
  - EGPA and GPA: can also present with granulomatous lung pathology. However, sarcoidosis rarely presents with atopy or positive ANCA titers.
  - Pneumoconiosis: can present with similar restrictive lung disease and reticular opacities on radiology. Can be distinguished by a careful social history.
- Steroids improve symptoms but do not affect pulmonary function or disease progression. For refractory disease, methotrexate, azathioprine, mycophenolate mofetil, cyclophosphamide, and anti–TNF-α agents can be effective.
  - **Others**
    - Systemic lupus erythematosus (SLE), Sjögren syndrome: Although not a defining feature, these connective tissue disorders can present with mild eosinophilia.
    - Eosinophilic myositis: rare disease spectrum with muscle pain, weakness, and swelling accompanied by tissue and, possibly, peripheral eosinophilia
    - Toxic oil syndrome: rare syndrome associated with a 1981 outbreak in Spain due to consumption of contaminated rapeseed oil intended for industrial use. There have been no additional cases since the original event.[56]
    - Eosinophilia–myalgia syndrome: rare syndrome associated with 1989 outbreak due to consumption of contaminated L-tryptophan supplements in the United States. Isolated cases have since occurred.[57]
- **Gastrointestinal disorders with eosinophilia**
  - EGIDs are **characterized** by a primary tissue eosinophilia of the GI tract and are classified by the anatomical region affected.
  - Except for the esophagus, eosinophils are normally present in healthy intestinal mucosa.
  - Normal tissue eosinophil values are not consistent, and there is debate regarding diagnostic cutoff values.
  - **Eosinophilic esophagitis (EoE)** (see Chapter 16 for further details)
    - Up to 50% of patients demonstrate peripheral eosinophilia of >300 cells/μL.[58]
    - Diagnosis requires tissue eosinophilia of >15 cells per high-power field.
    - Differential diagnosis
      - Gastroesophageal reflux disease (GERD): must be excluded. More likely to respond to proton-pump inhibitors (PPIs) and less likely to present with food impaction and atopy.
      - Crohn disease (CD): Esophageal manifestations are rare.
  - **Other EGIDs: eosinophilic gastritis (EG), eosinophilic gastroenteritis (EGE), and eosinophilic colitis (EC)** (see Chapter 16 for further details)
    - 80% of patients demonstrate at least mild peripheral eosinophilia.[59]
    - All EGIDs are diagnoses of exclusion requiring biopsy evidence of tissue eosinophilia. Consensus threshold values are lacking, but it is generally recognized that eosinophil numbers increase along the length of the GI tract.
  - **Other GI disorders associated with eosinophilia**
    - Celiac disease: Tissue eosinophilia on biopsy is associated with higher histological staging of celiac disease.[60]
    - Inflammatory bowel disease: Peripheral blood eosinophilia of >400 cells/μL occurs in 20–40% of patients and correlates with more severe disease, including higher rates of steroid usage, hospitalization, and surgical management.[61]

- **Hypereosinophilic syndrome (HES)**
  - There are six variants of HES, with molecular characteristics described in Table 19-2.[1,62]
  - **Etiology:** The etiology of HES is broad, including both reactive and primary clonal disorders. Reactive eosinophilia is usually caused by increased production of eosinopoietic cytokines, mostly IL-5, IL-3, and GM-CSF.
    - **Myeloproliferative (M-HES):** 10–14% of HES patients have clonal eosinophilia from an abnormal fusion of Fip1-like1 (*FIP1L1*) and platelet-derived growth factor receptor α (*PDGFRA*), or *FIPL1-PDGFR* (*F/P*). The *F/P* fusion protein results in production of a constitutively active tyrosine kinase, modifying hematopoietic stem cells, and leading to eosinophilia. Other variants associated with M-HES included *PDGFRB, PDGFRA, FGFR1,* and *PCM1-JAK2* rearrangements. The M-HES can be further classified to *PDGFRA*-associated chronic eosinophilic leukemia (CEL), CEL-NOS, and HES with myeloproliferative features but unproven clonality.[63]
    - **Lymphocytic (L-HES):** Patients develop aberrant T-cell populations that generate at least one eosinophil hematopoietin, resulting in marked peripheral eosinophilia.
    - **Overlap or organ-restricted HES**: This HES variant consists of organ-specific eosinophilic disorders associated with peripheral eosinophilia. The etiology depends on the distinct diagnosis such as EGID and eosinophilic pneumonia.
    - **Associated HES**: AEC >1,500 cells/μL associated with other conditions as described in previous sections. The etiology depends on the underlying conditions.
    - **Familial HES**: extremely rare, autosomal dominant condition
    - **Idiopathic HES**: symptomatic patients with negative workup for etiologies
  - **Epidemiology**
    - The incidence and prevalence of HES are not well characterized.[64]
    - Approximately 20% of patients with HES have features suggestive of M-HES. The M-HES subtype is more common in males aged 20–40 years.[65]
    - There is no gender predilection in L-HES.
  - **Presentation**
    - Common symptoms of HES include weakness, fatigue, cough, dyspnea, myalgias, angioedema, rashes, fever, and rhinitis.
    - The presentations of M-HES and L-HES are summarized in Table 19-8.
    - Episodic angioedema and eosinophilia (Gleich syndrome) is a subset of L-HES. Patients present with cyclic episodes of angioedema and urticaria occurring every 28–32 days.
    - Symptoms and signs of patients with overlap and associated HES variants vary based on the underlying disease.
  - **Distinct diagnostic features**
    - Patients with unexplained hypereosinophilia with organ involvement should undergo further evaluation for underlying conditions and exclusion of leukemia, as listed previously, including bone marrow aspiration and biopsy, molecular testing for *FIP1L1-PDGRFRA* mutations and *JAK2* abnormalities, and flow cytometry for T-lymphocyte phenotyping.[66] These steps require hematology consultation.
    - Laboratory findings differentiating M-HES and L-HES are listed in Table 19-8.
  - **Distinct treatment features**
    - Initial treatment with corticosteroids, 1 mg/kg prednisone to 1 g of methylprednisolone should be considered in patients with cardiac, neurologic or thromboembolic complications, and/or presence of extremely high AEC. The initial dose depends on the severity of the clinical manifestations. Consider administering ivermectin concomitantly to patients with a history of exposure to *Strongyloides* to prevent potentially fatal complications from steroid-induced hyperinfection syndrome.[67]

TABLE 19-8 FEATURES OF CLONAL EOSINOPHILIC DISORDERS, M-HES, AND L-HES

HES variant	Presentation	Unique diagnostic features	Unique treatment features
Myeloproliferative variant HES	• Male predominance • Splenomegaly • More likely to have cardiac manifestations	• Anemia, thrombocytopenia • Elevated vitamin B12 • Elevated tryptase level • Presence of dysplastic eosinophils and eosinophilic precursors in the blood • Bone marrow with hypercellularity and fibrosis • *PDGFR* mutations or other associated chromosomal abnormalities	• High mortality if untreated • Refractory to steroids • Imatinib used for patients with *PDGFR*-associated mutation • For *PDGFR*-negative patients, treatment should be guided by the underlying molecular abnormalities. • Patients with no abnormalities and not meeting criteria for leukemia should be treated with high-dose steroids
Lymphocytic variant HES	• Male = Female • Skin and soft-tissue manifestations including erythroderma, urticaria, and plaques	• CD3⁻CD4⁺ L-HES • Elevated IgE level • Elevated TARC level	• May require moderate- to high-dose steroids • Second line: interferon-α • Can progress to lymphoma (5–25%)

L-HES, lymphocytic variant hypereosinophilic syndrome; M-HES, myeloproliferative variant hypereosinophilic syndrome; *PDGFR*, platelet-derived growth factor receptor; TARC, thymus and activation regulated chemokine.

▪ Specific treatments for clonal eosinophilic disorders include hydroxyurea, interferon-α, imatinib mesylate, newer tyrosine kinase inhibitors, and other biologic agents. The drug of choice depends on the clinical presentation, HES variant, and molecular diagnosis of the patient.

▪ Treatment of associated HES and overlap HES depends on the underlying disease.

TABLE 19-9 GENERAL EOSINOPHILIA STARTING WORKUP

First line

- CBC
- CMP
- UA
- CXR
- ESR/CRP
- ANA/ANCA
- Serum IgE
- Serum tryptase
- Stool ova and parasites

Second line

- Flow cytometry
- Peripheral smear
- Vitamin B12
- HIV ELISA
- *Strongyloides*/*Schistosoma* serology

ANA, antinuclear antibody; ANCA, antineutrophil cytoplasmic antibody; CBC, complete blood count; CMP, complete metabolic panel; CRP, C-reactive protein; ELISA, enzyme-linked immunosorbent assay; ESR, erythrocyte sedimentation rate.

Diagnostic Testing

- In most cases, the history and physical examination will direct the clinician toward a specific workup for a patient's eosinophilia.
- In cases with no clear etiology, a limited screening workup may help direct further investigation (Table 19-9).
- The degree of peripheral eosinophilia has limited diagnostic utility, as counts can be highly variable within a disease. However, moderate-to-severe eosinophilia is more likely to be associated with HES or infection.

TREATMENT

- Glucocorticoids are first-line therapy for many eosinophilic disorders. However, infectious etiologies must first be ruled out to prevent worsening of symptoms.
- Additional cytotoxic and immunosuppressive agents are typically used in noninfectious causes of eosinophilia that are refractory to glucocorticoids and show evidences of organ involvement.
- Biological therapies targeting eosinophils via IL-5 and IL-5R could potentially be useful in the treatment of certain types of asthma, EoE, HES, and EGPA.
- Imatinib and other small molecule inhibitors have been used in clonal HES.

REFERENCES

1. Klion AD. Eosinophilia: a pragmatic approach to diagnosis and treatment. *Hematology Am Soc Hematol Educ Program.* 2015;2015:92–7.
2. Williams KW, Ware J, Abiodun A, et al. Hypereosinophilia in children and adults: a retrospective comparison. *J Allergy Clin Immunol Pract.* 2016;4(5):941–7.

3. Mejia R, Nutman TB. Evaluation and differential diagnosis of marked, persistent eosinophilia. *Semin Hematol*. 2012;49(2):149–59.
4. Kuruvilla M, Khan DA. Eosinophilic drug allergy. *Clin Rev Allergy Immunol*. 2016;50(2):228–39.
5. Watanabe H. Recent advances in drug-induced hypersensitivity syndrome/drug reaction with eosinophilia and systemic symptoms. *J Immunol Res*. 2018;2018:5163129.
6. Kodner CM, Kudrimoti A. Diagnosis and management of acute interstitial nephritis. *Am Fam Physician*. 2003;67(12):2527–34.
7. Svenningsen S, Nair P. Asthma endotypes and an overview of targeted therapy for asthma. *Front Med (Lausanne)*. 2017;4:158.
8. Casciano J, Krishnan JA, Small MB, et al. Burden of asthma with elevated blood eosinophil levels. *BMC Pulm Med*. 2016;16(1):100.
9. de Groot JC, ten Brinke A, Bel EHD. Management of the patient with eosinophilic asthma: a new era begins. *ERJ Open Res*. 2015;1:00024–2015.
10. Chung KF, Wenzel SE, Brozek JL, et al. International ERS/ATS guidelines on definition, evaluation and treatment of severe asthma. *Eur Respir J*. 2014;43:343–73.
11. Rodríguez-Jiménez JC, Moreno-Paz FJ, Terán LM, et al. Aspirin exacerbated respiratory disease: current topics and trends. *Respir Med*. 2018;135:62–75.
12. Shah NH, Schneider TR, DeFaria Yeh D, et al. Eosinophilia-associated coronary artery vasospasm in patients with aspirin-exacerbated respiratory disease. *J Allergy Clin Immunol Pract*. 2016;4:1215–9.
13. Fountain CR, Mudd PA, Ramakrishnan VR, et al. Characterization and treatment of patients with chronic rhinosinusitis and nasal polyps. *Ann Allergy Asthma Immunol*. 2013;111(5):337–41.
14. Liu FT, Goodarzi H, Chen HY. IgE, mast cells, and eosinophils in atopic dermatitis. *Clin Rev Allergy Immunol*. 2011;41(3):298–310.
15. Sonawane R, Ahire N, Patil S, et al. Study of eosinophil count in nasal and blood smear in allergic respiratory diseases. *MVP J Med Sci*. 2016;3:44–51.
16. Shah A, Panjabi C. Allergic bronchopulmonary aspergillosis: a perplexing clinical entity. *Allergy Asthma Immunol Res*. 2016;8(4):282–97.
17. Schulte C, Krebs B, Jelinek T, et al. Diagnostic significance of blood eosinophilia in returning travelers. *Clin Infect Dis*. 2002;34(3):407–11.
18. Pardo J, Carranza C, Muro A, et al. Helminth-related eosinophilia in African immigrants, Gran Canaria. *Emerg Infect Dis*. 2006;12(10):1587–9.
19. Bierman WFW, Wetsteyn JCFM, van Gool T. Presentation and diagnosis of imported schistosomiasis: relevance of eosinophilia, microscopy for ova, and serology. *J Travel Med*. 1999;12(1):9–13.
20. de Jesus AR, Silva A, Santana LB, et al. Clinical and immunologic evaluation of 31 patients with acute schistosomiasis mansoni. *J Infect Dis*. 2002;185(1):98–105.
21. Barrett J, Warrell CE, Macpherson L, et al. The changing aetiology of eosinophilia in migrants and returning travellers in the Hospital for Tropical Diseases, London 2002–2015: an observational study. *J Infect*. 2017;75(4):301–8.
22. Greaves D, Coggle S, Pollard C, et al. Strongyloides stercoralis infection. *BMJ*. 2013;347:f4610.
23. Hochedez P, Caumes E. Common skin infections in travelers. *J Travel Med*. 2008;15(4):252–62.
24. Ong RK, Doyle RL. Tropical pulmonary eosinophilia. *Chest*. 1998;113:1673–9.
25. Checkley AM, Chiodini PL, Dockrell DH, et al. Eosinophilia in returning travellers and migrants from the tropics: UK recommendations for investigation and initial management. *J Infect*. 2010;60(1):1–20.
26. Ella OHA, Kady E, Mohamed A, et al. Ascaris lumbricoides and other gastrointestinal helminthic parasites among Qena inhabitants with special concern to its relation to anemia and eosinophilia. *IOSR J Dent Med Sci Ver II*. 2015;14:98–105.
27. Bruschi F, Murrell KD. New aspects of human trichinellosis: the impact of new Trichinella species. *Postrad Med J*. 2002;78:15–22.
28. Moro P, Schantz PM. Echinococcosis: a review. *Int J Infect Dis*. 2009;13:125–33.
29. Al Mohajer M, Villarreal-Williams E, Andrade RA, et al. Eosinophilia and associated factors in a large cohort of patients infected with human immunodeficiency virus. *South Med J*. 2014;107:554–8.
30. Sawanyawisuth K, Chotmongkol V. Eosinophilic meningitis. *Handb Clin Neurol*. 2013;114:207–15.
31. Re VL, Gluckman SJ. Eosinophilic meningitis. *Am J Med*. 2003;114:217–23.
32. Belhassen-García M, Pardo-Lledías J, Pérez Del Villar L, et al. Relevance of eosinophilia and hyper-IgE in immigrant children. *Medicine*. 2014;93:1–8.
33. Yong PF, Freeman AF, Engelhardt KR, et al. An update on the hyper-IgE syndromes. *Arthritis Res Ther*. 2012;14(6):228.

34. Biggs CM, Keles S, Chatila TA. DOCK8 deficiency: insights into pathophysiology, clinical features and management. *Clin Immunol.* 2017;181:75–82.

35. Engelhardt KR, Gertz ME, Keles S, et al. The extended clinical phenotype of 64 patients with dedicator of cytokinesis 8 deficiency. *J Allergy Clin Immunol.* 2015;136:402–12.

36. Woellner C, Gertz EM, Schäffer AA, et al. Mutations in STAT3 and diagnostic guidelines for hyper-IgE syndrome. *J Allergy Clin Immunol.* 2010;125:424–32.

37. Shearer WT, Dunn E, Notarangelo LD, et al. Establishing diagnostic criteria for severe combined immunodeficiency disease (SCID), leaky SCID, and Omenn syndrome: the Primary Immune Deficiency Treatment Consortium experience. *J Allergy Clin Immunol.* 2014;133:1092–8.

38. Ulusoy E, Karaca NE, Azarsiz E, et al. Activating gene 1 deficiencies without Omenn syndrome may also present with eosinophilia and bone marrow fibrosis. *J Clin Med Res.* 2016;8:379–84.

39. Shah S, Wu E, Koneti Rao V, et al. Autoimmune lymphoproliferative syndrome: an update and review of the literature. *Curr Allergy Asthma Rep.* 2014;14(9):462.

40. Poppema S, Maggio E, Van den Berg A. Development of lymphoma in autoimmune lymphoproliferative syndrome (ALPS) and its relationship to Fas gene mutations. *Leuk Lymphoma.* 2004;45:423–31.

41. Rao VK, Oliveira JB. How I treat autoimmune lymphoproliferative syndrome. *Blood.* 2011;118:5741–51.

42. Oliveira JB, Bleesing JJ, Dianzani U, et al. Revised diagnostic criteria and classification for the autoimmune lymphoproliferative syndrome (ALPS): report from the 2009 NIH International Workshop. *Blood.* 2010;116:e35–40.

43. Bacchetta R, Barzaghi F, Roncarolo MG. From IPEX syndrome to FOXP3 mutation: a lesson on immune dysregulation. *Ann N Y Acad Sci.* 2018;1417(1):5–22.

44. Barzaghi F, Amaya Hernandéz LC, Neven B, et al. Long-term follow-up of IPEX syndrome patients after different therapeutic strategies: an international multicenter retrospective study. *J Allegy Clin Immunol.* 2018;141:1036–49.e35.

45. Masi AT, Hunder GG, Lie JT, et al. The American College of Rheumatology 1990 criteria for the classification of Churg-Strauss syndrome (allergic granulomatosis and angiitis). *Arthritis Rheum.* 1990;33:1094–100.

46. Neumann T, Manger B, Schmid M, et al. Cardiac involvement in Churg-Strauss syndrome: impact of endomyocarditis. *Medicine.* 2009;88:236–43.

47. Groh M, Pagnoux C, Baldini C, et al. Eosinophilic granulomatosis with polyangiitis (Churg-Strauss) (EGPA) Consensus Task Force recommendations for evaluation and management. *Eur J Intern Med.* 2015;26:545–53.

48. Wechsler ME, Akuthota P, Jayne D, et al. Mepolizumab or placebo for eosinophilic granulomatosis with polyangiitis. *N Engl J Med.* 2017;376:1921–32.

49. Ardila-Suarez O, Abril A, Gomez-Puerta JA. IgG4-related disease: a concise review of the current literature. *Reumatol Clin.* 2017;13:160–6.

50. Carruthers MN, Khosroshahi A, Augustin T, et al. The diagnostic utility of serum IgG4 concentrations in IgG4-related disease. *Ann Rheum Dis.* 2015;74:14–8.

51. Culver EL, Sadler R, Bateman AC, et al. Increases in IgE, eosinophils, and mast cells can be used in diagnosis and to predict relapse of IgG4-related disease. *Clin Gastroenterol Hepatol.* 2017;15:1444–52.

52. Pinal-Fernandez I, Selva-O' Callaghan A, Grau JM. Diagnosis and classification of eosinophilic fasciitis. *Autoimmun Rev.* 2014;13:379–82.

53. Wright NA, Mazori DR, Patel M, et al. Epidemiology and treatment of eosinophilic fasciitis: an analysis of 63 patients from 3 tertiary care centers. *JAMA Dermatol.* 2016;152:97–9.

54. Reich JM. Mortality of intrathoracic sarcoidosis in referral vs population-based settings: influence of stage, ethnicity, and corticosteroid therapy. *Chest.* 2002;121:32–9.

55. Renston JP, Goldman ES, Hsu RM, et al. Peripheral blood eosinophilia in association with sarcoidosis. *Mayo Clin Proc.* 2000;75:586–90.

56. Gelpí E, Posada de la Paz M, Terracini B, et al. The Spanish toxic oil syndrome 20 years after its onset: a multidisciplinary review of scientific knowledge. *Environ Health Perspect.* 2002;110:457–64.

57. Allen JA, Peterson A, Sufit R, et al. Post-epidemic eosinophilia-myalgia syndrome associated with L-tryptophan. *Arthritis Rheum.* 2011;63:3633–9.

58. Liacouras CA, Furuta GT, Hirano I, et al. Eosinophilic esophagitis: updated consensus recommendations for children and adults. *J Allergy Clin Immunol.* 2011;128:3–20.

59. Walker MM, Potter M, Talley NJ. Eosinophilic gastroenteritis and other eosinophilic gut diseases distal to the oesophagus. *Lancet Gastroenterol Hepatol.* 2018;3:271–80.

60. Brown IS, Smith J, Rosty C. Gastrointestinal pathology in celiac disease: a case series of 150 consecutive newly diagnosed patients. *Am J Clin Pathol.* 2012;138:42–9.
61. Click B, Anderson AM, Koutroubakis IE, et al. Peripheral eosinophilia in patients with inflammatory bowel disease defines an aggressive disease phenotype. *Am J Gastroenterol.* 2017;112:1849–58.
62. Simon HU, Rothenberg ME, Bochner BS, et al. Refining the definition of hypereosinophilic syndrome. *J Allergy Clin Immunol.* 2010;126(1):45–9.
63. Klion AD. Eosinophilic myeloproliferative disorders. *Hematology Am Soc Hematol Educ Program.* 2011;2011:257–63.
64. Gotlib J. World Health Organization-defined eosinophilic disorders: 2014 update on diagnosis, risk stratification, and management. *Am J Hematol.* 2014;89(3):325–37.
65. Legrand F, Renneville A, MacIntyre E, et al. The spectrum of FIP1L1-PDGFRA-associated chronic eosinophilic leukemia: new insights based on a survey of 44 cases. *Medicine (Baltimore).* 2013;92(5):e1–9.
66. Valent P. Pathogenesis, classification, and therapy of eosinophilia and eosinophil disorders. *Blood Rev.* 2009;23(4):157–65.
67. Klion AD. How I treat hypereosinophilic syndromes. *Blood.* 2015;126(9):1069–77.

Mastocytosis and Mast Cell Activation Disorders

20

Zhen Ren and H. James Wedner

GENERAL PRINCIPLES

- Mast cells (MCs) play a central role in acquired immediate hypersensitivity reactions mediated through IgE-mediated release of histamine and other inflammatory mediators.
- Mastocytosis is the pathologic proliferation of MCs resulting in uncontrolled release of inflammatory mediators, causing both cutaneous and systemic clinical manifestations.
- It is a rare disease that can occur at any age ranging from infancy to adulthood.

Classification

The classification of mastocytosis is presented in Table 20-1.[1]

Epidemiology

The exact prevalence of mastocytosis remains unclear. Based on a recent population-based epidemiology study in Denmark, the estimated prevalence of mastocytosis is approximately 1 case/10,000 persons.[2]

TABLE 20-1 CLASSIFICATION OF MASTOCYTOSIS		
Cutaneous mastocytosis (CM) (infiltration of mast cells limited to the skin)	Systemic mastocytosis (SM)	Mast cell sarcoma
• Maculopapular cutaneous mastocytosis (MPCM)	• Smoldering systemic mastocytosis (SSM)	
• Diffuse cutaneous mastocytosis (DCM)	• Indolent systemic mastocytosis (ISM)	
• Mastocytoma of skin	• Systemic mastocytosis with an associated hematologic neoplasm (SMAHN), previously known as **systemic mastocytosis with associated clonal, hematologic non–mast cell lineage disease (SM-AHNMD)**	
	• Aggressive systemic mastocytosis (ASM)	
	• Mast cell leukemia (MCL)	

Adapted from Valent P, Akin C, Metcalfe DD. Mastocytosis: 2016 updated WHO classification and novel treatment concepts. *Blood.* 2017;129:1420–7.

Pathophysiology

- MCs are widely distributed in tissues and generally found in the gastrointestinal (GI) tract, respiratory tract, lymphoid tissues, and skin. They are long-lived and do not generally circulate.
- Mature MCs have cytoplasmic granules containing preformed mediators, including histamine, heparin, proteases (e.g., tryptase, chymase, carboxypeptidase), tumor necrosis factor (TNF)-α, peroxidase, and phospholipases.
- Other components of granules are de novo synthesized lipid mediators (prostaglandin D2, leukotrienes C4, D4, E4), cytokines (interleukin [IL]-3, IL-5, IL-6, and IL-16), chemokines (eotaxin, monocyte chemoattractant protein-1, C-C chemokine ligand 5), and growth factors (transforming growth factor-β), and platelet-activating factor.[3,4]
- Mature MCs can be categorized into two subsets based on their protease content.
  - The MC_{TC} subset cells express tryptases, chymases, and carboxypeptidases in their granules, whereas MC_T express only tryptases.
  - MC_{TC} cells are found in the skin, lymph nodes, the lung, and gut submucosa, whereas MC_T cells reside in the intestinal and pulmonary mucosa.
- Symptoms associated with mastocytosis are **secondary to release of mast cell mediators** both within the tissues in which MCs reside and distantly via circulation of those mediators.[3]
- MCs also display a vast array of antigens on their cell surface that serve as regulators of cell activation/recognition as well as receptors of various cytokines.
  - The proto-oncogene c-Kit encodes a transmembrane tyrosine kinase receptor for stem cell factor (SCF) that is significantly expressed in MCs.
  - Point mutations of c-Kit, such as D816V (most common), V560G, D816Y, D816F, D816H, E839K, and F522C, are associated with around 93% of all patients with systemic mastocytosis (SM).[3]
  - Occasionally impaired antiapoptotic signaling pathways were reported to be associated with MC-related disorders, such as *TET* oncogene family member 2 (*TET2*) mutations and *PRKG2-PDGFRB* fusion gene.[5,6]

DIAGNOSIS

Clinical Presentation

- **The vast majority (up to 90%) of adult and pediatric patients with mastocytosis have dermatologic involvement.** Affected areas usually include the axilla, trunk, and thighs and spare the face.[7]
- **Cutaneous mastocytosis (CM)** is the most common form of mastocytosis that primarily affects the skin. CM can be classified by their characteristic presentation and appearance.
  - **Maculopapular cutaneous mastocytosis (MPCM),** previously known as **urticaria pigmentosa (UP)**
    - Small yellowish to reddish maculopapular lesions
    - May present as nodules or plaques
    - Spares the palms, soles, face, and scalp
    - Rubbing can lead to urtication and erythema (Darier sign).
    - Pruritus worsened by temperature change, local friction, hot beverages, spicy foods, and alcohol
  - **Diffuse cutaneous mastocytosis (DCM)**
    - A rare condition
    - No discrete lesions: diffuse infiltration of the dermis
    - Erythroderma of all the skin
    - Onset before 3 years old
    - Skin is prematurely aged, thickened with a yellowish-brown color, and peau d'orange texture.

○ Blisters can be associated with both MPCM and DCM in young children. In fact, blister formation is reported as a hallmark of DCM and mostly limited to the first few years of life.

○ Occasionally, DCM can be associated with systemic disease and can lead to complications such as hypotension and GI bleeding.

○ CM usually appears prior to the first year of life and is not associated with systemic disease. About half of the cases will resolve spontaneously by puberty.[8]

○ **Mastocytoma** of skin (uncommon) presents as one reddish-brown maculopapular lesion or nodule with a positive Darier sign. It often occurs during the first 3 months of life and usually resolves during childhood.

○ **Telangiectasia macularis eruptiva perstans (TMEP)** presents as telangiectatic macules that occur on tan-brown-colored skin typically in adults. These patients can also have maculopapular lesions at other body sites. In 2016, World Health Organization (WHO) suggests to remove TMEP as a separate form of CM.[1]

• **SM** clinical manifestations are the result of MC mediator release and MC infiltration into involved organs with or without cutaneous involvement. SM is more common in adults than in children.

○ Most common site of involvement in SM is in the bone marrow.

○ Owing to MC infiltration, organomegaly may be present (liver, spleen, and lymph nodes), and cytopenias can occur.

○ **Symptoms are nonspecific but can include flushing, dyspepsia, diarrhea, recurrent syncope, recurrent anaphylaxis, bone pain, and fatigue**.

○ Patients with severe anaphylaxis to stings should be screened for mastocytosis.

○ In aggressive forms of SM or in comorbid non-MC hematologic malignancies, symptoms of weight loss and fever may be present.

○ Mastocytosis needs to be considered in the evaluation of flushing syndromes, especially with associated hypotension.

○ Systemic symptoms can occur in the absence of cutaneous symptoms.

○ GI symptoms can be triggered or worsened by spicy foods, alcohol, or stress and are the second most common symptom compared to cutaneous symptoms.[3]

  ▪ Abdominal pain, diarrhea, nausea, and vomiting can occur.

  ▪ One-third of SM patients experience malabsorption.[9]

  ▪ Caused by urticarial lesions in the GI tract, hypermotility, altered intestinal secretion, or peptic ulcer disease

  ▪ Hepatic involvement may result in elevated alkaline phosphatase and γ-glutamyl transferase, but rarely leads to serious disease.[3]

○ Splenic involvement usually results in trabecular, fibrotic thickening.

○ Musculoskeletal manifestations include osteoporosis, pathologic fractures, and nonspecific pains of unclear etiology. Bone discomfort usually involves the long bones and can be associated with pathologic fractures.

○ Neuropsychiatric symptoms often reported in adults with mastocytosis include poor attention span, irritability, headache, and memory impairment.

• **Systemic mastocytosis with associated hematologic neoplasm** (SM-AHN), previously known as **systemic mastocytosis with associated clonal, hematologic non–mast cell lineage disease (SM-AHNMD)**, can be seen in association with hypereosinophilic syndromes as well as other hematologic disorders.

• **Aggressive systemic mastocytosis** (ASM) and **mast cell leukemia** (MCL) are very rare and carry a poor prognosis.

Diagnostic Testing

The WHO diagnostic criteria for mastocytosis are presented in Table 20-2.[1]

TABLE 20-2	2016 WORLD HEALTH ORGANIZATION DIAGNOSTIC CRITERIA FOR MASTOCYTOSIS

- **Cutaneous mastocytosis:** Typical skin lesions associated with Darier sign and one of the following on skin biopsy:
  - Focal dense (>15 mast cells per cluster) or diffuse mast cell infiltrates
  - c-Kit D816V mutation in lesional skin
- **Systemic mastocytosis:** One major and one minor or three minor criteria
  - **Major: Multifocal dense** infiltrates of mast cell (>15 mast cells in aggregates) in the bone marrow (BM) or in sections of other extracutaneous organs
  - Minor
    - Mast cell infiltrates with >25% spindle-shaped, immature, or atypical morphology detected on sections of visceral organs
    - Mutation in c-Kit at codon 816 in the BM or another extracutaneous organ
    - CD2 and/or CD25 expression on CD117+ (encoded by c-Kit) cells
    - Tryptase level in serum >20 ng/mL

Adapted from Valent P, Akin C, Metcalfe DD. Mastocytosis: 2016 updated WHO classification and novel treatment concepts. *Blood.* 2017;129:1420–7.

Laboratories
- **Persistently elevated total serum tryptase level** (>20 ng/mL) is the most commonly used marker of SM.
- Elevated plasma/urine histamine or histamine metabolites (*N*-methylhistamine, methylimidazole acetic acid), and urine prostaglandin D2 metabolites
  - Increased *N*-methylhistamine levels can be seen in patients taking monoamine oxidase inhibitors (MAOIs). Histamine-rich diet can increase *N*-methylhistamine levels up to 30%.
  - Aspirin or NSAIDs inhibit the production of prostaglandins. Patients should be off aspirin or NSAIDs before taking urine prostaglandin D2 metabolites test.
- **Histamine level can be highly variable** between different individuals.
- Complete blood count (CBC) is useful to evaluate for cytopenias, thrombocytosis, eosinophilia, lymphocytosis, leukocytosis, and immature leukocytes.
- Alkaline phosphatase and serum aminotransferases can be elevated when there is hepatic involvement.
- Genetic testing for c-Kit mutation and flow cytometry testing for coexpression of CD2 and/or CD25 in CD117(KIT)-positive MCs are used to support the diagnosis of SM.
- Urine levels of 5-hydroxyindoleacetic acid and metanephrines are used to rule out carcinoid and pheochromocytomas as other possible causes of flushing and vascular instability.

Imaging
- Dual-energy x-ray absorptiometry (DEXA), skeletal survey, and bone scans are often done for the evaluation of bone involvement. Osteoporosis is a common sequela of indolent systemic mastocytosis (ISM).
- When there is concern of liver or splenic involvement, abdominal ultrasound and/or CT may be done.

Diagnostic Procedures

- Suspected mastocytosis should be confirmed by tissue biopsy.
- **Skin biopsy** is usually preferred if the patient has cutaneous symptoms.
  - Histologically, mastocytosis is characterized by **diffuse infiltration of MCs in the dermis.**
  - MCs stain positive with toluidine blue or Wright–Giemsa as well as tryptase immuno-histochemical analysis.
- **Bone marrow biopsy** should be considered in all adult patients with MPCM because the incidence of SM is high.
  - Multifocal dense infiltrates of MCs ($\geq$15 MCs in aggregates) detected in sections of bone marrow are one of the major diagnostic criteria in SM.
  - Bone marrow biopsy is also recommended for patients with unexplained hypotension episodes, syncope, pathologic bone fractures, splenomegaly, or the detection of a KIT D816V mutation in peripheral blood.[10]

TREATMENT

Medications

- The mainstay of therapy is directed at control of symptoms from mediator release.
- **Antihistamines**
  - H1 antagonists: hydroxyzine, diphenhydramine, loratadine, fexofenadine, and cetirizine
  - H2 antagonists: ranitidine, cimetidine, and famotidine
  - An option would be to give one nonsedating antihistamine during the day and a more potent sedating antihistamine at night.
- **Mast cell stabilizers**
  - Gastric cromolyn formulations inhibit MC degranulation and are effective in reducing GI symptoms.[11]
  - Ketotifen is an antihistamine and an MC stabilizer that can be used, but antihistamine properties are not more efficacious than hydroxyzine.[12]
- **Leukotriene modifying agents** may have some benefit.
- **Aspirin** may be helpful in improving flushing symptom through blockade of prostaglandin synthesis but should be used with caution, given the risk of triggering anaphylaxis.
- Patients with reactions involving hypotension must be taught how to use self-administered IM epinephrine injections (0.3 mg, 1:1,000) and must carry it with them at all times.
- **Oral glucocorticoids** can be most effective in treating malabsorption, ascites, hepatic fibrosis, and other GI symptoms but should be reserved for refractory disease or acute episodes.[13]
- Topical steroids may be used for cutaneous symptoms.
- **8-Methoxypsoralen with ultraviolet A (PUVA) phototherapy** can be used for cutaneous disease.[14]
- Surgical excision of a solitary lesion may also be an option.
- Given osteoporosis is the most prevalent bone manifestation in SM, patients should be monitored for osteoporosis and treated accordingly.
- **Cytoreductive therapy** is only indicated for patients who present with target organ damage from aggressive systemic disease.
  - **Interferon-α2b** is the first-line agent.[15]
  - **Cladribine** is a nucleoside analog that decreases MC burden.[15,16]
  - **Tyrosine kinase inhibitors**
    - Imatinib mesylate is approved by the U.S. Food and Drug Administration (FDA) for ASM without D816V c-KIT mutation (only <10% of all cases). In vitro studies demonstrate that D816V c-KIT mutations confer resistance to imatinib.[17]
    - Imatinib should also be used for patients who have concomitant eosinophilia with the FIP1L1-PDGFRA fusion oncogene.[17]

- ○ Midostaurin, a multikinase/Kit inhibitor that blocks the growth and survival of MCs, demonstrated effectiveness in treating advanced SM, regardless of *KIT* D816V mutation status.[18] Midostaurin is approved by the FDA for the treatment of ASM, SM-AHN, and MCL.
- ○ Allogeneic hematopoietic stem cell transplantation (HSCT) is considered in patients with advanced SM, such as acute MCL, ASM, and SM-AHN.[19]

Other Nonpharmacologic Therapies

- The first step in the therapeutic management of mastocytosis consists of patient counseling and education regarding the disease and **avoidance of triggers that may lead to MC degranulation.**
- Physical stimuli include intense exercise, excessive sunlight, friction, extreme temperatures, excessive pressure, and friction.[20]
- Emotional distress can trigger degranulation.[20]
- Multiple anesthetic agents have been implicated, including lidocaine, succinylcholine, D-tubocurarine, metocurine, doxacurium, atracurium, mivacurium, rocuronium, thiopental, etomidate, enflurane, and isoflurane.[20] If possible, preoperative medications should be limited to those previously tolerated.
- Other medications to consider include NSAIDs, opiates, alcohol, vancomycin, α-blockers, thiamine, aspirin, amphotericin B, quinine, and polymyxin-B.[20]
- **Contrast agents** can provoke nonallergic reactions with immunologic manifestations (anaphylactoid), so all mastocytosis patients should be premedicated with steroids and antihistamines before receiving contrast. Gadolinium is not associated with MC degranulation.

SPECIAL CONSIDERATIONS

- **Mast cell activation syndrome (MCAS)** is a term newly emerged in the past decade. It refers to patients who exhibit the signs and symptoms of MCA, response to therapies targeting MCs, but fail to meet mastocytosis diagnostic criteria.
- The diagnosis criteria for MCAS were proposed as follows[21]:
  - ○ Episodic multisystem symptoms consistent with MCA
  - ○ Appropriate response to medications targeting MCA
  - ○ Increase in serum total tryptase by at least 20% above baseline plus 2 ng/mL during or within 4 hours after a symptomatic period
  - ○ Documented increase in validated markers of MCA on at least two occasions
- MCASs are classified into three types, namely, primary MCAS, secondary MCAS, and idiopathic MCAS.
  - ○ Primary MCAS is applied to patients who are found to meet one or two minor mastocytosis diagnostic criteria but fail to meet full diagnostic criteria for SM. Hymenoptera-induced anaphylaxis or idiopathic anaphylaxis is increasingly recognized in this category.
  - ○ Secondary MCAS refers to patients who have allergy or another underlying disease causing MCA.
  - ○ Idiopathic MCAS refers to patients who meet MCA criteria, but no disease is identified.
- The mainstays of treatment for MCAS are antihistamines, MC stabilizers, leukotriene modifying agents, glucocorticoids, and omalizumab.
- It is crucial for patients to receive a comprehensive evaluation when the criteria for MCAS are not met. The differentials of MCAS include cardiovascular disorders, certain endocrine disorders, neoplasmas, GI disease, infectious disease, or psychiatric conditions.[21]
- Germline duplication and triplications in the *TPSAB1* gene encoding α-tryptase were reported in familiar hypertryptasemia.[22] The affected individuals reported symptom complexes, including flushing, pruritus, dysautonomia, chronic pain, and connective

tissue abnormalities including joint hypermobility. It is unclear if these symptoms are caused by MC mediator release or due to other pathologic process. More research will need to address this area.

OUTCOME/PROGNOSIS

- **CM has the best prognosis;** most children with isolated UP will have resolution by adulthood.[8]
- The prognosis of ISM is generally good, and patients can have normal life expectancy. The probability of leukemic transformation is very low.[20,23]
- **The prognosis for ASM is generally poor,** with median survival of 41 months.[20,23]
- For SM-AHNMD, the prognosis is poor—median survival of 24 months, but this depends on the associated hematologic disorder.[20,23] MCL has a very poor prognosis, with mean survival ranging from only 2 to 12 months.[23]

REFERENCES

1. Valent P, Akin C, Metcalfe DD. Mastocytosis: 2016 updated WHO classification and novel treatment concepts. *Blood.* 2017;129:1420–7.
2. Cohen SS, Skovbo S, Vestergaard H, et al. Epidemiology of systemic mastocytosis in Denmark. *Br J Haematol.* 2014;166:521–8.
3. Metcalfe DD. Mastocytosis. In: Adkinson NF, Bochner BS, Busse WW, et al., eds. *Middleton's Allergy Principles & Practice.* 7th ed. Philadelphia, PA: Mosby-Elsevier, 2009.
4. D'Ambrosio D, Akin C, Wu Y, et al. Gene expression analysis in mastocytosis reveals a highly consistent profile with candidate molecular markers. *J Allergy Clin Immunol.* 2003;112:1162–70.
5. Tefferi A, Pardanani A, Lim K-H, et al. TET2 mutations and their clinical correlates in polycythemia vera, essential thrombocytopenia, and myelofibrosis. *Leukemia.* 2009;23:905–1.
6. Lahortiga I, Akin C, Cools, J, et al. Activity of imatinib in systemic mastocytosis with chronic basophilic leukemia and a PRKG2-PDGFRB fusion. *Haematologica.* 2008;93:49–56.
7. Hartmann K, Escribano L, Grattan C, et al. Cutaneous manifestations in patients with mastocytosis: consensus report of the European Competence Network on Mastocytosis; the American Academy of Allergy, Asthma & Immunology; and the European Academy of Allergology and Clinical Immunology. *J Allergy Clin Immunol.* 2016;137:35–45.
8. Carter MC, Metcalfe DD. Paediatric mastocytosis. *Arch Dis Child.* 2002;86:315–9.
9. Cherner JA, Jensen RT, Dubois A, et al. Gastrointestinal dysfunction in systemic mastocytosis: a prospective study. *Gastroenterology.* 1988;95:657–67.
10. Theoharides TC, Valent P, Akin C. Mast cells, mastocytosis, and related disorders. *N Engl J Med.* 2015;373:163–72.
11. Horan RF, Sheffer AL, Austen KF. Cromolyn sodium in the management of systemic mastocytosis. *J Allergy Clin Immunol.* 1990;85:852–5.
12. Kettelhut BV, Berkebile C, Bradley D, et al. A double-blind, placebo-controlled, crossover trial of ketotifen versus hydroxyzine in the treatment of pediatric mastocytosis. *J Allergy Clin Immunol.* 1989;83:866–70.
13. Wilson TM, Metcalfe DD, Robyn J. Treatment of systemic mastocytosis. *Immunol Allergy Clin North Am.* 2006;26:549–73.
14. Godt O, Proksch E, Streit V, et al. Short-and long-term effectiveness of oral and bath PUVA therapy in urticaria pigmentosa and systemic mastocytosis. *Dermatology.* 1997;195:35–9.
15. Lim KH, Pardanani A, Butterfield JH, et al. Cytoreductive therapy in 108 adults with systemic mastocytosis: outcome analysis and response prediction during treatment with interferon-alpha, hydroxyurea, imatinib mesylate or 2-chlorodeoxyadenosine. *Am J Hematol.* 2009;84:790–4.
16. Kluin-Nelemans HC, Oldhoff JM, Van Doornaal JJ, et al. Cladribine therapy for systemic mastocytosis. *Blood.* 2003;102:4270–6.
17. Ustun C, DeRemer DL, Atkin C. Tyrosine kinase inhibitors in the treatment of systemic mastocytosis. *Leuk Res.* 2011;35:1143–52.

18. Gotlib J, Kluin-Nelemans HC, George TI, et al. Efficacy and safety of midostaurin in advanced systemic mastocytosis. *N Engl J Med.* 2016;374:2530–41.

19. Ustun C, Reiter A, Scott BL, et al. Hematopoietic stem-cell transplantation for advanced systemic mastocytosis. *J Clin Oncol.* 2014;32:3264–74.

20. Bains SN, Hsieh FH. Current approaches to the diagnosis and treatment of systemic mastocytosis. *Ann Allergy Asthma Immunol.* 2010;104:1–41.

21. Valent P, Akin C, Arock M, et al. Definitions, criteria and global classification of mast cell disorders with special reference to mast cell activation syndromes: a consensus proposal. *Int Arch Allergy Immunol.* 2012;157:215–25.

22. Lyons JJ, Yu X, Hughes JD, et al. Elevated basal serum tryptase identifies a multisystem disorder associated with increased TPSAB1 copy number. *Nat Genet.* 2016;48:1564–9.

23. Pardanani A, Tefferi A. Systemic mastocytosis in adults: a review on prognosis and treatment based on 342 Mayo Clinic patients and current literature. *Curr Opin Hematol.* 2010;17:125–32.

Primary Immunodeficiency Diseases

21

Ofer Zimmerman and Caroline Horner

GENERAL PRINCIPLES

- Primary immunodeficiency diseases (PIDs) are inherited disorders of the immune system that predispose affected subjects to a range of diseases including **recurrent and severe infections** with common pathogens, **opportunistic infections**, **immune dysregulation, autoimmune disease**, and solid and hematologic **malignancies**.[1]
- PIDs comprise **354 distinct disorders with 344 different gene** defects listed as of February 2017. Advances in molecular biology and increased availability of genetic testing allow the recognition of both many new disorders and milder variants of known PIDs.[2]
- Most cases of PIDs are diagnosed during infancy and childhood; however, **most children with PIDs now reach adulthood**.[3] Common variable immunodeficiency (CVID), GATA2 haploinsufficiency, immunodeficiency associated with autoantibodies, or immunodeficiency disorders presenting with a milder phenotype **can present in adulthood**.[1,4]
  - The early involvement of an immunologist in the management of newborns and infants with suspected PID is highly recommended. For older children and adults with suspected immune disorders, an immunologist should also be consulted to assist with diagnosis and ongoing care.[1]
  - The diagnosis and care of patients with PIDs is often challenging and requires the involvement of experts from different medical fields and subspecialties (infectious disease, genetics, pulmonary, gastroenterology, hematology, and endocrinology). Consider referral of complex cases to institutions with experience in managing PIDs.

Classification

PIDs are classified according to the component of the immune system that is primarily involved, as adopted by the International Union of Immunological Societies (IUIS)[2]:

- Immunodeficiencies affecting **cellular and humoral** immunity
- Predominantly **antibody** deficiencies
- Combined immunodeficiencies (CIDs) with associated or **syndromic features**
- Diseases of immune **dysregulation**
- Congenital defects of **phagocyte** number or function
- Defects in intrinsic and **innate immunity**
- **Autoinflammatory** disorders
- **Complement** deficiencies
- Phenocopies of inborn errors of immunity

Epidemiology

- Registry and survey data from a variety of sources suggest an **incidence for all symptomatic PIDs** ranging from **1 in 10,000 to 1 in 2,000 live births** and a **prevalence** of **1 in 12,000 to 1 in 10,000** in the general population.[1]
- **The most common PID is selective IgA (SIgA) deficiency** occurring in as many as 1 of 300–700 live births in American white subjects (although it is rarer in other ethnic groups, such as Asians).[1] However, most patients with IgA deficiency are asymptomatic.

- The incidence of severe combined immunodeficiency (SCID) is approximately 1:58,000 live births in the United States.[1]
- A much higher rate of PIDs is observed among populations with high consanguinity rates or among genetically isolated populations.
- **The male/female ratio of PIDs is approximately 5:1** in infants and children but approaches 1:1 in adults.[1]

DIAGNOSIS

Clinical Presentation

History

- Detailed history taking is essential for establishing the clinical suspicion that a patient might have PID and for choosing the most appropriate diagnostic tests. Particular defects in the immune system are often associated with certain infectious organisms (see Table 21-1).[5,6]
- Patterns and types of infections that should prompt further evaluation of PID include the following:
  - **Recurrent or chronic** respiratory infections; an often-cited guideline is **>6 upper respiratory tract infections (URIs) per year in the first decade of life or >1 episode of pneumonia per decade in adults.** It is important to note, however, that children exposed to frequent daycare and/or tobacco smoke may have up to 10 URIs/year.
  - Any serious infection (e.g., sepsis, meningitis) occurring twice in a child or once in an adult should raise suspicion of a PID.
  - **Prolonged duration** of infections and infections that require prolonged antibiotic treatment
  - **Severe or complicated infections.** For example, severe varicella complicated by pneumonia, hepatitis, or bronchiectasis
  - Chronic or recurrent mucocutaneous candidiasis
  - Recurrent skin or visceral organ abscesses or nonhealing wounds
  - **Infection with an opportunistic** organism or with **live attenuated vaccine (viruses or bacteria).** This includes *Pneumocystis jirovecii* (formerly *carinii*) pneumonia, *Cryptococcus neoformans* infections in the absence of HIV/AIDS as well as invasive *Nocardia* infection. Vaccine-related infections include disseminated varicella vaccine (chicken pox) or Bacillus Calmette-Guérin (BCG).
- Elements of the history that are suggestive of PID:
  - Failure to thrive (FTT), developmental delay, wasting
  - Delayed separation of umbilical cord
  - Chronic diarrhea and malabsorption
  - Recurrent periodontitis; conical or widely spaced teeth; retained primary teeth with frequent need for dental extractions to allow eruption of normal secondary teeth
  - Consanguinity
  - Family member with documented PID or recurrent infections
  - Family history of unexplained early infant death
  - Adverse reaction to blood or plasma transfusions (graft-vs.-host; anaphylaxis in IgA deficient patients)
  - Autoimmune disease (cytopenia, endocrinopathies, colitis, hepatitis)
  - Lymphoma in infancy
- The presence of certain constellations of signs should prompt suspicion of specific PID, such as:[2,5]
  - Cardiac disease, micrognathia, and hypocalcemia (DiGeorge syndrome)
  - Thrombocytopenia and eczema (Wiskott–Aldrich syndrome)
  - Hypohidrosis, dental anomalies, alopecia (NEMO [nuclear factor-κ-B essential modulator] mutation, hypohidrotic ectodermal dysplasia with immunodeficiency)

TABLE 21-1	COMMON PRESENTATIONS AND INFECTIOUS AGENTS CLASSIFIED BY THE TYPE OF THE PRIMARY IMMUNODEFICIENCY	
Affected arm of the immune system	**Clinical presentation/ site of infection**	**Etiologic agent**
B-cell deficiencies	Sinusitis	*Streptococcus pneumoniae*
	Pneumonia	*Haemophilus influenzae*
	Pharyngitis	*Pseudomonas* spp.
	Otitis	*Giardia lamblia*
	Meningitis	Campylobacter
	Bacteremia	Salmonella
	Encephalitis (enteroviral)	Enterovirus
	Colitis (giardiasis)	*Norovirus*
		Mycoplasma (including *Ureaplasma urealyticum*)
Combined T- and B-cell deficiencies	Opportunistic infections	*Candida albicans Pneumocystis jirovecii*
	Failure to thrive	
	Diarrhea	Mycobacterial species (Bacillus
	Dermatitis	Calmette-Guérin [BCG])
	Sepsis	Respiratory syncytial virus (RSV)
		Rotavirus
		Cytomegalovirus
		Herpes simplex
		Herpes zoster
		Epstein–Barr virus
Phagocytic cell disorders	Invasive skin infections/ abscesses	*Staphylococcus aureus, Burkholderia cepacia*
	Visceral abscesses	*Serratia marcescens,*
	Poor wound healing	*Aspergillus* spp.
	Lymphadenitis	*Nocardia* spp.
	Periodontitis	*Salmonella*
	Colitis	*Pseudomonas* species
		Mycobacterial species
Complement deficiencies	Recurrent bacteremia	*Neisseria species*
	Recurrent meningitis	*Streptococcus pneumoniae*
	Pyogenic infections	
TLR pathway	Recurrent meningitis	*Streptococcus pneumoniae*
	Bacteremia	*Neisseria meningitidis*
	Lack of fever	*Staphylococcus aureus*
		Herpes simplex virus

TLR, toll-like receptor.

○ Ataxia plus oculocutaneous telangiectasias (ataxia-telangiectasia syndrome)
○ Chronic mucocutaneous candidiasis, hypoparathyroidism, and adrenal gland insufficiency (APECED [autoimmune polyendocrinopathy-candidiasis-ectodermal dystrophy])

Physical Examination

Physical examination can yield findings suggestive of specific PID and can help in forming a differential diagnosis and choosing the appropriate tests.[5]

- The examination should focus on
  - Weight and height
  - Facial features (e.g., nasal size and shape, palpebral slant, philtrum)
  - Oropharyngeal findings (e.g., thrush, ulcers, gingivitis, retained primary teeth)
  - Cardiovascular system (e.g., cardiac anomalies)
  - Abdomen (e.g., organomegaly)
  - Musculoskeletal (e.g., kyphoscoliosis)
  - Skin and hair (e.g., sheen and pigmentation, dystrophic scars, telangiectasia, eczema, abscesses, and warts)
- Physical examination findings typical for different PIDs are presented in Table 21-2.

Diagnostic Testing

The diagnostic testing for immunodeficiency disorders includes phenotypic tests, functional tests, and genetic testing.[7]

- Tests can also be categorized according to the arm of the immune system that they evaluate (e.g., innate vs. adaptive or humoral vs. cellular).[7]
- Advances in genetic testing have led to a rapid recognition of many new genetic disorders. Genetic testing has become more available and affordable in recent years, and it is now one of the cornerstones of the immune system workup.[8]
- The choice of laboratory test should be tailored to each patient's clinical presentation and differential diagnosis. However, because the diagnosis of PIDs is often challenging, and because in many PIDs multiple arms of the immune system are involved, the following tests should be included in most initial immune workups:
  - Complete blood count (CBC) with differential
  - Basic metabolic panel
  - HIV serology (fourth-generation test)
  - Serum immunoglobulin levels
  - Specific antibody titers
- There are many other additional tests that should be considered. Some are reviewed here.

Laboratories

- **General tests**
  - A **CBC with differential** should be ordered in all cases of suspected immunodeficiency.
    - A CBC may indicate lymphopenia; however, a normal white blood cell (WBC) does not exclude lymphopenia. This value consists of both lymphocytes and granulocytes, which is why a differential is required.
    - Total lymphocyte count should be >1,200 cells/μL in adults and >3,000 cells/μL in infants.
    - Because T cells make up approximately 75% of the total lymphocyte count, lymphopenia typically implies a decreased number of T cells.
    - Alternatively, **leukocytosis** may be present, which could indicate infection or a sign of leukocyte adhesion defects.
    - **Eosinophilia** ($>0.5 \times 10^9$/L) is often present in hyper-IgE syndromes and Omenn syndrome.[1,5]
    - **Thrombocytopenia** (<70,000/μL) is seen in Wiskott–Aldrich syndrome (**small platelets**), STAT1 gain of function, IPEX syndrome, X-linked hyper-IgM syndrome, and other syndromes.[2]

TABLE 21-2	PHYSICAL EXAMINATION FINDINGS IN DIFFERENT PRIMARY IMMUNODEFICIENCY DISEASES

Finding	Association
Short stature, low weight	**Severe combined T- and B-cell deficiencies**; chronic granulomatous disease (**CGD**); **endocrinopathies** with growth hormone deficiency, hypoadrenalism or hypothyroidism such as seen in **APECED** (autoimmune polyendocrinopathy-candidiasis-ectodermal dystrophy), **STAT1 gain of function**, and **IPEX**
Neurologic impairment	**PNP** deficiency, adenosine deaminase (**ADA**) deficiency, **Chédiak–Higashi syndrome, Kostmann disease**
Atypical facies	**DiGeorge syndrome**: hypertelorism, shortened philtrum, and downslanting palpebral fissures; **STAT3 loss of function** (AD hyper-IgE syndrome): broad nose and a triangular mandible. **Kabuki syndrome**: microcephaly, arched eyebrows, long eyelashes, long openings of the eyelids (long palpebral fissures), a flat, broadened tip of the nose, and large protruding earlobes
Periodontitis	Phagocyte disorders
Small or absent tonsillar, adenoidal, peripheral lymph nodes	T-cell and B-cell deficiencies
Lymphadenopathy, splenomegaly, and hepatomegaly	**Omenn syndrome, hyper-IgM syndrome, CVID, ALPS**
Mucocutaneous candidiasis	Severe combined T- and B-cell deficiencies; **APECED** (autoimmune polyendocrinopathy-candidiasis-ectodermal dystrophy), **STAT1 gain of function, STAT3 loss of function (AD hyper-IgE), CRAD9, DOCK8 deficiency; IL17F/IL17RA mutations**
Atopic dermatitis	**Wiskott–Aldrich syndrome**; hyper-IgE syndromes—both **STAT3 loss of function and DOCK8 deficiency**
Cutaneous abscesses	Phagocyte disorders; **STAT3 loss of function** (AD hyper-IgE syndrome)
Telangiectasias (eye involvement)	**Ataxia-telangiectasia syndrome**
Urticaria	**Familial cold autoinflammatory syndrome 1 and 2, PLAID: PLCG2-associated antibody deficiency and immune dysregulation, STAT5b somatic mutation**
Albinism (oculocutaneous)	**Chédiak–Higashi syndrome**
Arthritis	Antibody deficiencies (**CVID, X-linked agammaglobulinemia**), **Wiskott–Aldrich syndrome, complement deficiencies**
Delayed umbilical cord detachment	**Leukocyte adhesion defects**

AD, autosomal dominant; ALPS, autoimmune lymphoproliferative syndrome; CVID, common variable immune deficiency.

TABLE 21-3	IMMUNOGLOBULIN RANGE IN HEALTHY ADULTS
IgG (mg/dL)	700–1,600
IgA (mg/dL)	70–400
IgM (mg/dL)	40–230

Adapted from Dati F, Schumann G, Thomas L, et al. Consensus of a group of professional societies and diagnostic companies on guidelines for interim reference ranges for 14 proteins in serum based on the standardization against the IFCC/BCR/CAP Reference Material (CRM 470). International Federation of Clinical Chemistry. Community Bureau of Reference of the Commission of the European Communities. College of American Pathologists. *Eur J Clin Chem Clin Biochem.* 1996 Jun;34(6):517–20.

○ **HIV testing** (fourth generation), which includes both p24 antigen and antibodies to HIV-1 and -2, is the test of choice; however, in infants <18 months with perinatal and postnatal exposure, in adult patients with suspected acute infection, or in patients with combined or antibody deficiency immune disorders, HIV polymerase chain reaction (PCR; DNA or RNA) assay is part of the diagnostic algorithm.[9–12]

○ **Quantitative immunoglobulins** (IgG, IgA, IgM, IgE) should be interpreted according to age-related standards (see immunoglobulin range in healthy adults; Table 21-3[13]). Hypogammaglobulinemia is defined by immunoglobulin levels two standard deviations below age-adjusted normal.[8]

○ **Lymphocyte subpopulations:** $CD3^+$ T cells, $CD4^+$ T cells, $CD8^+$ T cells, $CD19^+$ B cells, $CD16^+CD56^+$ natural killer (NK) cells should be measured by a laboratory that provides age-matched normal control values.[7] Please see Tables 21-4 and 21-5.[14,15]

○ **T-cell phenotype,** or CD45RA/RO status, can help in the diagnosis of maternal or blood product lymphocyte engraftment in patients with SCID, because maternal or other oligoclonal foreign T cells would usually have a predominantly memory $CD45RO^+$ phenotype, whereas in a healthy infant most T cells should have a naïve $CD45RA^+$ phenotype.[7]

○ **B-cell phenotype** may assist in defining prognostic factors and known complications in patients with CVID. CVID patients with low total memory ($CD27^+$), and low switched memory cells (IgD^-CD27^+) are more likely to develop bronchiectasis, colitis, splenomegaly, and autoimmunity.[1]

TABLE 21-4	CELL-SUBSET COUNTS OF PERIPHERAL BLOOD LYMPHOCYTES IN HEALTHY ADULTS	
Normal range	**(%)**	**Absolute numbers**
CD3 (T cell)	60–88	661–1,963
CD4 (helper T cell)	31–64	365–1,294
CD8 (cytotoxic T cell)	12–40	187–781
CD19 (B cell)	6–25	86–488
CD16/CD56 (NK cell)	5–25	76–467

NK cell, natural killer cell.

Adapted from Barnes-Jewish Hospital. Lymphocyte Subpop 7. Last Accessed 8/27/20. https:// bjhlab.testcatalog.org/show/LAB3042-1

TABLE 21-5 CELL-SUBSET COUNTS OF PERIPHERAL BLOOD LYMPHOCYTES IN HEALTHY CHILDREN

Subset	N	0–3 months	3–6 months	6–12 months	1–2 years	2–6 years	6–12 years	12–18 years
White blood cell	800	10.60	9.20	9.10	8.80	7.10	6.50	6.00
Normal range		(7.20–18.00)	(6.70–14.00)	(6.40–13.00)	(6.40–12.00)	(5.20–11.00)	(4.40–9.50)	(4.40–8.10)
Lymphocyte	800	5.40	6.30	5.90	5.50	3.60	2.70	2.20
Normal range		(3.40–7.60)	(3.90–9.00)	(3.40–9.00)	(3.60–8.90)	(2.30–5.40)	(1.90–3.70)	(1.40–3.30)
CD3	699	3.68	3.93	3.93	355	2.39	1.82	1.48
Normal range		(2.50–5.50)	(2.50–5.60)	(1.90–5.90)	(2.10–6.20)	(1.40–3.70)	(1.20–2.60)	(1.00–2.20)
CD19	699	0.73	1.55	1.52	1.31	0.75	0.48	0.30
Normal range		(0.30–2.00)	(0.43–3.00)	(0.61–2.60)	(0.72–2.60)	(0.39–1.40)	(0.27–0.86)	(0.11–0.57)
CD16/56	770	0.42	0.42	0.40	0.36	0.30	0.23	0.19
Normal range		(0.17–1.10)	(0.17–0.83)	(0.16–0.95)	(0.18–0.92)	(0.13–0.72)	(0.10–0.48)	(0.07–0.48)
CD4	699	2.61	2.85	2.67	2.16	1.38	0.98	0.84
Normal range		(1.60–4.00)	(1.80–4.00)	(1.40–4.30)	(1.30–3.40)	(0.70–2.20)	(0.65–1.50)	(0.53–1.30)
CD8	699	0.98	1.05	1.04	1.04	0.84	0.68	0.53
Normal range		(0.56–1.70)	(0.59–1.60)	(0.50–1.70)	(0.62–2.00)	(0.49–1.30)	(0.37–1.10)	(0.33–0.92)
CD4/45RA/62L	694	2.25	2.23	2.10	1.64	0.96	0.56	0.39
Normal range		(1.20–3.60)	(1.30–3.60)	(1.10–3.60)	(0.95–2.80)	(0.42–1.50)	(0.31–1.00)	(0.21–0.75)
CD8/45RA/62L	696	0.73	0.74	0.70	0.76	0.54	0.41	0.30
Normal range		(0.38–1.30)	(0.45–1.20)	(0.33–1.20)	(0.40–1.40)	(0.26–0.85)	(0.20–0.65)	(0.17–0.56)
CD4/45RA	694	2.27	2.32	2.21	1.65	0.98	0.57	0.40
Normal range		(1.20–3.70)	(1.30–3.70)	(1.10–3.70)	(1.00–2.90)	(0.43–1.50)	(0.32–1.00)	(0.23–0.77)
CD8/45RA	696	0.87	0.91	0.87	0.94	0.67	0.54	0.40

	N							
Normal range		(0.45–1.50)	(0.55–1.40)	(0.48–1.50)	(0.49–1.70)	(0.38–1.10)	(0.31–0.90)	(0.24–0.71)
CD4/DR/38	694	0.08	0.11	0.10	0.10	0.06	0.04	0.03
Normal range		(0.03–0.18)	(0.05–0.26)	(0.04–0.22)	(0.05–0.25)	(0.03–0.14)	(0.02–0.08)	(0.01–0.06)
CD8/DR/38	697	0.05	0.07	0.09	0.18	0.11	0.06	0.04
Normal range		(0.02–0.16)	(0.03–0.17)	(0.04–0.27)	(0.05–0.54)	(0.05–0.34)	(0.03–0.18)	(0.02–0.13)
CD4/DR	694	0.10	0.15	0.12	0.13	0.09	0.07	0.06
Normal range		(0.04–0.18)	(0.06–028)	(0.05–0.26)	(0.07–0.28)	(0.05–0.18)	(0.04–0.12)	(0.03–0.10)
CD8/DR	697	0.05	0.08	0.09	0.18	0.14	0.09	0.07
Normal range		(0.02–0.16)	(0.03–0.17)	(0.04–0.29)	(0.06–0.60)	(0.07–0.42)	(0.04–0.27)	(0.03–0.18)
CD4/38	694	2.54	2.77	2.55	2.02	1.21	0.75	0.57
Normal range		(0.16–3.90)	(1.60–4.00)	(1.20–4.10)	(1.20–3.30)	(0.59–2.00)	(0.48–1.20)	(0.33–1.00)
CD8/38	697	0.93	0.94	0.93	0.95	0.67	0.48	0.31
Normal range		(0.55–1.60)	(0.53–1.50)	(0.45–1.60)	(0.57–1.90)	(0.39–1.10)	(0.24–0.74)	(0.16–5.70)
CD4/28	695	2.56	2.65	2.58	2.12	1.33	0.94	0.79
Normal range		(1.60–3.80)	(1.60–4.00)	(1.20–4.20)	(1.30–3.40)	(0.69–2.00)	(0.63–1.50)	(0.49–1.20)
CD8/28	696	0.71	0.73	0.67	0.72	0.50	0.40	0.29
Normal range		(0.35–1.30)	(0.35–1.20)	(0.28–1.10)	(0.40–1.30)	(0.28–0.87)	(0.21–0.70)	(0.16–0.52)
CD4/95	695	0.29	0.41	0.51	0.50	0.42	0.36	0.40
Normal range		(0.16–0.58)	(0.23–0.62)	(0.29–0.82)	(0.27–0.91)	(0.27–0.65)	(0.25–0.62)	(0.25–0.66)
CD8/95	696	0.12	0.16	0.22	0.34	0.30	0.25	0.21

(continued)

TABLE 21-5 CELL-SUBSET COUNTS OF PERIPHERAL BLOOD LYMPHOCYTES IN HEALTHY CHILDREN (continued)

Subset	N	0–3 months	3–6 months	6–12 months	1–2 years	2–6 years	6–12 years	12–18 years
Normal range		(0.05–0.31)	(0.06–0.39)	(0.08–0.66)	(0.10–0.85)	(0.11–0.58)	(0.08–0.53)	(0.08–0.45)
CD3/4/45RO	644	0.32	0.33	0.34	0.40	0.36	0.35	0.38
Normal range		(0.06–0.90)	(0.12–0.63)	(0.16–0.80)	(0.21–0.85)	(0.22–0.66)	(0.23–0.63)	(0.24–0.70)
CD3/4-/45RO	644	0.10	0.12	0.12	0.23	0.19	0.21	0.16
Normal range		(0.03–0.33)	(0.03–0.29)	(0.04–0.33)	(0.06–0.57)	(0.09–0.44)	(0.07–0.39)	(0.06–0.31)
CD3/45RO	644	0.48	0.46	0.47	0.65	0.57	0.59	0.56
Normal range		(0.09–1.20)	(0.15–086)	(0.22–1.10)	(0.30–1.30)	(0.33–1.00)	(0.32–0.95)	(0.34–0.97)
CD3⁻/19/38	655	0.60	1.20	1.29	1.04	0.56	0.28	0.03
Normal range		(0.12–2.00)	(0.00–2.80)	(0.02–2.20)	(0.00–2.20)	(0.01–1.20)	(0.00–0.67)	(0.00–0.35)
CD3⁻/19	655	0.62	1.26	1.33	1.10	0.67	0.34	0.04
Normal range		(0.12–2.10)	(0.00–2.80)	(0.02–2.30)	(0.00–2.30)	(0.02–1.40)	(0.00–0.74)	(0.00–0.39)

Reprinted with permission Shearer WT, Rosenblatt HM, Gelman RS, et al. Lymphocyte subsets in healthy children from birth through 18 years of age: the Pediatric AIDS Clinical Trials Group P1009 study. J Allergy Clin Immunol. 2003;112:973–80.

○ **CD4⁺ T-Cell Recent Thymic Emigrants (RTE):** evaluating thymic output in patients with established or suspected DiGeorge syndrome or other cellular immunodeficiencies[16]

○ **T-Cell Receptor Excision Circles (TREC): PCR assay** can be performed on both dry blood or fresh blood; TRECs are extrachromosomal DNA by-products of T-cell receptor (TCR) rearrangement, which are nonreplicative. TRECs are expressed only in T cells of thymic origin and serve as a biomarker for naïve T-cell production. The dry blood TREC assay is used to perform DNA-based newborn screening for severe combined immunodeficiency (SCID).[1] As of 2018, TREC screening is being performed in all 50 states in the United States. **For an algorithm for the evaluation of infants with a positive SCID screen, see Figure 21-1.**

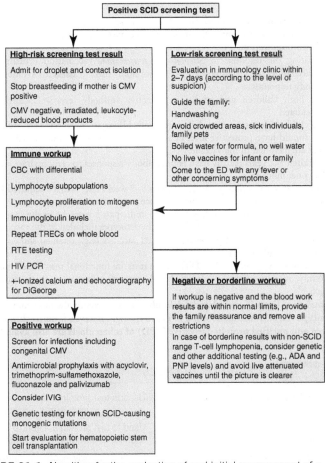

FIGURE 21-1 Algorithm for the evaluation of and initial management of a patient with suspected SCID with a positive SCID screen. ADA, adenosine deaminase; CBC, complete blood count; CMV, cytomegalovirus; ED, emergency department; PNP, purine nucleoside phosphorylase; RTE, recent thymic emigrants; SCID, severe combined immunodeficiency; TREC, T-cell receptor excision circles.

○ **Total hemolytic complement** (CH50) is a screening test for the functional integrity of the classical component of the complement cascade from C1 through the membrane attack complex (C5–C9). The **alternative pathway hemolytic complement** (AH50) tests the alternative pathway of complement activation. Patients with C1, C2, or C4 deficiency will have a low CH50 but normal AH50. Patients with a low AH50 but normal CH50 suggest a deficiency of factor B, factor D, or properdin.[1] A decrease in both CH50 and AH50 suggests a deficiency in a shared complement component, C3 or C5–C9.[17] In order to confirm a suspected complement defect, one can assess individual complement levels or function.

○ Fluorescence in situ hybridization (FISH) for 22q11 deletion is used in the diagnosis of **DiGeorge syndrome**. The rate of false negative is 5%.[18] A new PCR-based test is now available with high sensitivity and specificity.[19]

- **Functional assays**
  ○ **Antibody response to immunization** is a functional test for the immune system. Pre- and post-immunization antibody titers should be measured at baseline and 4–6 weeks after the immunization.
    ■ Measuring the response to *Streptococcus pneumoniae* vaccination (Pneumococcal polysaccharide, e.g., Pneumovax 23™) is commonly used to assess for T-independent antibody responses.
      □ For both children and adults, a protective antibody level >1.3 mg/mL[1] is considered.
      □ If a child ≤6 years received the recommended Prevnar 13™ vaccine schedule, he or she should have protective level of antibodies to at least 50% of the 13 serotypes that are included in the vaccine.
      □ Children <2 years usually have poor antibody responses to carbohydrate antigens, like pneumococcus.
      □ Booster immunizations with repeat titers 4–8 weeks later may be required in children and in adults with long intervals since previous vaccination.[1]
      □ If an adult received a Pneumovax vaccine in the past 5 years, he or she should have protective level of antibodies to 70% of the serotypes included in the vaccine.
    ■ Response to protein and protein-conjugated vaccines (e.g., tetanus) should also be confirmed,[1] see Table 21-6.
  ○ **Delayed-type hypersensitivity (DTH) skin tests** are functional tests of cell-mediated immunity, measuring the cellular-mediated memory response to a previously seen antigen.[1,5,7]
    ■ *Candida* antigen (Candin) and **Trichophyton** are currently the only commercially available reagents intended for use in DTH testing. However, **mumps skin test antigen and purified protein derivative (PPD) of tuberculosis are also available.**

TABLE 21-6 VACCINATION RESPONSE

Haemophilus influenzae type B antibody >1.0 µg/mL	Used to test protein antigen-specific responses in immunized individuals
Tetanus >0.1 units/mL	Used to test protein antigen responses in immunized individuals
Streptococcus pneumoniae Serotype-specific IgG: 1.3 µg/mL in >50% response in children and >70% in adults	Used to test polysaccharide antigen responses in immunized individuals

- These antigens are injected intradermally and evaluated 48–72 hours later. Cutaneous induration of 5 mm or more is considered positive (some accept 2 mm as positive). **Erythema alone does not indicate a positive reaction.**
- There are some caveats when using this modality of testing, which should be considered.
  - DTH testing requires that there has been previous exposure to the antigen prior to testing.
  - It is not recommended to perform DTH testing on children <12 months of age as they are frequently unresponsive due to immunologic immaturity.
  - Various infections and medications are associated with false-negative test results.
  - Finally, a positive test to some antigens does not ensure normal cellular immunity to all antigens.
  - The main advantages of DTH testing are its ease and economy. It is a useful screening test in many instances of suspected cellular immunodeficiency.
  - A negative DTH should be followed by measurement of lymphocyte populations by flow cytometry, combined with in vitro assays of T-cell function, which are less sensitive to interference during intercurrent illnesses or by drugs.
- **Lymphocyte in vitro proliferation to mitogens and antigens** are functional tests of immune cells that are performed in tissue culture. Proliferation is impaired in immunodeficiencies such as complete DiGeorge syndrome, SCID, Wiskott–Aldrich syndrome, and ataxia telangiectasia.
  - **Mitogen proliferation** assesses the ability of immune cells to respond to an antigen-independent stimulus. *Escherichia coli* lipopolysaccharide (LPS) induces only B-cell proliferation; pokeweed mitogen (PWM) induces both B-cell and T-cell proliferation; and phytohemagglutinin (PHA), concanavalin A (ConA), and anti-CD3 antibody are selective T-cell proliferation inducers.[7]
  - **Antigen proliferation** tests the ability of lymphocytes to respond to specific antigens, such as *Candida albicans*, tetanus toxoid, or tuberculin antigens.
- **Dihydrorhodamine (DHR)** test is a reliable screening test for chronic granulomatous disease (CGD). Neutrophils are incubated with DHR and then activated with phorbol myristate acetate (PMA) or *N*-formyl-methionyl-leucyl-phenylalanine (fMLP).[7] DHR testing can indicate and detect abnormalities in any of the protein components of the oxidative respiratory burst (gp91, p22, p40, p47, and p67), female carriers of the X-linked form (gp91/CYBB) as well as patients with Rac2 deficiency and complete myeloperoxidase (MPO) deficiency.
- **Additional testing: There are many specialized tests to detect** very specific defects in the immune system **that are not discussed here.**[7]
  - Genetic testing is being increasingly utilized to assist in making a rapid and accurate diagnosis of PID. Genetic testing can also help in genetic counseling for patients and their families.[7] Numerous "targeted" and "untargeted" sequencing techniques and technologies exist to help diagnose PID.
    - Targeted sequencing methods identify abnormalities of single genes. These methods can be used to analyze abnormalities in exons, introns, deletion/duplication analysis. Multiple genes can be analyzed in the same assay to screen multiple genes simultaneously.
    - Untargeted methods include whole exome sequencing (WES) or whole genome sequencing (WGS). These methods differ from targeted methods in that they are designed to identify abnormalities from any gene, not just a preselected panel. Sending an NGS gene panel or even a WES can be more cost-effective and more efficient compared with a single gene sequence approach.[8]
  - Testing for cystic fibrosis (CF) and primary ciliary dyskinesia. Nonimmune conditions that can result in severe, recurrent, or chronic sinopulmonary infections should also be ruled out.

- CF presents with recurrent episodes of bronchitis, sinusitis, and pneumonia and is associated with malnutrition, FTT, and steatorrhea.[20] Newborn screening for CF is now performed routinely in all 50 states. Newborn screening typically employs two serial assays; infants with abnormal results for the first assay are retested with a second assay.[21]
- Primary ciliary dyskinesia is an autosomal recessive condition with recurrent upper and lower respiratory infections and bronchiectasis. Diagnosis is made by measuring nasal nitric oxide levels (available only as a research test), ciliary motion and ultra-structure tests, and genetic testing.[22,23]

Selected PID Diseases

We review here the general concept of the diagnosis and treatment of two prototypical PIDs, SCID and CVID. It is beyond the scope of this book to provide an in-depth review of the 354 known clinical and laboratory features of PID. Table 21-7 summarizes the immunologic profile and genetic defects associated with some PIDs.[1,2,5]

Severe Combined Immunodeficiency

- SCID is a group of heterogeneous disorders arising from a defect in the development and function of both T and B cells, affecting both cellular and humoral immunity, which leads to significant morbidity and mortality, usually starting during the first year of life.[1]
- SCID is caused by mutations in genes crucial for the development of both T and B cells. In some cases, the mutations affect only T-cell function. However, severe T-cell dysfunction leads to impaired humoral immunity because B cells require signals from T cells to produce antibody. More than half of the patients with SCID also suffer from NK-cell dysfunction.
- There are approximately 18 known genetic mutations associated with SCID and 32 mutations associated with less profound CID phenotype.[1,2]
  - Most SCID cases are due to X-linked mutations in IL2RG gene that encodes interleukin-2 receptor γ. All other causes are autosomal recessive and the most prevalent mutations are in genes encoding JAK3 (Janus kinase 3 gene), IL7RA (interleukin-7 receptor alpha gene), RAG1 and RAG2 (recombination-activating genes 1 and 2), DCLRE1C (DNA cross-link repair protein 1C gene or Artemis), and ADA (adenosine deaminase gene). **In 25% of SCID patients, the genetic defect is unknown.**
  - **Leaky SCID** refers to CIDs that are often but not always caused by a hypomorphic mutation in a typical SCID gene that allows development of low numbers of usually poorly functioning T cells.[1] These patients have some T cells (300–1,500 cells/µL) and have a milder phenotype with a late presentation.
- The classic presentation of babies with SCID is recurrent severe infections, chronic diarrhea, and FTT. Maternal-derived IgG provides patients some protection and may delay the diagnosis.[1]
- Physical examination might reveal thrush or lack of lymphoid tissue (tonsils or lymph nodes). The lack or presence of thymic shadow on chest X-ray can neither confirm nor rule out the diagnosis of SCID. However, an absence of thymic shadow should prompt an immune evaluation.[1]
  - Common infections in patients with SCID are mucocutaneous candidiasis, viral pathogens, such as adenovirus, cytomegalovirus (CMV), Epstein–Barr virus (EBV), rotavirus, norovirus, respiratory syncytial virus (RSV), varicella zoster virus (VZV), herpes simplex virus (HSV), measles, influenza, and parainfluenza (all are frequently fatal). Opportunistic infections such as *Pneumocystis jirovecii* (formerly *carinii*) may occur. Attenuated vaccine organisms, such as oral polio vaccine virus, rotavirus, varicella, and BCG, may cause severe or fatal infection.[1,5]

TABLE 21-7 SUMMARY OF IMMUNOLOGIC PROFILE AND GENETIC DEFECTS OF SELECTED PIDS

Disease	Genetic defect/ inheritance	T-cell levels	B-cell levels	NK cells	Ig levels	Important features
Combined T- and B-cell deficiencies						
γc deficiency (common γ chain SCID, CD132 deficiency)	IL2RG/XL	Very low	Normal to high	Low	Low	Males with severe lymphopenia and hypogammaglobulinemia
Jak3 kinase deficiency	JAK3/AR	Very low	Normal to high	Low	Low	Progressive immune abnormalities. Cognitive defects, bone defects, may have pulmonary alveolar proteinosis
Adenosine deaminase deficiency	ADA/AR	Very low	Low, decreasing	Low	Low, decreasing	
Purine nucleoside phosphorylase deficiency	PNP/AR	Progressive decrease	Low, decreasing	Low, decreasing	Normal or low	Progressive immune abnormalities ranging from severe to nonsevere combined immunodeficiency with neurologic impairment and autoimmunity (hemolytic anemia)
MHC II deficiency	CIITA/RFXANK/ RFX5/RFXAP—all AR	Low CD4	Normal	Normal	Normal or low	Respiratory and gastrointestinal infections, liver/biliary tract disease
ZAP-70 deficiency (ZAP70 LOF)	ZAP70/AR	Low CD8, Nl CD4 number but poor function	Normal	Normal	Normal	May have immune dysregulation, autoimmunity. SCID newborn screening might be negative
Recombinase-activating gene (RAG1, RAG2) deficiency	RAG1/2, both AR	Low	Low	Normal	Decreased	Hypomorphic or leaky RAG1/RAG2 defects can give rise to Omenn syndrome with proliferation of oligoclonal T cells, severe erythroderma and desquamation, splenomegaly, eosinophilia, and elevated IgE.

(continued)

Disease	Genetic defect/ inheritance	T-cell levels	B-cell levels	NK cells	Ig levels	Important features
CD40 ligand deficiency (CD154)	CD40LG (TNFSF5)/XL	Normal to low	sIgM+, IgD+ cells present, absent sIgG+, IgA+, and IgE+ cells	IgM normal or high, other Ig isotypes low		Neutropenia, thrombocytopenia, hemolytic anemia, opportunistic infections, biliary tract and liver disease, *Cryptosporidium* infection
Antibody deficiencies						
Agammaglobulinemia BTK deficiency, XL agammaglobulinemia (XLA)	BTK/XL	Normal	Very low (<2%) to absent	Normal	Low to absent	Severe bacterial infections, normal numbers of pro-B cells
μ heavy chain deficiency	IGHM/AR	Normal	Very low to absent	Normal	Low to absent	Severe bacterial infections, normal numbers of pro-B cells
BLNK deficiency	BLNK/AR	Normal	Absent pre-B or mature B cells	Normal	All isotypes decreased	Severe bacterial infections, normal numbers of pro-B cells
NFKB1 deficiency	NFKB1/AD	Normal	Low or normal B cells, low memory B cells	Normal	Normal or low IgG, IgA, IgM	Recurrent sinopulmonary infections, COPD, EBV proliferation, autoimmune cytopenias, alopecia, and autoimmune thyroiditis
NFKB2 deficiency	NFKB2/AD	Normal	Low	Normal	Low serum IgG, IgA, and IgM	Recurrent sinopulmonary infections, alopecia, and endocrinopathies
IKAROS deficiency	IKZF1/AD	Normal	Low or normal B cells, potentially reducing levels with age	Normal	Low IgG, IgA, IgM	Recurrent sinopulmonary infections

Disease	Genetics	T cells	B cells	Serum Ig	Antibody	Associated features
Selective IgA deficiency	Unknown	Normal	Normal	Normal	Very low to absent IgA with other isotypes normal, normal subclasses and specific antibodies	Bacterial infections, autoimmunity mildly increased
Specific antibody deficiency with normal Ig levels and normal B cells	Unknown	Normal	Normal	Normal	Reduced ability to produce antibodies to specific antigens	May have recurrent or severe sinopulmonary infections
Transient hypogammaglobulinemia of infancy	Unknown	Normal	Normal	Normal	Decreased IgG	A transient disorder with normal ability to produce antibodies to vaccine antigens, usually not associated with significant infections
Combined immunodeficiencies with associated or syndromic features						
EDA-ID due to NEMO/IKBKG deficiency (ectodermal dysplasia, immune deficiency)	NEMO (IKBKG)/XL	Normal or decreased, TCR activation impaired	Normal Low memory and isotype-switched B cells	Low function	Decreased, some with elevated IgA, IgM, poor specific antibody responses, absent antibody to polysaccharide antigens	Anhidrotic ectodermal dysplasia (in some), various infections (bacteria, mycobacteria, viruses, and fungi), colitis, conical teeth, variable defects and infections of skin, hair and teeth, monocyte dysfunction
Wiskott-Aldrich syndrome (WAS LOF)	WAS/XL	Progressive decrease in numbers, abnormal lymphocyte responses to anti-CD3	Normal	Normal (some low IgM)	Low IgM and antibody responses to polysaccharides, often high IgA and IgE	Thrombocytopenia with small platelets, recurrent bacterial and viral infections, bloody diarrhea, eczema, lymphoma, autoimmune disease, IgA nephropathy, vasculitis

(continued)

TABLE 21-7 SUMMARY OF IMMUNOLOGIC PROFILE AND GENETIC DEFECTS OF SELECTED PIDS (continued)

Disease	Genetic defect/ inheritance	T-cell levels	B-cell levels	NK cells	Ig levels	Important features
Ataxia telangiectasia	ATM-AR	Progressive decrease, abnormal proliferation to mitogens	Normal	Normal	Often low IgA, IgE, and IgG subclasses, increased IgM monomers, antibodies variably decreased	Ataxia, telangiectasia, pulmonary infections, lymphoreticular and other malignancies, increased alfa fetoprotein, increased radiosensitivity, chromosomal instability and chromosomal translocations
Bloom syndrome	BLM (RECQL3/ AR	Normal	Normal	Normal	Low	Short stature, dysmorphic facies, sunsensitive erythema, marrow failure, leukemia, lymphoma, chromosomal instability
AD-HIES STAT3 deficiency (Job syndrome)	STAT3/AD loss of function	Normal overall, Th-17 and T-follicular helper cells decreased	Normal, reduced switched and non-switched memory B cells, BAFF expression increased	Normal	High IgE, specific antibody production decreased	Distinctive facial features (broad nasal bridge), bacterial infections (boils and pulmonary abscesses, pneumatoceles) due to Staphylococcus aureus, pulmonary aspergillosis, Pneumocystis jirovecii, eczema, mucocutaneous candidiasis, hyperextensible joints, osteoporosis and bone fractures, scoliosis, retention of primary teeth, coronary and cerebral aneurysm formation
Cartilage hair hypoplasia (CHH)	RMRP/AR	Varies from severely decreased (SCID) to normal, impaired lymphocyte proliferation	Normal	Normal	Normal or reduced, antibodies variably decreased	Short-limbed dwarfism with metaphyseal dysostosis, sparse hair, bone marrow failure, autoimmunity, susceptibility to lymphoma and other cancers, impaired spermatogenesis, neuronal dysplasia of the intestine

Diseases of immune dysregulation

IPEX, immune dysregulation, polyendocrinopathy, enteropathy X-linked	FOXP3/XL	Normal	Normal	Normal	Normal	Lack of (and/or impaired function of) CD4$^+$ CD25$^+$ FOXP3$^+$ regulatory T cells (Tregs). Autoimmune enteropathy, early-onset diabetes, thyroiditis, hemolytic anemia, thrombocytopenia, eczema, elevated IgE, IgA
CTLA4 deficiency (ALPSV)	CTLA4/AD	Decreased	Decreased	Normal	Reduced IgG, IgA, or IgM levels and impaired responses to polysaccharide vaccinations	Impaired function of Tregs. Autoimmune cytopenias, enteropathy, interstitial lung disease, extra-lymphoid lymphocytic infiltration, recurrent infections
LRBA deficiency	LRBA/AR	Normal or decreased CD4 numbers, T-cell dysregulation	Low or normal numbers of B cells	Normal	Reduced IgG and IgA in most	Recurrent infections, inflammatory bowel disease, autoimmunity, EBV infections
STAT3 GOF mutation	STAT3/AD gain of function	Decreased	Decreased	Decreased	Decreased	Enhanced STAT3 signaling, leading to increased Th17 cell differentiation, lymphoproliferation and autoimmunity. Decreased Tregs and impaired function. Lymphoproliferation, solid organ auto-immunity, recurrent infections

(continued)

TABLE 21-7 SUMMARY OF IMMUNOLOGIC PROFILE AND GENETIC DEFECTS OF SELECTED PIDS (continued)

Disease	Genetic defect/ inheritance	T-cell levels	B-cell levels	NK cells	Ig levels	Important features
APECED (APS-1), autoimmune poly-endocrinopathy with candidiasis and ecto-dermal dystrophy	*AIRE* both AR and AD	Normal	Normal	Normal	Naturalizing autoantibodies against IL-17 and other cytokines	AIRE serves as checkpoint in the thymus for negative selection of autoreactive T cells and for generation of Tregs. Autoimmunity: hypoparathyroidism, hypothyroidism, adrenal insufficiency, diabetes, gonadal dysfunction and other endocrine abnormalities, chronic mucocutaneous candidiasis, dental enamel hypoplasia, alopecia areata, enteropathy, pernicious anemia, lung disease
Congenital defects of phagocyte number or function						
Elastase deficiency (SCN1)	ELANE/AD	Normal	Normal	Normal	Normal	Myeloid differentiation. Susceptibility to MDS/leukemia. Severe congenital neutropenia or cyclic neutropenia
Chronic granuloma-tous disease (CGD)	CYBB (XD); CYBA, NCF1, NCF2 and NCF4 (AR)	Normal	Normal	Normal	Normal	Impaired phagocytic cell oxidative metabolism with defective bacterial and fungal killing in all forms of CGD. Pulmonary, cutaneous, lymphatic, and hepatic infections; abscesses are frequent. Gingivitis is common. Most prevalent pathogens are: *Staphylococcus aureus*, *Burkholderia cepacia* complex, *Serratia marcescens*, *Nocardia* spp., and *Aspergillus* spp.

Disease	Gene/Inheritance					Associated features
Leukocyte adhesion deficiency type 1 (LAD1)	ITGB2/AR	Normal	Normal	Normal	Normal	Adherence, chemotaxis, endocytosis, T/NK cytotoxicity. Recurrent bacterial skin infections, sepsis, and pneumonia with absent pus formation at the site of infection. Delayed cord separation, skin ulcers, periodontitis, leukocytosis (50-100K)
Leukocyte adhesion deficiency type 2 (LAD2)	SLC35C1/AR	Normal	Normal	Normal	Normal	Rolling, chemotaxis. Mild LAD type 1 features with hh-blood group, mental retardation, microcephaly, growth retardation
Leukocyte adhesion deficiency type 3 (LAD3)	FERMT3/AR	Normal	Normal	Normal	Normal	Adherence, chemotaxis. LAD type 1 plus bleeding tendency
Defects in intrinsic and innate immunity						
IFN-γ receptor 1/2 deficiency	IFNGR1/AR and AD IFNGR2/AR	Normal	Normal	Normal	Normal	IFN-γ binding and signaling. Susceptibility to mycobacteria and *Salmonella*
WHIM (warts, hypogammaglobulinemia, infections, myelokathexis) syndrome	CXCR4/AD GOF	Normal	Low	Low	Low	Increased response of the CXCR4 chemokine receptor to its ligand CXCL12 (SDF-1). Warts and neutropenia
CARD9 deficiency	CARD9/AR	Normal	Normal	Normal	Normal	CARD9 signaling pathway. CMC and invasive candidiasis infection, deep dermatophytoses, other invasive fungal infections
STAT1 GOF	STAT1/AD GOF	Normal/low	Normal/low	Normal/low	Normal/low	CMC, various fungal, bacterial, and viral (HSV) infections, autoimmunity (thyroiditis, diabetes, cytopenias), enteropathy

(continued)

TABLE 21-7   SUMMARY OF IMMUNOLOGIC PROFILE AND GENETIC DEFECTS OF SELECTED PIDS (continued)

Disease	Genetic defect/ inheritance	T-cell levels	B-cell levels	NK cells	Ig levels	Important features
IRAK-4 deficiency	IRAK4/AR	Normal	Normal	Normal	Normal	TIR-IFAK4 signaling pathway. Recurrent invasive bacterial infections (cellulitis, sepsis, meningitis, osteomyelitis) mainly with Staphylococcus aureus and Streptococcus pneumoniae. High mortality in the first decade of life but infections decrease significantly with age
MyD88 deficiency	MYD88/AR	Normal	Normal	Normal	Normal	TIR-MyD88 signaling pathway. Bacterial infections (pyogenes)
TLR3 deficiency	TLR3/AD or AR	Normal	Normal	Normal	Normal	Impaired TLR3-dependent IFN-α, β, and γ response. HSV1 encephalitis
Autoinflammatory disorders						
Familial Mediterranean fever	MEVF/AR or AD	Normal	Normal	Normal	Normal	Decreased production of pyrin permits ASC-induced IL-1 processing and inflammation following subclinical serosal injury, macrophage apoptosis decreased. Recurrent fever, serositis, and inflammation responsive to colchicine, with a long-term complication of amyloidosis and renal failure
Complement deficiencies						
Complement deficiencies	Multiple genes—AR, AD, and XL	Normal	Normal	Normal	Normal	C1, C2, C4, and C3 deficiencies associated with autoimmunity and pyogenic infections. C5–9 and properdin deficiencies associated with recurrent and disseminated Neisserial infections

AD, autosomal dominant; AR, autosomal recessive; CMS, chronic mucocutaneous candidiasis; COPD, chronic obstructive pulmonary disease; EBV, Epstein–Barr virus; HSV, herpes simplex virus; IFN, interferon; IL, interleukin; NEMO, nuclear factor-κ-B essential modulator; NK, natural killer; PID, primary immunodeficiency; SCID, severe combined immunodeficiency; TCR, T-cell receptor; XL, X-linked.

- **Graft-vs.-host disease (GVHD)**: Transfusion of blood products containing viable lymphocytes or transplacental passage of alloreactive maternal T cells can lead to rapidly fatal GVHD.[1]
- **SCID patients have increased rates of malignancy.** The majority are hematologic malignancies such as EBV-induced lymphoproliferative disease, lymphoma, and leukemia.
- Laboratory findings are typically low absolute lymphocyte count, low to absent T-cell number with **low T-cell proliferation to mitogens.** Antigen proliferation testing is not part of the standard evaluation for SCID.
  - Normal lymphocyte count or T-cell absolute number can be seen in patients with high number of B cells or in patients with engraftment of maternal T cells.
  - IgG level can be normal due to the presence of maternal IgG. Serum levels of IgM, IgA, and IgE are usually very low. Specific antibody response should be impaired, but it is not part of the workup of babies with suspected SCID, because most patients have not been vaccinated.
- Early diagnosis of SCID improves outcomes.[1] Although newborn screening is in place in all 50 U.S. states, every infant, toddler, or a child with the alarming symptoms and findings, without explained etiology, should undergo evaluation for SCID.
- SCID definitions:
  - **Definite SCID:** Less than 300 T cells/μL **or** absence of naïve CD45RA T cells **with one of the following:**
    - Male with deleterious IL2RG mutations
    - Male or female with deleterious homozygous mutation or compound heterozygous mutations in a known SCID-causing geneá
    - ADA activity of <2%
    - Engraftment of maternal T cells
  - **Probable SCID:** CD3+ T cells <20%, absolute lymphocytic count <3,000 cells/μL, and impaired mitogen-induced lymphocyte proliferation (<10%) **or** the presence of maternal lymphocytes in circulation[24]
- For the initial management of a patient with suspected SCID, refer to Figure 21-1.
- Hematopoietic cell transplantation (HCT) is the most common curative therapy for all forms of SCID.[1] Tailored therapies have been developed for specific disorders and conditions such as enzyme replacement therapy for ADA deficiency, gene therapy for X-linked SCID, or **adoptive T-cell virus-specific immunotherapy for life-threatening CMV or EBV infections.**[1,25]

Common Variable Immunodeficiency

- CVID is a PID characterized by impaired B-cell differentiation and defective immunoglobulin production. It is the **most prevalent form of severe antibody deficiency affecting both children and adults.**
- CVID is a collection of syndromes resulting from many genetic defects, both monogenic and polygenic. Specific monogenic disorders can currently be identified only in a subset of patients. In most cases, the genetic causes are currently unknown.[26,27]
- Although there is no universally agreed definition of CVID, most patients will demonstrate[1]
  - Markedly reduced (two standard deviations below the age-appropriate normal range) serum concentrations of IgG, plus low levels of IgA and/or IgM
  - Absent or poor response to vaccination
  - No other identifiable cause for immunodeficiency[1]
- CVID has **heterogeneous clinical manifestations**, which include[1,2,5,7]
  - **Recurrent infections**
  - **Chronic lung disease** (bronchiectasis, obstructive, restrictive, granulomatous disease, and lymphoid hyperplasia)

- ○ **Autoimmune disorders** (cytopenias, rheumatoid arthritis and rheumatoid-like arthritis, pernicious anemia, thyroiditis, and vitiligo)
- ○ **Gastrointestinal disease** (inflammatory bowel-like disease, sprue-like illness with flat villi, nodular lymphoid hyperplasia, and more)
- ○ Increased susceptibility to **lymphoma**
- **The most common infections in CVID are sinopulmonary** infections with encapsulated bacteria, especially *Streptococcus pneumoniae* and *Haemophilus influenzae*, and *Mycoplasma* spp.
  - ○ Patients also have frequent **acute and chronic gastrointestinal infections** with **norovirus, *Campylobacter jejuni*, or Salmonella**. Chronic **giardiasis** causing refractory diarrhea, malabsorption, and weight loss has been reported in patients with CVID. Other infections causing chronic diarrhea include **CMV, or *Cryptosporidium*** and norovirus. Many gastrointestinal symptoms cannot be attributed to an infectious etiology.
  - ○ Other infectious disorders reported in patients with CVID include septic arthritis, meningitis (both bacterial and viral), and sepsis.[1,5]
- CVID is estimated to affect as many as 1 in 30,000 individuals. The majority of patients are diagnosed between the ages of 20 and 45 years. Up to a third of the patients are diagnosed before the age of 10 years. **The diagnosis of CVID should not be made definitively before the age of 4 years.**[1]
- Physical examination may reveal diminished lymph nodes and tonsillar tissue, although there may be signs of lymphoid hyperplasia with lymphadenopathy and/or splenomegaly. Nasal discharge or congestion due to chronic sinusitis, scarring of the tympanic membrane, clubbing due to lung disease, arthritis, or conjunctivitis may be present.
- B-cell subpopulations are typically normal in CVID, but patients with low levels of isotype-switched memory B cells have worse prognosis and lung and colon involvement.
- **Immune globulin replacement** either intravenously or subcutaneously is the cornerstone of **treatment in CVID**. A typical approach is to begin therapy with intravenous immune globulin (**IVIG 400–600 mg/kg**, every 3–4 weeks). The SC route may be substituted after 2 or more months on IVIG. If the patient received their first dose during an acute infection, a second dose can be given within days.[28]
  - ○ Premedication with diphenhydramine and acetaminophen is commonly used and in some cases, a glucocorticoid is also given.
  - ○ Adverse effects include fever, nausea, vomiting, and back pain. Severe **anaphylactic reactions rarely occur** (possibly due to trace amounts of IgA in the IVIG. Low IgA content IVIG products are available for use in patients with IgA deficiency and history of anaphylactic reaction to IVIG). Aseptic meningitis and hemolytic anemia are also rare complications.
  - ○ **Monitoring therapy:** Steady-state IgG levels are usually achieved after 3–6 months of therapy. Trough levels of IgG can be measured 6 months after the first dose and every 6 months thereafter. The level of IgG in the blood on therapy should be at least near the middle of the normal range, and the patient should experience a significant decrease in major infections. Dosing may need to be adjusted periodically, as patient weight and endogenous production or clearance may change over time.
  - ○ **Indications for higher dosing:** Continued major infections, chronic lung disease (600 mg/kg), or enteropathy may prompt increased dosing. Very high doses of IVIG (≥ 1 g/kg) may be helpful in patients already on standard therapy who develop autoimmune hematologic disorders.[1,29]
  - ○ **Subcutaneous immunoglobulin** (SCIG) is usually administered weekly, or every 3–4 weeks using a preparation containing hyaluronidase. In children, preparations with hyaluronidase are not approved for clinical use, and children should receive SCIG every 1–2 weeks. SCIG is particularly helpful for patients with reactions to IVIG or difficult intravenous access and can be self-infused at home.[28]

- ○ **Prophylactic antimicrobials**: There is lack of conclusive evidence supporting the use of antibiotic prophylaxis in patients on IVIG. However, adding antibiotic prophylaxis may be considered in patients with recurrent infections despite appropriate IVIG treatment, such as patients with chronic lung disease and recurrent bronchiectasis infection.[1]
- As with other PIDs, early and judicious use of empiric antibiotics followed by culture-directed specific antibiotic treatment should be employed to treat infections in CVID.
- **Vaccinations**—In general, **live vaccines are not recommended for patients with CVID** (e.g., oral polio, smallpox, live attenuated influenza vaccine, yellow fever, or live oral typhoid vaccines), particularly those with significantly impaired T-cell function. Although antibody responses will be impaired, killed or inactivated vaccines can be given safely to patients with CVID. Vaccination might reinforce T-cell immunity to viral agents, in addition to inducing the formation of specific antibodies. Guidelines recommend administration of yearly influenza vaccine to CVID patients. Immunocompetent healthy family members and household contacts of patients with CVID may receive live vaccines, except oral polio vaccine.[30]
- **Prognosis:** Immunoglobulin therapy significantly reduces the incidence of death associated with acute bacterial infection in CVID patients.
  - ○ Lung disease and malignancies are currently the leading cause of death. Other poor prognostic factors are gastrointestinal disease, liver disease, lower levels of serum IgG, increased serum IgM, and lower percentages of circulating B cells.
  - ○ Patients who suffer only from infectious complications have excellent prognosis.[1,31,32]

REFERENCES

1. Bonilla FA, Khan DA, Ballas ZK, et al. Practice parameter for the diagnosis and management of primary immunodeficiency. *J Allergy Clin Immunol.* 2015;136:1186–205.e1–78.
2. Picard C, Bobby Gaspar H, Al-Herz W, et al. International Union of Immunological Societies: 2017 Primary Immunodeficiency Diseases Committee Report on Inborn Errors of Immunity. *J Clin Immunol.* 2018;38:96–128.
3. Barlogis V, Mahlaoui N, Auquier P, et al. Physical health conditions and quality of life in adults with primary immunodeficiency diagnosed during childhood: A French Reference Center for PIDs (CEREDIH) study. *J Allergy Clin Immunol.* 2017;139:1275–81.e7.
4. Hsu AP, McReynolds LJ, Holland SM. GATA2 deficiency. *Curr Opin Allergy Clin Immunol.* 2015;15:104–9.
5. Holland SM, Gallin JI. Evaluation of the patient with suspected immunodeficiency. In: Bennett JE, Dolin R, Blaser M, eds. *Mandell, Douglas, and Bennett's Principles and Practice of Infectious Diseases.* 8th ed. Philadelphia, PA: Elsevier/Saunders, 2015:134–45.
6. Hernandez-Trujillo VP. Approach to children with recurrent infections. *Immunology and Allergy Clinics of North America*, 2015;35:625–36.
7. Locke BA, Dasu T, Verbsky JW. Laboratory diagnosis of primary immunodeficiencies. *Clin Rev Allergy Immunol.* 2014;46:154–68.
8. Heimall JR, Hagin D, Hajjar J, et al. Use of genetic testing for primary immunodeficiency patients. *J Clin Immunol.* 2018;38:320–9.
9. Centers for Disease Control and Prevention. 2018 Quick reference guide: Recommended laboratory HIV testing algorithm for serum or plasma specimens. Last Accessed 7/27/18. https://stacks.cdc.gov/view/cdc/50872
10. Stekler J, Maenza J, Stevens CE et al. Screening for acute HIV infection: lessons learned. *Clin Infect Dis.* 2007;44:459–61.
11. U.S. Department of Health and Human Services. AIDS info. *Diagnosis of HIV in infants and children.* Last Accessed on 7/27/18. https://clinicalinfo.hiv.gov/en/guidelines/perinatal/diagnosis-hiv-infection-infants-and-children
12. Padeh YC, Rubinstein A, Shliozberg J. Common variable immunodeficiency and testing for HIV-1. *N Engl J Med.* 2005;353:1074–5.
13. Dati F, Schumann G, Thomas L, et al. Consensus of a group of professional societies and diagnostic companies on guidelines for interim reference ranges for 14 proteins in serum based on the

standardization against the IFCC/BCR/CAP Reference Material (CRM 470). International Federation of Clinical Chemistry. Community Bureau of Reference of the Commission of the European Communities. College of American Pathologists. *Eur J Clin Chem Clin Biochem.* 1996 Jun;34(6):517–20.

14. Mayo Foundation for Medical Education and Research. Lymphocyte subpop 7. Last Accessed 8/27/20. https://bjhlab.testcatalog.org/show/LAB3042-1

15. Shearer WT, Rosenblatt HM, Gelman RS, et al. Lymphocyte subsets in healthy children from birth through 18 years of age: the Pediatric AIDS Clinical Trials Group P1009 study. *J Allergy Clin Immunol.* 2003;112:973–80.

16. Ravkov E, Slev P, Heikal N. Thymic output: assessment of CD4+ recent thymic emigrants and T-Cell receptor excision circles in infants. *Cytometry B Clin Cytom.* 2017;92:249–57.

17. Oliveira JB, Fleisher TA. Molecular- and flow cytometry-based diagnosis of primary immunodeficiency disorders. *Curr Allergy Asthma Rep.* 2010;10:460–7.

18. Stachon AC, Baskin B, Smith AC, et al. Molecular diagnosis of 22q11.2 deletion and duplication by multiplex ligation dependent probe amplification. *Am J Med Genet A.* 2007;143A:2924–30.

19. Tomita-Mitchell A, Mahnke DK, Larson JM, et al. Multiplexed quantitative real-time PCR to detect 22q11.2 deletion in patients with congenital heart disease. *Physiol Genomics.* 2010;42A:52–60.

20. Boyle MP. Nonclassic cystic fibrosis and CFTR-related diseases. *Curr Opin Pulm Med.* 2003;9:498–503.

21. Wells J, Rosenberg M, Hoffman G. A decision-tree approach to cost comparison of newborn screening strategies for cystic fibrosis. *Pediatrics.* 2012;129:e339–47.

22. Afzelius BA. A human syndrome caused by immotile cilia. *Science.* 1976;193:317–9.

23. Lobo LJ, Zariwala MA, Noone PG. Primary ciliary dyskinesia. *QJM.* 2014;107:691–9.

24. Picard C, Al-Herz W, Bousfiha A, et al. Primary immunodeficiency diseases: an update on the classification from the International Union of Immunological Societies Expert Committee for Primary Immunodeficiency 2015. *J Clin Immunol.* 2015;35:696–726.

25. Naik S, Nicholas SK, Martinez CA, et al. Adoptive immunotherapy for primary immunodeficiency disorders with virus-specific T lymphocytes. *J Allergy Clin Immunol.* 2016;137:1498–505.e1.

26. de Valles-Ibáñez G, Esteve-Solé A, Piquer M, et al. Evaluating the genetics of common variable immunodeficiency: monogenetic model and beyond. *Front Immunol.* 2018;14:636.

27. Kienzler AK, Hargreaves CE, Patel SY. The role of genomics in common variable immunodeficiency disorders. *Clin Exp Immunol.* 2017;188:326–32.

28. Perez EE, Orange JS, Bonilla F. Update on the use of immunoglobulin in human disease: a review of evidence. *J Allergy Clin Immunol.* 2017;139(3S):S1–46.

29. Wang J, Cunningham-Rundles C. Treatment and outcome of autoimmune hematologic disease in common variable immunodeficiency (CVID). *J Autoimmun.* 2005;25:57–62.

30. Rubin LG, Levin MJ, Ljungman P, et al. 2013 IDSA clinical practice guideline for vaccination of the immunocompromised host. *Clin Infect Dis.* 2014;58:309–18.

31. Chapel H, Lucas M, Lee M, et al. Common variable immunodeficiency disorders: division into distinct clinical phenotypes. *Blood.* 2008;112:277–86.

32. Quinti I, Agostini C, Tabolli S, et al. Malignancies are the major cause of death in patients with adult onset common variable immunodeficiency. *Blood.* 2012;120:1953–4.

Index

Note: Page locators followed by *f* and *t* indicate figure and table, respectively.